WHAT CAUSES ADHD?

WHAT CAUSES ADHD?

Understanding What Goes Wrong and Why

JOEL T. NIGG

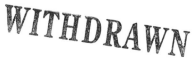
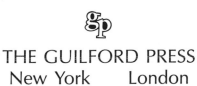

THE GUILFORD PRESS
New York   London

KH

Library of Congress Cataloging-in-Publication Data
Nigg, Joel T.
  What causes ADHD?: understanding what goes wrong and why / Joel T.
Nigg.
    p. cm.
  Includes bibliographical references and index.
  ISBN-10: 1-59385-267-3   ISBN-13: 978-1-59385-267-2 (hardcover)
  1. Attention-deficit hyperactivity disorder. I. Title.
  RJ506.H9N52 2006
  618.92′8589–dc22

                                                    2006000722

2/8/07

About the Author

Joel T. Nigg, PhD, is a licensed clinical psychologist and an active scientist in the Department of Psychology at Michigan State University. His research on the etiology of and mechanisms involved in attention-deficit/hyperactivity disorder (ADHD) has been funded by the National Institutes of Health continuously since 1997. Dr. Nigg is best known for his work in helping to characterize the neuropsychological features of ADHD and its subtypes; he also studies temperamental and personality characteristics related to ADHD. He has published over 50 scientific articles on ADHD and related topics, and has presented his work at numerous national and international scientific meetings in the field of children's mental health. Dr. Nigg also serves as a reviewer for grants for the National Institute of Mental Health, and is on the editorial boards of several major scientific journals, including the *Journal of Abnormal Psychology, Development and Psychopathology,* and the *Journal of Child Psychology and Psychiatry.*

Acknowledgments

This book represents the confluence of several lines of thought and the culmination of numerous ongoing conversations with colleagues in the field, not all of whom can be recognized here. However, I am especially grateful for criticisms of key sections of this book by Russell A. Barkley (who, in addition to helpful criticism of early drafts of key chapters, provided crucial encouragement in the early decision to go forward with the book), Naomi Breslau, Karen Friderici (who also generously offered the use of Figure 9.2), Kelly Klump, Tony Nunez, David Hambrick, David Hay, Joseph Jacobson, Sandra Jacobson, Jeff Measelle, and Erik Willcutt. I am uniquely indebted to the very generous work of Timothy Goth-Owens, who read and commented in detail on the entire manuscript in an effort to render it more accessible to clinicians. Stephen P. Hinshaw, Cynthia Huang-Pollock, and Thomas H. Carr collaborated with me on articles that overlapped with sections of this book, so I doubtless have derived benefits from this collaboration that are not noted elsewhere. However, of particular note is that Chapter 4 benefited a great deal from the advice of Cynthia Huang-Pollock; the discussion of psychosocial influences draws upon exchanges with Stephen P. Hinshaw. Benjamin B. Lahey, Joseph Sergeant, Erik Willcutt, and many other colleagues provided invaluable discussion and encouragement related to the ideas in various parts of the book. Kitty Moore at The Guilford Press provided crucial suggestions and encouragement at key junctures in the process. As always, despite the sharp eyes of these generous colleagues, some errors have doubtless survived; I retain sole responsibility for those and for any other shortcomings in this work.

Work on this book was made possible by a sabbatical leave provided by Michigan State University and supported by the generous efforts of my colleagues in the Department of Psychology, who covered my teaching and administrative obligations during the sabbatical. The data from my research described in this book were obtained with the support of funds from the National Institute of Mental Health, including Grant Nos. R01-MH63146 (in collaboration with John Henderson and Fernanda Ferreira) and R01-MH59105. No other financial support or vested interest undergirds my research or my work on this book. Collection of those data would not have been possible without the support of the Lansing community, including the Lansing School District and in particular Marion Philips of the Office of Evaluation Services in Lansing. Several undergraduate students as well as many dedicated graduate students in clinical psychology and in cognitive psychology at Michigan State worked long hours with families and children to collect and help analyze those data. I am indebted to them all.

Contents

| PART IV |

INTEGRATION

PART I

CONCEPTUAL CONTEXT

ADHD's Controversies

Attention-deficit/hyperactivity disorder (ADHD—also still known by its somewhat misleading former name, attention deficit disorder or ADD) has become a household word, yet it remains poorly understood. The purpose of this book is twofold. The first purpose is to describe the present state of knowledge about "what's wrong" in children with ADHD, as seen through the lens of neuropsychological mechanisms. The second purpose is to begin to map a direction forward in terms of a multipathway model of ADHD, and to make suggestions for what I call "high-risk/high-payoff" research investments to generate break-throughs in understanding that can lead to meaningful prevention.

The need for this discussion is not hard to find: ADHD often pro-vokes heated controversies in our society, and these controversies show little sign of abating (for historical overviews of the decades of disputes about ADHD in the United States, see Barkley, 2006, and Safer & Krager, 1992). This first chapter addresses the sources of the controversies. It underscores the need for the sorts of understanding this book calls for by addressing prevalence, treatment rates, and the concepts of medicalization and reductionism. First, however, I outline key terms and definitions, and describe the book's plan in a bit more detail.

TWO MEANINGS OF "VALIDITY"
AND THE AIMS OF THIS BOOK

Periodically, this controversy takes the form of questions about the "validity" of ADHD as a medical disease construct or disorder (Barkley et al., 2002; Brown, 2003). Thus teachers, parents, or the general public may ask, "Does ADHD really exist?" "Is it valid to diagnose it in a child?" "Is it really a disease?"

Two kinds of validity can be identified for present purposes. "Clinical validity" is the extent to which a disorder hangs together statistically (as a syndrome), is exhibited by impaired children who need help, responds to treatment, and has other meaningful external correlates (such as family or biological findings, differential long-term outcomes, and differential treatment response) at the group level. This is a very practical kind of validity, and perhaps the most important criterion for disease or disorder concepts in our society is that they attain it. Establishing clinical validity is also usually the first stage in evaluating a presenting problem. Scientists generally agree that ADHD has good clinical validity (Faraone, 2005; Lahey & Willcutt, 2002), despite the continued need for refinement of its operational criteria (Achenbach, 2000) and better integration with ongoing empirical analyses.

The second kind of validity can be called "etiological validity." This is the extent to which we know what caused the disorder/disease and why it developed, in every case. ADHD has not achieved this status—but, then again, neither have most psychiatric disorders. We have many clues to causes, but these findings mostly apply at the group level. We do not yet know for each individual child where the disorder (or the impairing behavior) came from.

To address etiological validity, we must distinguish (1) within-child mechanisms and (2) etiologies (causes). Put another way, to understand a disorder's etiological validity, we have to understand two things. The first is "What is different about this child?" Is what is wrong inside the child—let's call him Tommy—best understood as his memory, his attention, his blood pressure, the level of neurotransmitter activity in his brain, his sleep quality? These internal mechanisms or "markers" of disorder help provide further validation. They may be clues to the syndrome's causes, or they may themselves be part of the cause. In other words, they may be additional symptoms of the disorder (analogy: fever and high white blood cell count as clues to what is wrong), or they may be causal (analogy: blood clot as source of fainting, torn ligament as source of pain). The second thing we have to understand is "What led to this problem?" That is, what has caused it beyond Tommy's current condition— for example, genes, prenatal injury, or unusual early stress? Although Chapter 2 points out that nonlinear causality is likely, key causal effects must be sought.

Even though groups of children with ADHD show characteristic deficits on a range of neurological and neuropsychological measures, debate continues as to the core deficit(s)—and these measures are generally absent from clinical decision making. Identifying these *within-child* mechanisms (i.e., "What is different about this child?") more clearly, and linking them to originating etiologies (i.e., "What caused this problem?"), therefore remain crucial goals of current research. Again, this book both provides an update on the status of knowledge about these causal mechanisms and points to directions forward from here.

These directions forward include potentially speculative yet promising ideas for new research. I call these speculative ideas "high-risk/high-payoff" research ideas. They are "high-risk" because they will cost society time and money to carry out, yet their chances of paying off may be judged less than certain (or perhaps less than 50%). They are "high-payoff" because if they were to succeed, they would fundamentally alter our ability to understand, treat, and prevent the condition. For example, I explore in some detail the potential role of environmental pollutants. As it becomes increasingly apparent, their role can provide clear direction for prevention, should prevention become a priority to society. All of us have a stake in the national research agenda on ADHD, because (1) as taxpayers, we pay both for the research and for the unsolved problems in society that the research tries to address (Chan, Zhan, & Homer, 2002); and (2) as clinicians or educators, we daily struggle with difficult problems in our clients, and are eager to utilize new discoveries that may bring relief to these children. Whether research dollars are productively invested is thus a cross-cutting public concern for clinicians, parents, educators, and scientists, as well as society as a whole.

Clarification of current knowledge is timely for several other reasons, despite a steady stream of books about ADHD (see Nigg, 2003a, for a guide to such books). A wealth of new research appears every year (over 2,700 new journal articles or book chapters on ADHD were published from 2001 through 2005 alone), making frequent consolidation of the state of the field essential. Medication rates for children are climbing rapidly in the United States (Zito et al., 2003), generating a press for answers by the U.S. Congress, parents, and the public (Brown, 2003). Claims and counterclaims about this and other issues abound, creating confusion and the need for cogent analyses of where we are and where we should go.

In the meantime, professionals face a steady stream of questions about ADHD from parents, teachers, and the public, and need to be able to provide current, up-to-date, and sophisticated answers. Indeed, in the midst of a proliferation of papers and studies, even specialists may have difficulty keeping up with the latest findings and may feel unsure of what to think. Advances in genetics or neuroscience related to ADHD can be especially difficult to evaluate, and their clinical relevance may not always be apparent (for a cogent earlier review, see Tannock, 1998). This leads to a complex state of affairs. Even as scientists are refining theories of neurobiology in ADHD, clinicians and other professionals are reading arguments that ADHD is not a valid disorder, is overdiagnosed, is excessively treated with medication, or represents a dangerous reductionism that mistakenly views all behavioral and adjustment problems merely in terms of biology (see Safer & Krager, 1992).

In spite of the urgency and concern in society about ADHD (and in spite of allegations that ADHD research has moved ahead too quickly to a medical formulation), research and clinical practice usually move ahead conservatively and cautiously. There is good reason for caution in clinical practice: "Do no harm" is the first mandate! At the same time, on the research front, Congress, the National Institutes of Health, and the public are voicing a growing interest in integrative, cross-cutting suggestions that carry the potential for breakthroughs in understanding—breakthroughs that can lead to real prevention of disability and improvement of children's health. Yet such suggestions will inevitably entail the risk of failure—and of loss of the research investment.

In this book, I combine current thinking on the neuropsychology of ADHD with an analysis of the relatively underexplored issue of etiological mechanisms (causes). I argue for far greater study of a targeted set of high-payoff (and high-risk) experiential causes of ADHD (i.e., for research that moves outside the mainstream), informed by the latest genetic and toxicological findings. Research on the disorder that integrates these perspectives must rely on yet-to-be-developed *multipathway* approaches to understanding the causal mechanisms in this syndrome.

This book therefore has two big-picture aims. To achieve the first aim—that of describing what is presently known about ADHD's causal mechanisms, in light of recurrent (and at times ill-informed) controversies over the disorder's nosological status—Part II of this book evaluates knowledge about *within-child* differences that may reflect causal mechanisms, or breakdowns in functioning of key abilities. This discussion follows a systematic model of candidate neural systems that are under active investigation. Understanding the nature of the within-child dysfunction in ADHD is essential to its eventual full validation. In other words, for ADHD to achieve full etiological validity, we seek to describe for each individual child what the systemic breakdown is in the child, or how that child developed the disorder (the label by itself hardly does so). Currently we cannot do this for any psychopathologies except certain types of mental retardation. Yet understanding within-child dysfunction is also essential to eventual improved objectivity of assessment. Unsurprisingly, therefore, this first topic is at the heart of a vigorous contemporary scientific discussion in the field, and I try to provide a current update that reflects today's thinking in the field.

To achieve the second aim—that of exploring potential etiologies (often confused with within-child dysfunction), in order to point out integrative research directions for the future—Part III of this book considers factors beyond the individual child that may cause the within-child dysfunctions we observe in the laboratory. In this section of the book, I first discuss the concept of multiple pathways and explain recent genetic findings. I then turn to experiential causes that receive too little discussion in the scientific literature, the consulting room, or the public policy discussions of child health. These include causes that are already fairly well established (and could be targets of more aggressive prevention efforts at the policy level), as well as emerging evidence for other causes that warrant study in a high-risk/high-payoff approach, including environmental toxins.

Although generalizations do not come easily to those who examine the ADHD literature closely, in Part IV of this book I draw some conclusions from the trends in this literature concerning both what scientists have learned so far and what remains to be worked out. I note at each step the answers to commonly asked questions about ADHD as well as clinical implications, thus drawing the scientific findings back to their real-world significance. A theme running throughout the book is that ADHD reflects multiple conditions, arising from multiple pathways of causal action. I do little more than begin to sketch what those pathways might be, in hopes of stimulating thinking by others. Yet that sketching will nonetheless carry potential implications for clinical understanding of the diversity of ADHD's presentations—a diversity that has led to some confusion in the clinical and public arenas.

BACKGROUND ISSUES ABOUT ADHD

Diagnostic Criteria and Comorbidity

What tools will readers need to follow my analysis, to place it in context, and to understand its relevance? First, this book assumes that readers are acquainted with or can easily access a range of clinically relevant background issues. ADHD's diagnostic criteria are available in current and past versions of the *Diagnostic and Statistical Manual of Mental Disorders* (now in the text revision of its fourth edition, or DSM-

IV-TR; American Psychiatric Association [APA] 1980, 1987, 1994, 2000), and the criteria for hyperkinetic disorder (HKD) are available in the *International Classification of Diseases* (now in its 10th revision, or ICD-10; World Health Association [WHO], 1993). Alternative methods of empirically measuring and defining the symptom cluster are explained by Achenbach (2000) and pertain to well-normed clinical assessment scales that diverge somewhat from the DSM-IV-TR criteria (although convergence across these methods also supports clinical validity).

As well, the discussion assumes familiarity with the fact that ADHD often co-occurs with other disorders, particularly conduct disorder (CD) and oppositional defiant disorder (ODD) (see Angold, Costello, & Erkanli, 1999; Caron & Rutter, 1991; Hinshaw, 1987; and Patterson, De Garmo, & Knutson, 2000, for discussions of conceptual and taxonomic issues); gender ratios in prevalence and referral (Gaub & Carlson, 1997); and long-term outcomes of ADHD with and without comorbidity. These topics raise important clinical considerations, but expert discussions of them are readily available in other sources. For overviews of ADHD's clinical and descriptive features, see Barkley (2006), Weiss and Hechtman (1993), and Wender (2000). For discussions of clinical issues related to comorbidity, see Brown (2000) and Pliszka, Carlson, and Swanson (1999). Most of the current book emphasizes the ADHD syndrome in childhood and its early precursors. Yet much of this discussion is also applicable to ADHD in adults (see Wasserstein, Wolf, & Lefever, 2001; Wilens, Faraone, & Biederman, 2005).

Assessment and Treatment Issues

It is also assumed that readers are familiar with standard assessment and treatment approaches for ADHD. For discussions of assessment, see Achenbach (1998, 2000) and Barkley (2006). For detailed treatment guidelines, see Barkley (2006), Hinshaw (1999), Jensen and Cooper (2002), and the other volumes just cited. Although I do not cover these issues here, I explore later why treatments may work the way they do.

This point about familiarity with established assessment and treatment approaches is important, because I highlight treatment implications of various findings about ADHD throughout this book. Those implications are to be seen as potential supplements to, not replacements for, existing practice parameters and descriptions of empirically established treatments Practice parameters for ADHD assessment and treatment have been published by the American Academy of Pediatrics (2000; also available at www.aap.org) and the American Academy of Child and Adolescent Psychiatry (1997; also available at www.aacap.org). In addition, following an extensive formal evaluation of the evidence for various treatments for child disorders (Chambless et al., 1996; Chambless & Ollendick, 2001), the Society for Clinical Child and Adolescent Psychology tabulates evidence-based treatments for ADHD at www.effectivechildtherapy.com.

Moreover, although my focus is on the neuropsychological level of analysis, other factors are also important in clinical assessment of children. These include anxiety level, self-esteem, attachment security, defensive style, goals and motivation to achieve them, and relative intangibles (e.g., a child's morale). These domains are mostly beyond the scope of this book, but receive some acknowledgment later when I consider temperament and personality style.

Subtypes of ADHD

The DSM-IV-TR provides for three subtypes of ADHD: combined type (ADHD-C), predominantly inattentive type (ADHD-PI), and predominantly hyperactive–impulsive type (ADHD-PHI). ICD-10's HKD is a narrower concept. Children with HKD are most likely to meet criteria for DSM-IV-TR's ADHD-C type, whereas a few would have ADHD-PI; however, many children with ADHD by DSM-IV-TR definitions would fail to meet the more stringent HKD criteria at all.

A key theme of this book is the heterogeneity of the ADHD construct (see Chapter 8 in particular). However, most of this book pertains to ADHD-C, simply because we have the most data on it. Periodically I comment on the other two subtypes. ADHD-PI, often erroneously referred to as "ADD" (the old term for ADHD), is of considerable interest, but data on it are limited. It may be somewhat more common in girls and more often associated with internalizing disorders. ADHD-PHI is often assumed to be closely related to ADHD-C, but that assumption is not made here. ADHD-PHI is relatively uncommon in clinical samples after preschool, and appears to have etiological determinants distinct from those of ADHD-C in childhood (Willcutt, Pennington, & DeFries, 2000). When identified in preschool, it often, but not always, is a precursor to the later ADHD-C (Lahey, Pelham, Loney, Lee, & Willcutt, 2005).

There has been substantial debate as to whether ADHD-PI is a completely distinct disorder from ADHD-C (Milich, Balentine, &

Lynam, 2001; Lahey, 2001; Hinshaw, 2001). The reasons for disagreement here are understandable. On the one hand, these two subtypes tend to have somewhat distinct external correlates. On the other hand, one subtype can develop into the other over time (Lahey et al., 2005) and neuropsychological deficits are sometimes similar in these two types (Hinshaw, Carte, Sami, Treuting, & Zapan, 2002). Children diagnosed with ADHD-PI probably include some who have a milder version of ADHD-C, and others who have a more distinct condition characterized by underactivity rather than overactivity (Carlson & Mann, 2002; McBurnett, Pfiffner, & Frick, 2001). A meta-analysis of family psychiatric studies of ADHD subtypes supports this conclusion. It shows that relatives of children with ADHD-C tend to have both ADHD-C and ADHD-PI, whereas relatives of children with ADHD-PI tend only to have ADHD-PI (Stawicki, Nigg, & von Eye, in press).

In view of these controversies, I treat the subtypes (1) as though they have some etiologies in common (i.e., the heterogeneity of causes to be explored in this book cuts across the three existing subtypes), yet also (2) as if they provide clues to some of the preliminary distinctions among etiological pathways that we can make at this juncture. The decision to allow some etiological relationship between subtypes in my conceptual model of ADHD only affects the argument slightly, for two reasons. First, nearly all research is on ADHD-C or its proxies, so it would be the focus of discussion in any case. Second, the main impact of treating the subtypes as entirely distinct disorders would be to alter the working prevalence rate of ADHD, which would change risk magnitudes (but only slightly) in the later chapters of the book.

Whereas most research pertains to ADHD-C (and hence it dominates this volume), ICD-10's HKD describes a subgroup of children who do not have mood or anxiety disorders or CD. A recent reexamination of the Multimodal Treatment Study of ADHD (MTA) data set suggested that about 25% of children with ADHD-C would meet strict criteria for HKD (see Swanson et al., 2004). We (Swanson et al., 2004) have suggested that clearer etiologies might emerge for HKD as a refined phenotype. However, the appropriate boundaries of the phenotype for ADHD research remain in dispute. In other words, will we get a clearer signal in relation to various etiologies (genes, contaminants, or brain differences) if we define the disorder very narrowly, or if we define it more broadly? Very little research has examined children with HKD; the vast majority of studies look at children with ADHD-C or versions of it (e.g., children with high rating scale scores on measures of inattention and hyperactivity).

TABLE 1.1. Basic Operational Definitions and Types of ADHD

Type name	Description
ADHD–combined type (ADHD-C; DSM-IV-TR)	Both inattentive and hyperactive–impulsive
ADHD–primarily inattentive type (ADHD-PI; DSM-IV-TR)	Inattentive, but below threshold for hyperactive–impulsive
ADHD–primarily hyperactive–impulsive type (ADHD-PHI; DSM-IV-TR)	Hyperactive–impulsive, inattention below cutoff
Hyperkinetic disorder (HKD; ICD-10)	Some each of inattentive, hyperactive, impulsive
Attention deficit disorder (ADD; DSM-III)	Old term no longer in official use

Table 1.1 outlines the three DSM-IV-TR ADHD subtypes, as well as ICD-10's HKD and DSM-III's ADD (now superseded).

ENSUING TOPICS

The importance of identifying causal mechanisms is driven in part by public concern about three issues concerning which details are often lacking in publications about ADHD: (1) ADHD's reputed variable prevalence, (2) its rapidly increasing rate of medication treatment, and (3) concern about the growing "medicalization of behavior" in U.S. society. I address those three issues in this opening chapter. The brief reviews of prevalence and treatment data underscore the need to characterize causal processes associated with the behavioral syndrome. Likewise, taking time to outline the conceptual critique of "medicalization of behavior" provides a context for understanding why this ADHD controversy is important and why identification of causal mechanisms is so actively sought after by the nation's scientists as well as by Congress (Brown, 2003).

Furthermore, it is important that we work from some common ground with regard to how we define "disorder," or else much of the discussion may be confusing. Related to this is the need to appreciate multilevel, transactional accounts of developmental psychopathology and, in that appreciation, to avoid false reductionism. Those reflections on disorder and transactional accounts of development are provided in Chapter 2, where the concepts of "clinical validity" versus "etiological validity," with which I have opened this chapter, should become clear.

The key conclusion from Chapter 2 is that contemporary definitions of disorder require both kinds of validity. For clinical validity, the disorder construct must accurately identify impaired individuals who need clinical intervention. ADHD is well supported in this regard (Lahey & Willcutt, 2002; Hinshaw, 2002a; Johnston, 2002), despite ongoing refinement of the symptom lists, and so this book does not delve long into that "noncontroversy." The requirement of etiological validity is more challenging. Modern theory requires an established "dysfunction in the child" to validate a disorder's status as etiologically valid (Wakefield, 1992). Yet doing so is not straightforward. For example, it is now clear that at the group level various neuropsychological and biological deficits can be reliably identified in ADHD (Barkley et al., 2002; Swanson & Castellanos, 2002). This fact encourages belief that the disorder can be validated etiologically. Yet debate continues as to just how those performance deficits can be best characterized, and how they should be understood. Furthermore, and crucially, these neurocognitive dysfunctions remain unclear at the all- important *individual* level, at which they must be applied in clinical practice. The *group* level findings do not apply to all of the children designated as having ADHD according to the current definitional formats of DSM-IV-TR and ICD-10. As a result, they are diagnostically inconclusive at present.

This consideration is a key focus of later chapters in this book. In all, describing what is known about within-child neurocognitive mechanisms remains a primary focus for the field, and for that reason is the focus of this book's Part II. However, a full picture of where the field needs to go requires integrative thinking about etiology and in particular about multiple etiological pathways, which become the focus of Parts III and IV.

Finally, several areas of controversy about ADHD are bypassed in this book, because they have been well addressed by others or because too few data exist to do much more than speculate about them. I highlight many of these in the final section of Chapter 2.

These preliminary conceptual points (in Chapters 1–2) set the context for why we need to continue illuminating the status of within child dysfunctional mechanisms in ADHD if we are to eventually give some rest to the debates about "validity" in ADHD. They also provide a perspective to prevent misunderstanding and/or misuse of the material that follows in the heart of this book. I now move directly to an overview of prevalence and treatment data.

PREVALENCE, INCIDENCE, AND TREATMENT RATES: DRIVERS OF CONTROVERSIES

Prevalence and Incidence Rates

Key questions often asked about ADHD include "Is there more ADHD now than in the past?" "How common is it?" "Is it more common in the United States than everywhere else?" "Is it assessed totally differently in different countries?" These widely asked questions are addressed here to the extent possible. First, I supply a few quick definitions. "Incidence" refers to onset of new cases over time (e.g., in a new birth cohort). It can only be assessed via prospective cohort designs, which are lacking for ADHD. "Prevalence" refers to the percentage of cases in the population at a given point in time; it can be estimated from cross-sectional surveys. Therefore, we must rely on existing prevalence estimates to gauge what the incidence might be. I return to the issue of incidence after describing what we know about prevalence.

The official prevalence estimate is that 3–7% of children in the United States are affected by ADHD at any one time (APA, 2000). Numerous studies have relied on parent or teacher survey data alone and yielded prevalence estimates in the double digits in various nations, with total estimates ranging from 2.3% to 19.8% (Airaksinen, Michelsson, & Jokela, 2004; Baumgaertel, Wolraich, & Dietrich, 1995; Bu-Haroon, Eapen, & Bener, 1999; Magnússon, Smári, Grétarsdottir, & Prándardóttir, 1999; Gadow et al., 2000; Meyer, 1998; Nolan, Gadow, & Sprafkin, 2001; Wolriach, Hannah, Pinnock, Baumgaertel, & Brown, 1996). However, such studies really assess screening prevalences, not prevalence of disorder. They are unable to consider the essential criterion of impairment, other criteria (such as cross-situational display of problems or duration of symptoms), or alternative explanations (such as learning disabilities). Therefore, studies that rely only on rating scale scores from a single informant cannot be considered estimates of the prevalence of ADHD as defined in DSM-IV and its text revision, or considered to assess disorder in any meaningful sense. Attempting to combine these screening estimates with those from studies that relied on other methods or on multiple informants is inappropriate.

Unsurprisingly, prevalence estimates are much lower when more rigorous methods are used such as structured interviews or multiple informants, and when even some of the DSM-IV(-TR) criteria (in particular, impairment; see Gordon et al., 2005) are considered. I computed

unweighted median prevalence estimates across five studies that utilized either structured ratings or parent plus teacher ratings and
impairment criteria to assess DSM-IV criteria (Rohde et al., 1999, in
Brazil; Pineda, Lopera, Palacio, Ramirez, & Henao, 2003, in Colombia;
Gomez, Harvey, Quick, Scharer, & Harris, 1999, in Australia; Graetz,
Sawyer, Hazell, Arney, & Baghurst, 2001, in Australia; Wolraich,
Hanna, Baumgaertel, & Feurer, 1998, in Tennessee). The results were
2.9% for ADHD-C, 3.2% for ADHD-PI, and 0.6% for ADHD-PHI, yielding a total of 6.8%. The median ratio of boys to girls was 2:1. The only
study in the United States (Wolraich et al., 1998) yielded figures nearly
identical to this median value. Rates were quite similar across the
nations studied—with the exception of the study in Colombia, which,
despite using the same methods as the other studies, yielded a prevalence rate about twice that in the United States, Australia, or Brazil.
Only three studies were located that surveyed prevalence rates for
HKD (Leung et al., 1996, in China; Liu et al., 2000, in Hong Kong;
Gosden, Kramp, Gabrielsen, & Sestoft, 2003, in Denmark), all yielding
rates of about 1%.

As these citations make apparent, no comprehensive survey of
ADHD prevalence using full DSM-IV(-TR) criteria in the United States
exists. Even the studies cited here did not consider all of the possible
rule-outs, confounds, and comorbid disorders that affect actual ADHD
diagnosis. Even if some of the DSM-IV(-TR) criteria (such as age of
onset) prove needless, these estimates are still certainly too high, due to
failure to consider these other issues. Thus 6% can be viewed as a "high
estimate" of ADHD prevalence across all subtypes. Note that (1) variation on these estimates is less than 10-fold worldwide, and (2) the existence of ADHD-PI adds appreciably to overall ADHD prevalence.

The varying definitions of ADHD over time, exemplified by the
changing definitions from DSM-III (APA, 1980) to DSM-III-R (APA,
1987) to DSM-IV and its text revision (APA, 1994, 2000), have contributed to uncertainty about incidence and prevalence. Lahey, Miller,
Gordon, and Riley (1999) and Bird (2002) provide thorough summaries of past prevalence research on child disruptive behavior problems
defined by various dimensional systems, as well as by the different version of the DSM and ICD. Lahey et al.'s (1999) appendices catalogue
dozens of such studies to that time, but those reviews identified very
few studies using the now-current DSM-IV(-TR) or ICD-10. Lahey et al.
(1999) noted that when methodological, definitional, and age effects
across studies were ignored, prevalence estimates ranged from 0% to
16%, with a median of 2.0%. That figure is not far from the median fig-

ure of 2.9% for ADHD-C that I have drawn above from studies using DSM-IV.

Aside from the problem of single-rater surveys versus multi-informant or structured-interview approaches to identifying ADHD, several other methodological issues make it difficult to rely on a single summary number across these studies—a caution noted by Lahey et al. (1999) that still holds true. I note here the most obvious issues, because they underscore the value of an eventual definition of ADHD that includes not only behavioral descriptors but also within-child mechanisms or dysfunctions, and eventually causal sources in development. What are these methodological issues?

First, when the prevalence of ADHD viewed as a *categorical* syndrome is considered, DSM-IV has yielded higher rates of ADHD case identification than DSM-III or DSM-III-R (Baumgaertel et al., 1995; Wolraich et al., 1996), and markedly higher rates than HKD as defined in ICD-9 or ICD-10 (Leung et al., 1996). Higher rates are due in substantial part to the operational definition of ADHD-PI, which is at least as common as ADHD-C in population surveys and was not included in earlier DSMs or in the ICD formulation. Higher rates in relation to HKD derive from three additional differences in criteria (Prendergast et al., 1988): (1) CD is a rule-out for HKD but not for ADHD (Liu et al., 2000, identified 1% with HKD, but an additional 1% with HKD plus CD); (2) HKD is not diagnosed if a mood disorder is present, contrary to DSM-IV and its text revision; and (3) HKD requires symptoms in three domains (hyperactivity, impulsivity, inattention) whereas even ADHD-C requires only two domains (it is possible to diagnose ADHD-C with six symptoms of hyperactivity from the nine hyperactive–impulsive symptoms in the criterion set). Thus, even though the most reasonable comparison to ICD-10's syndrome of HKD is DSM-IV's syndrome of ADHD-C, we might expect at least a 2:1 ratio of cases of ADHD-C versus HKD if about half of ADHD-C cases are associated with CD or mood disorder (Lahey et al., 1999). As noted before, the ratio may be even greater, on the order of 4:1 (Swanson et al., 2004).

Second, rates of diagnosis may change with development. For example, although data are inconsistent (see Lahey et al., 1999), prevalence is probably lower in adolescence than in childhood (Achenbach, 2000). In part this may be due to reductions in hyperactive behaviors during that developmental period (Hart, Lahey, Loeber, Applegate, & Frick, 1995). By the same token, ADHD-PHI is most easily identified in preschoolers, but ADHD-PI tends to appear later in development. Thus the entire epidemiological profile may be moderated by age and developmental period. Such age-related changes would be expected if, as is currently the case, diagnostic criteria are not adjusted for age (Achenbach, 2000).

Third, population incidence and prevalence should not be confused with administrative incidence and prevalence, or the rate at which the disorder is recognized or treated by educators and clinicians (Taylor, Sandberg, Thorley, & Giles, 1991). As Swanson et al. (1998) have described, administrative incidence or prevalence can change rapidly, simply because of changes in laws, norms, or other practices. For example, when the United States changed its educational rules in 1990 to allow ADHD to qualify as a separate category for special services, administrative prevalence quickly doubled. This increased willingness to identify the syndrome obviously has no direct relation to its actual rate of occurrence in the population.

In short, the median estimates of prevalence that I have calculated from studies discussed here are 6.8% for all types of ADHD, 2.9% for ADHD-C, 3.2% for ADHD-PI, and 0.6% for ADHD-PHI. These values provide an "upper-bound" estimate of point prevalence in North and South America, Western Europe, and Australia, all based on very limited evidence. Although we cannot rule out true differences in prevalence across regions or nations, differences in survey methodology remain the most likely explanation for the modest variation in estimates across these studies to date. Note that these estimates mask somewhat higher estimates for boys (i.e., they are the average of higher rates for boys and lower rates for girls).

How do prevalence estimates relate to the incidence (or rate of onset of new cases) of ADHD? This requires a moment's comment, because later in the book many of our questions about etiology will oblige us to ask about incidence. In general, prevalence = incidence × duration (so if 10 in 1,000 people get a disease per year and each has the disease for 10 years, then prevalence will be 100/1,000). Thus a "low estimate" of incidence for the ages of 6–18 would be 6% divided by 12, or an incidence rate of 0.5%. However, for ADHD, the rate of new cases drops off dramatically after the initial elementary school years, and studies of children with ADHD tend to yield similar prevalence estimates regardless of ages studied. These findings suggest that the prevalence within each age is about the same through childhood (although medication rates vary by age). Thus, for the sake of simplicity, let us assume the following: (1) 6% of first graders develop ADHD each year (incidence is 6%); (2) no new cases occur among children ages 7–17; and (3) 18-year-olds are no longer children with ADHD.

These assumptions would yield a prevalence of 6% (the same as the assumed incidence), both within each age cohort and in the population of children ages 6–17. In reality, of course, not all cases emerge in first grade; some children recover; and some new cases emerge at each age during the elementary school years. However, if rates of recovery and new diagnoses during the elementary years are assumed to be roughly similar to one another, then this scenario still would approximately hold. Therefore, in the absence of actual incidence data, I rely on these simplifying assumptions and utilize an incidence rate of 6% in this book. (Note that a lower incidence estimate—e.g., 1% or even 0.5%—would generally have little effect on the estimates of the magnitude of environmental risk effects discussed later in the book; see note 1 to Chapter 10 for more details.)

Despite the relatively good agreement across the studies cited above, prevalence estimates underscore the dissatisfaction with how ADHD is defined, because they depend on the inclusiveness of its operational or behavioral definition—which varies from study to study. A stronger conclusion about prevalence and incidence could be drawn if the syndrome were anchored in a causal definition. If within-child breakdown of psychological or cognitive mechanisms were added to the definition, it is unknown what the incidence or even the prevalence would be (presumably it would be lower), or whether it would vary across cultures or nations. The current estimates of incidence and prevalence are, from an etiological perspective, therefore preliminary. They doubtless will be refined in future years (or decades) as the syndrome is better characterized by causal mechanisms.

Treatment Rates

Are more children being treated for ADHD than in the past? The answer here is clear: yes. Whereas the secular trajectory of incidence or prevalence rates over time is unknown (and may be fairly constant), treatment rates are rising rapidly in the United Stated. Prescriptions for methylphenidate (i.e., Ritalin and related medications), the majority of which are for children (Rappley, Gardiner, Jetton, & Houang, 1995), have risen steadily.

Methylphenidate use in the United States nearly doubled from 1981 to 1987; leveled off for a period of several years in the late 1980s, due in part to public controversy, negative publicity, and threatened lawsuits (Safer & Krager, 1992); then doubled again from 1990 to 1995 (Robison, Skaer, Sclar, & Galin, 1999; see reviews of Drug Enforcement

Administration data by Cooper, 2002, and Feussner, 2002). Other stimulant prescriptions also increased sharply during the 1990s (Cooper, 2002). During the 1990s the ADHD diagnoses made in primary care physician office visits more than doubled among boys and nearly tripled among girls (population rate increase-adjusted), while the rate of prescription of stimulant medication in the United States to children in that time period increased by the same amounts (Robison et al., 1999)—indicating that the increased medication usage is not mainly due to higher dosages in bigger or more disturbed children. Moreover, other medications are also used to treat ADHD. Overall, one recent review estimated that between 2 and 2.5 million U.S. children are receiving psychotropic medication for ADHD (Safer & Zito, 1999), or about 3% of children in the nation. Another recent survey found that among insured patients, 4.3% of children are prescribed stimulant medication (Cox, Motheral, Henderson, & Mager, 2003). These rates vary by age; among 11-year-old boys (the most frequently treated group), rates were at 9%. Although rates of prescription worldwide are unclear, prescription rates in the United States are likely to be significantly higher than in other nations. For example, prescription of stimulants has been long accepted in the United States, and clinical guidelines recommend a stimulant trial. By contrast, in the United Kingdom stimulant prescription was long restricted by law.

Moreover, there is noticeable regional variation in treatment rates within the United States (Cox et al., 2003). Rates of children medicated for ADHD are estimated at 1.39% in portions of Utah (Goldstein & Turner, 2001), and as high as 10% in some counties in Virginia (LeFever, Dawson, & Morrow, 1999). Cox et al. (2003) found rates ranging from 6.5% in Louisana to 1.6% in the District of Columbia. Within my home state of Michigan, we see a 10-fold variation in rates of stimulant prescription from county to county, ranging from 0.25% to 2.8% among all children, and from 0.9% to 11.7% among 10- to 11-year-old boys (the most frequently medicated group) (Rappley et al., 1995). Thus, within the United States, the rate of stimulant prescription is highly variable from region to region and from county to county within a given region, ranging from about 1% to over 10%.

Because of differences in the way sampling is handled across studies, it is difficult to determine whether these *local* study results are consistent with the estimated *national* average treatment rate of 2.8% in the United States (Robison et al., 1999). Nonetheless, it is striking that we see variation in treatment rates within the United States that are at least as great as the variation in diagnostic prevalence estimated across different nations. At least in part, this is doubtless attributable to the fact that in clinical practice, widely varying diagnostic methodologies and clinical procedures are in use, leading to varying rates of diagnosis and treatment from region to region and nation to nation.

Some of this variation may reflect failure to follow best clinical practices consistently. For example, the large-scale MTA found that medication treatment (with stimulants) as practiced in routine community care was associated with some improvement, but that it was relatively ineffective compared with medication treatment implemented according to a best-practices approach (double-blind, placebo-controlled, multidose, multidrug trial)—or, for that matter, compared with well-implemented albeit costly behavioral and psychosocial intervention (Jensen et al., 2001). The medication practice in MTA entailed double-blind ratings by teachers at three different dosages and placebo, so that the best dose was systematically identified.

Key cautions qualify the treatment rate data as well. Exact figures on the number of children prescribed stimulant medication are unavailable, so these have to be estimated indirectly. Furthermore, some of this increase in total medication use is attributable to longer-duration treatment of children as they grow older (Cox et al., 2003); to recent new evidence of the utility of the medications in adolescents and adults; to changes in the DSM-IV that provided diagnostic criteria for ADHD-PI, enabling children with this subtype to be identified and treated; and to growing recognition of the ADHD syndrome in girls (Rowland et al., 2002; Safer & Zito, 1999). In addition, some increase is to be expected because of population increases (although some studies have taken this into account).

Although it brings little comfort to those alarmed by growing stimulant usage in children, it is important to recognize that the use of all medications for children, not just psychostimulants, has increased by about the same amount during the past two decades in the United States (Zito et al., 2003). Thus, whereas stimulant medication rates have raised concerns, stimulants are not special in their rate of increased use; numerous psychiatric medications show the same pattern. The rising medication of children for ADHD is part of a larger pattern in U.S. society of increasing use of psychiatric medicines, both with children and with adults. The many social and economic factors that may account for that phenomenon (Zito et al., 2003) are beyond the scope of the discussion. The upshot, however, is that ADHD is not necessarily a unique phenomenon in regard to either medication use or the medicalization of behavior.

Finally, the percentage of children thought to be receiving treatment for ADHD in the United States (just under 3%) remains less than half of the estimated point prevalence of ADHD, all subtypes (6.8%). On the other hand, treatment rates apparently approach 9% within certain age and gender groups (e.g., 10- to 11-year-old boys; Cox et al., 2003), and these appear to be higher than expected. The regional, age, and gender variations in rates of treatment have led to suggestions that both undertreatment and overtreatment may be occurring (Cox et al., 2003; Jensen et al., 1999).

In all, the increases in medication treatment and wide regional variations in rates of medication treatment give some observers pause because of the unknown extent to which they may reflect sociological phenomena, including the rapid medicalization of behavior (see below), rather than valid medical practice or treatment of a bona fide medical condition. The concern centers around what are perceived to be the "soft" diagnostic boundaries of the syndrome (again, an issue shared with many if not all other psychiatric conditions), enabling substantial variation in how the diagnosis is operationally established in clinical practice. This state of affairs, though amenable to correction by more consistent operational definitions of the behavioral criteria, may be exacerbated by lack of a uniformly defined and measured causal mechanism or marker. In contrast, few observers question the legitimacy of cancer or even asthma, despite their rising incidences—perhaps because they have better within-child markers of pathophysiology than does ADHD.

The bottom line is that whereas many assumptions are made in both popular and academic critiques of ADHD, the real reasons for the rising and highly variable rates of medication treatment are unknown. For example, from a logical/analytic point of view, we must consider the possibility that prevalence varies from region to region more than expected. Although that may be judged unlikely (especially in view of the smaller range of estimates across nations for prevalence than within the United States for treatment rates), it is a logical possibility.

In fact, several possibilities exist, and data to sort them out are not at hand. Table 1.2 summarizes several possibilities (varying in likelihood). It underscores the occasional tendency of commentators to choose their personal favorite rather than to evaluate all in an even-handed manner. For example, as the table illustrates, rising treatment rates could be due to changes in medical practice, and/or to genuine increases in rates of child problems. As we will see in Chapters 9–11, this last possibility deserves consideration. Because it is unclear

TABLE 1.2. Why Would Treatment or Prevalence Rates of ADHD Vary with Time or Location?

Treatment rates could vary (increase) because:

1. Physicians are more willing to write prescriptions as evidence of medications' safety and efficacy mounts.

2. More children meet diagnostic criteria, due to changes in DSM-IV.

3. Reduction in health care coverage for many families means that psychological evaluation and behavioral intervention are not available, so medication is used now for problems previously given psychotherapy.

4. Schools are required to provide programming for children with problems, placing enormous cost pressures on them which lead to the use of less costly medical intervention.

5. Pharmaceutical company advertising, together with competitive pressure on kids and parents, lead more parents to push for medication; physicians comply due to lack of time and resources for alternative interventions.

6. Varying acceptance of medication in different local communities.

7. Physician practices, including diagnostic thresholds, vary across local communities.

8. Rates of behavior problems really do vary regionally (see below).

Prevalence rates could vary (or appear to vary) because of variation in:

1. The perception of the meaning of the DSM-IV(-TR) or ICD-10 behavioral symptoms.

2. Willingness to endorse problem symptoms on ratings or interview in studies.

3. Definition of impairment, either implicit or explicit.

4. Study procedures (e.g., examiner threshold for marking symptoms present).

5. Changes in risk factors that potentiate or maintain expression of behavior problems (e.g., school funding, family distress, socioeconomic pressures).

6. Environmental etiological potentiators (e.g., environmental contaminants such as pollutants; poor vs. strong prenatal care, leading to varying survival rates of low-birthweight children).

7. Population genetic variations, leading to variation in liability to disorder.

whether there is a change over time in actual rates of ADHD problems, data on that question would be very useful and would inform etiological theories. Achenbach and Howell (1993) and Achenbach, Dumenci, and Rescorla (2002) provide initial data on variation over time in children's rates of behavioral and emotional problems generally. They suggest some increase in problems over time, although this increase is apparently not linear. Once again, the need for a definition of the syndrome that includes markers of disorder within the child (markers of dysfunction, or of causal process) is underscored by these various possibilities.

MEDICALIZATION OF BEHAVIOR?

With the rapid increase in prescription not only of methylphenidate, but of many other psychotropic medications to young children (Zito et al., 2003), concern has risen in our society about excessive reliance on medications for a wide array of ills, particularly in children. Thus "medicalization" (used in the sense of viewing a behavior as coming under the purview of medicine) as a phenomenon of concern extends well beyond ADHD. Adding to the stakes, pharmaceutical companies have begun marketing drugs directly and aggressively to consumers in the past decade (Barsky & Borus, 1995), raising concerns among sociologists, media muckrakers, and citizen advocacy groups (Wolfe, 2003). Indeed, the drug companies' aggressive involvement in the research enterprise itself has become a sensitive and controversial area in the entire mental health field, as attested in book-length critiques by such knowledgeable commentators as the former editors of the *New England Journal of Medicine* (Angell, 2004; Kassirer, 2004).

Concern about medication of children for ADHD thus mirrors wider concerns nationally about whether pharmacology is overutilized as a solution to life's problems, perhaps combined with blame directed at the drug companies' aggressive advertising and alleged involvement in scientific thinking. Indeed, concerns about the marketing powers of the "medical–industrial complex" are long-standing (Relman, 1980). Critics can point to the growing number of diagnoses in the DSM over the years, and the growing list of conditions to be treated by pharmacological tools, to support their view that the pharmaceutical industry's profits are driving this approach. Even medical writers have worried about the number of conditions that medical professionals are now expected to address (Barsky & Borus, 1995; Conrad, 1992). Sociological and scholarly critics of these phenomena have found ADHD a ready exemplar both in the past (Smith & Kronick, 1979) and more recently (Searight & McClaren, 1998). In view of the importance of these concerns, it is unfortunate that in publications for popular consumption they are sometimes stated in extreme form—causing scientists and clinicians to dismiss them, and leaving many laypeople and educators confused.

What is the core of this concern, from the point of view of a *scientific* understanding of ADHD? As described by Searight and McClaren (1998), it can be paraphrased as follows: Although larger contextual processes in society, or in children's development, may partially account for the observed problems in at least some substantial subset of cases, those processes may be overlooked by an excessive research and clinical focus on intrinsic (within-child) factors. This focus is driven by overreliance on a medical metaphor to understand the problems (medicalization). In other words, clinicians, scientists, and educators may be overlooking important clues about the phenomena that constitute ADHD. This is a noteworthy concern, and it will be important when reading Chapters 4–7 to recall that we will be taking up possible causal agents in Chapters 9–11.

From this perspective, "overtreatment" is likely, due to a confluence of societal, economic, and/or policy factors unrelated to disease. These include popular media attention to ADHD, which may lead to referral and diagnosis by parents (or, in the case of adults with ADHD, by the individuals themselves); increased expectations of children, due to competitive demands in school and society; fiscal pressure on school districts that are unable to provide services for growing numbers of children diagnosed with learning problems and ADHD; fiscal pressure on health care systems, including capitated systems that discourage thorough assessment as well as more costly behavioral or psychological treatment for child disorders; and the recent lifting of the taboo against pharmaceutical companies' marketing their products directly to consumers (Searight & McClaren, 1998). These are important societal and policy issues, pointing to (among other issues) a lack of appropriate support services for children and families in need. However, for our purposes, we can note again that determination of specific diagnostic or causal mechanisms in affected children would contribute to clarifying the appropriate extent of such concerns.

In the meantime, clinicians may often be asked to speculate as to whether the incidence or prevalence of ADHD is increasing, or whether the condition is overtreated. In fact, neither is clear. However, it *is* clear that (1) administrative prevalence has increased, due to legal changes in the United States; (2) medication rates have risen rapidly over the past generation, for multiple reasons; and (3) medication rates in the United States vary widely from region to region. Recognizing that medicalization reflects multiple dynamics in society concerning health care and educational services may enable clinicians to avoid facile conclusions and consequent treatment mistakes.

OTHER IMPORTANT ISSUES

A number of other important issues about the definition of ADHD ultimately need consideration. First, should ADHD be understood as a categorical (taxonic) entity, or as an extreme of a trait (dimension)? In other words, do children with ADHD have a true clinical disease, with unique determinants (in the same way that an infectious disease has the unique determinants of viral or bacterial invasion)? Or do they have an extreme level of a trait that is simply present in lower levels in the typically developing population (in much the same way that hypertension is defined by a somewhat arbitrary, but statistically meaningful, cutoff on the blood pressure continuum)? Dimensional assessment tools (Achenbach, 2000) provide an empirically defensible alternative to a DSM-IV-TR or ICD-10 formulation clinically, and imply a distinct conceptualization of the phenomenon (although it is not unrelated to the DSM and ICD views).

Clinical decisions require labeling a child with a disorder, and clinicians must naturally weigh whether the benefits of doing so (e.g., access to needed care) outweigh the risks (e.g., stigma). As a result, the field continues to debate the appropriate threshold for diagnosis. If cutoff points are too narrow, many children needing services are excluded, but if they are too broad, many typically developing children will be labeled. This quest again underscores the effort to clarify within-child mechanisms or markers that might better define the disorder or its types, as well as the search for definable causal agents.

This practical question is an important one. Yet it rests on a theoretical question: At the level of causal structure, does ADHD reflect distinct causes (e.g., the IQ distribution contains many single-gene disorders of mental retardation at its low end)? Sophisticated behavior genetic analyses (DeFries & Fulker, 1988) represent a key method here. Studies using those approaches tend to suggest that ADHD is best viewed as an extreme of an underlying trait dimension (Levy, Hay, McStephen, Wood, & Waldman, 1997; Willcutt et al., 2000), although other, equally sophisticated taxometric methods have yet to be employed (Meehl, 1995; Waller & Meehl, 1999). Yet this does not negate the utility of the syndrome definition to identify extreme problems in need of intervention related to impairments (Hinshaw, 2002a; Johnston, 2002), which is a judgment clinicians must make each day. Indeed, because categorical studies of extreme groups (e.g., children meeting criteria for ADHD) seem most applicable to clinical problems, those types of studies remain the norm.

Gender and Cultural Issues

Second, causes and outcomes for ADHD may depend on children's gender (Gaub & Carlson, 1997) or on cultural variation. Yet these effects are still poorly understood. For example, it is unclear whether girls may be more protected than boys from expression of the ADHD syndrome, or whether the syndrome may reflect a more consistent neural injury in girls versus wide temperament variation in boys (James & Taylor, 1990). Most of the etiological research available pertains to boys, and nearly all pertains to largely white samples in the United States, Canada, Australia, Great Britain, the Netherlands, and Germany. The extent to which conclusions about mechanisms will generalize to girls is unclear (Hinshaw, 2002b). Likewise, the extent to which conclusions can be generalized to other nations, or to other ethnic groups within these well-studied countries (e.g., lower-income black and Hispanic populations in the United States), remains unclear and constitutes an important gap in knowledge.

Developmental Changes

Third, nearly all research treats ADHD in static fashion, rather than as an unfolding developmental pathway. The expression of ADHD symptoms apparently changes with development. Specifically, there is greater display of hyperactivity in the preschool years, whereas more prominent difficulties with inattention, disorganization, and impulsivity are seen in adolescence and adulthood (Hart et al., 1995)—even as some individuals show recovery at those later ages (Mannuzza & Klein, 2000). The diagnostic nosology completely ignores the appropriate and most relevant symptoms to assess in adolescents and adults (see Wender, 1995).

CLINICAL IMPLICATIONS

The key points for clinicians here are several. First, it is important to recognize that there are both utilities and limits to assuming a medical disease approach to ADHD. Many children with ADHD do have neuropsychological weaknesses, which a full assessment can identify. A thorough evaluation—including assessment of cognitive functioning and assessment of comorbid or "mimic" conditions—is the best protection against misdiagnosis.

Second, effective treatments for ADHD are available, and these include both medication and psychotherapy (see the Society for Clinical Child and Adolescent Psychology's list of empirically validated treatments at www.effectivechildtherapy.com). Often a combination of psychotherapy and medication may provide the greatest probability of a child's recovering from behavior problems (Swanson et al., 2001b). In light of the medicalization critique, an important note is that the efficacy of medication is often dramatic, especially when carefully applied in the context of a data-based monitoring of progress. It therefore would be as much of a mistake (and a disservice to children and families) to rule out medication use a priori in all cases (as some clinicians do on self-described "philosophical" grounds) as it would to use it almost automatically without thorough evaluation, with virtually every child who apparently has ADHD (as sometimes seems to happen out of necessity when adequate treatment or assessment resources are lacking in a given practice locale).

Third, understanding each child's context is important. There may be cases wherein lack of sufficient supports for the child is a powerful issue that can be addressed by family counseling or teacher guidance. Realizing the need for such supports and providing them may require advocacy and some creativity when resources at home or at school are already sharply stretched. Unfortunately, evidence for the clinical efficacy of such interventions is unclear, because no intervention studies have separated children with ADHD into those with high and low levels of family distress or neuropsychological impairment. Thus careful monitoring of each child's adjustment will remain essential, along with a willingness to try other interventions if the first approach is not working.

Fourth, perhaps the most important point in this chapter for clinicians is to avoid settling for a caricatured, simplistic, or misguided critique of ADHD as a "myth," while at the same time recognizing the real possibility of overreliance on a medical metaphor in some cases. This obliges the clinician to remember to differentiate his or her personal stance from theory, and thus to *make use of* theoretical perspectives, rather than to adopt a theoretical perspective uncritically. A clinician who is able to think of a case through a medical disease lens (a biological lens), as well as a developmental lens and a systems lens, will stand children in good stead.

Finally, from a clinical viewpoint, concerns about prevalence and medicalization are double-edged swords. On the one hand, clinicians may wish to avoid too easily labeling a child with a medical condition (ADHD) without an understanding of how doing so is going to lead to improvements in the child's life (e.g., increased parental understanding, needed support in school, etc.). On the other hand, medicalizing children's behavior problems can also provide relief, support, energy,

TABLE 1.3. Frequently Asked Questions about ADHD Incidence and Treatment

Question	Answer
Is the incidence of ADHD rising?	Unknown in terms of true population level. However, rates of administrative identification have risen sharply in the United States, due to changes in legal and educational rules in the past 15 years.
Is ADHD far more common in the United States?	No. Rates of ADHD are roughly similar, at least across "First World" or developed Western nations.
Are drugs more frequently prescribed?	Yes. Rates of medication of children have risen dramatically in the United States in the past two decades.
Are too many children getting medicines?	Yes and no. In some areas, very few are medicated; in other areas, a large number are. Both under- and overtreatment may be occurring.

and direction to families (see the incisive discussion by Klasen, 2000). Thus clinical judgment may suggest in which instances one will be properly "biased" toward medicalizing or not medicalizing. In future chapters, I look more closely at relevant assessment angles that should move this decision beyond values and give it some empirical grounding. One good protection against over- or undermedicalizing in practice is to utilize thorough and empirically supported assessment strategies (Achenbach, 1998, 2000; Pelham, Fabiano, & Massetti, 2005; Barkley, 2006).

Table 1.3 summarizes some of the most commonly asked questions that clinicians may be asked to address in their daily practice.

CONCLUSION

In outlining basic foundational issues and facts concerning ADHD's prevalence, treatment, and conceptualization, this chapter has in many respects emphasized concerns (most notably, medicalization) that are found in the sociology literature, in the popular media, and in some alternative views of ADHD. These views are not widely reflected in the clinical science literature, even though clinical and developmental scientists are doubtless aware of these concerns. Indeed, a large group of scientists recently issued a consensus statement about ADHD to counter unbalanced claims in the popular media (Barkley et al., 2002). Thus there is a degree of disconnection between the concerns of some social critics and those of the clinical scientific community. Table 1.4 describes, with the aid of some caricature (i.e., one could certainly point to many exceptions to the all-or-nothing views depicted in the table), discrepant views in U.S. society and perhaps much of the Western world.

Yet, despite the caricature in both directions here, it is clear that our society is seriously concerned about the possible medicalization of behavior. That is, many people fear that clinical interventions and scientific investigations alike may be unduly guided by assumptions of medical disorder and insufficiently attentive to contextual moderators of child behavior problems. These concerns could be applied to most child psychopathologies, but the prominent use of psychotropic treatment for children with ADHD fuels particular concern about it. Were we to discover a biological, neural, or other marker within a child that could be reliably measured as an indicator of disorder, many (though certainly not all) of the questions about this condition would be addressed. We might speculate that in the end, some youngsters—perhaps only a subset of children currently identified with ADHD—will exhibit such a causal marker. This book outlines ways in which that evidence might emerge, and instances in which it is already in hand.

The societal criticisms of the ADHD construct can be healthy for deepening our understanding. Certainly it is healthy for scientific discussion to be reminded that the medical perspective is not the only way to view a phenomenon such as ADHD. Likewise, readers are cautioned

TABLE 1.4. Implicit Assumptions about ADHD

Issue	Mainstream clinical scientists	Social critics
Problem locus	In the child	In society, outside the child
Status as a disorder	Valid	Invalid
Diagnostic tools	Partially objective	Entirely subjective
Rate of medication use	Underused or misused	Overused
Basic etiology	Biologically based syndrome	Inadequate support context for child
Role of poor parenting	Rarely the cause	Often the cause
Role of poor teaching	Rarely the cause	Often the cause
Reason for medicating	Stimulants work	Marketing works
Validity of ADHD	Established	Debatable at best

that even though I emphasize the neuropsychological level of analysis, other levels of analysis may in time prove as important. At the same time, the neuropsychological and biological findings are striking and must be grasped in order to form a complete picture of this phenomenon. The neuropsychological level currently provides the most likely arena of a future breakthrough in establishing a within-child causal mechanism or marker in ADHD; in turn, it may then be possible to link this marker to etiological mechanisms, such as those to be described in this book's final chapters.

Defining "Disorder"

We cannot decide whether ADHD is a "valid disorder" unless we first know what we mean by the concept of "disorder." Many parents, students, and others may ask clinicians to explain why ADHD is a disorder, and not merely exuberance or a problem of insufficient tolerance or skill on the part of teachers or parents. Scientists are often asked this and similar questions at a conceptual level. Indeed, the entire medicalization controversy outlined in Chapter 1 brings us to the question of the definition of a disorder (Wakefield, 1992). If ADHD merely reflects a difficulty of adapting to modern life, based on traits that may be adaptive in some cultures (see Jensen et al., 1997b, for discussion), then it is not a disorder. If it is a disorder, what are the criteria for saying so?

Mental disorders are commonly referred to as "open concepts" (Meehl, 1995), which means that they are not precisely defined and are still undergoing construct validation. They are also often referred to as constructions based on social need, values, and context (Gaines, 1992; Kirmayer & Young, 1999)—a critique that applies to medicine generally, as the prior discussion of medicalization indicates (Kirmayer, 1988).

Much like taxonomic classifications in the biological sciences, categories of psychopathology are seen as imposed on nature by scientists, not inherent in nature (Lilienfeld & Marino, 1999). Mental disorders are indeed constructions created to impose meaning on clinical problems. They can do so usefully, as illustrated in the relatively efficient identification of children with serious attention and impulsivity problems in need of assistance (Lahey & Willcutt, 2002; Hinshaw, 2002a), and the relatively consistent neuroimaging findings in samples of children defined by the ADHD criteria (Swanson & Castellanos, 2002). In short, the *utility* of a category or disorder concept for advancing understanding and intervention is one crucial index of "clinical validity," as defined in Chapter 1.

Yet, because clinical and other utility decisions are made dangerously if made on the basis of values or utility alone, concern remains that science must try to determine the *factual basis* for observed syndromes (Wakefield, 1999), both to aid understanding and to guide intervention. Science cannot provide a value-free judgment about the nature of ADHD, but it can contribute to informing those judgments.

Thus, in terms of clinical validity, the current ADHD construct performs respectably despite some ongoing issues. These issues include the need for continued refinement of the behavioral criteria due to overlapping and inefficient symptoms (Hartman et al., 2001), and their further rectification with empirically based child syndromes emanating from the factor-analytic tradition (Achenbach, 2000). Recent quantitative studies have tended to build support for the internal validity of the DSM-IV(-TR) ADHD syndrome or something close to it (Molina, Smith, & Pelham, 2001; Pillow, Pelham, Hoza, Molina, & Stultz, 1998) although more investigation of internal validity will be needed. Moreover, the syndrome receives substantial clinical validation on a range of criteria, including a reliable symptom structure, developmental predictions, outcomes, and impairment/need for intervention (reviewed by Barkley, 2006; Barkley et al., 2002; Hinshaw, 2002a; Lahey & Willcutt, 2002). Indeed, these reviews underscore the massive cost to society of the impairments children with ADHD experience. In short, regardless of how we understand ADHD, the phenomenon is real in terms both of impaired children and of its economic and social burden (Kelleher, 2002; Hinshaw, 2002a). Because these recent reviews amply document ADHD's relatively firm footing in terms of these indicators of clinical validity, this book does not repeat such information.

Instead, the remaining focus here is on the "etiological validity" of the syndrome. That is, how far have we come in understanding the causal structure of the disorder, and identifying those causes in individual cases? This is a difficult test for mental disorders (or even many modern diseases) to pass, but it is a test that ultimately must be addressed—especially when public concern runs high.

The psychopathology field shifted course in the mid-20th century and embraced a "disease" or "medical" model of psychopathology as the basis for the DSM. Subsequently, theorists and skeptics alike have given the topic of how to define "disorder" renewed thought (Kendell, 1986; Klein, 1978, 1999; Lilienfeld & Marino, 1995, 1999; Scadding, 1967; Sedgwick, 1982; Spitzer, 1999; Spitzer & Endicott, 1978; Szasz, 1974; Taylor, 1971; Wakefield, 1992, 1999). The difficulty of the topic rests in the tension between the role of value judgments and scientific facts (Wakefield, 1992), or, to describe it another way, between an objectivist and a constructivist vision of human language (Kirmayer & Young, 1999). These philosophical issues leave ample room for personal preference, and the tension that exists here is probably healthy for eventual clinical and scientific understanding. Yet a consequence is that a consensus on the best approach to conceptualizing "disease" (and thus ADHD or other psychiatric or psychological problems, if they are to be thought of as disorders) is lacking.

As noted in the medicalization discussion in Chapter 1, historical arguments have waxed and waned about the use of a medical perspective for psychopathology. Historically, one position has been that a properly defined medical metaphor provides the only solid way forward to evaluating conditions such as ADHD. An opposing view has been that the medical metaphor carries deterministic connotations and thus fails to empower people or to address systemic social injustices that might contribute to particular behavioral and emotional problems (Szasz, 1974; Menzies, 1997). We will see later that in the case of ADHD, systemic social injustices or ecological problems may in fact cause a neuropsychological disease syndrome; in other words, both views can be true. In the meantime, surveying all of these various philosophical issues would be the topic of another book. Interested readers are referred to a special issue of the *Journal of Abnormal Psychology* (1999, Vol. 108, No. 3).

I draw on those philosophical discussions while bypassing the nuances. My goal is to create a workable blend of objectivist and constructivist viewpoints with which to enable readers to evaluate the current state of knowledge about ADHD. Obviously, in so doing I am granting the ADHD construct legitimacy and siding with those who favor syndrome definition as a way toward clearer understanding of these child difficulties. However, the syndrome approach adopted here, and in most of the field today, is tempered by recognition of systemic interactions across multiple levels of analysis—a recognition informed by the recent developmental psychopathology perspective. In short, instead of tracing the somewhat intractable conceptual issues centering around a philosophical meaning of disorder, I outline a "working" understanding of disorder or disease, such that if ADHD is a disorder, we will have a basis for saying why and a proper context for interpreting its meaning. Such an understanding provides a sufficient framework for the material to be covered in the book.

In the classical nosology of medicine, a "syndrome" is an observed constellation of signs and symptoms. An "illness" is an expression of disease, whereas a "disease" is a core pathognomonic process. I use the terms "disease" and "disorder" rather interchangeably in much of what follows, recognizing that others draw distinctions between those concepts. However, I distinguish "syndrome" from "disease," since the latter connotes a known causal process operating in every case of an illness.

TRADITIONAL CRITERIA FOR DISEASE

Scientifically, all disease, disorder, or psychopathology requires some basic criteria for its validity. Traditionally, several such criteria are suggested. For example, there should be evidence of regularly co-occurring patterns of signs and symptoms (the syndrome), which is established in modern research by statistical methods. These types of evidence involve factor analysis of the symptom structure and internal reliability. As noted earlier, such initial criteria are generally supportive for ADHD despite remaining caveats (Lahey & Willcutt, 2002) and are not reviewed herein.

Second is evidence of external validity, such as the syndrome's tending to occur with itself rather than with other syndromes in families. Here, ADHD is again on relatively solid footing, in that it clearly occurs in families well beyond chance levels and distinctly from other disorders, including CD and antisocial personality disorder (Cantwell, 1972; Faraone, Biederman, & Friedman, 2000a; Faraone et al., 2000b; Levy, McStephen, & Hay, 2001; Frick, Lahey, Christ, Loeber, & Green, 1991; Nigg & Hinshaw, 1998; Lahey et al., 1988), although questions remain about the validity of the subtype distinctions in this regard (Faraone et al., 2000a, 2000b) and generally (Lahey et al., 2005). Third is evidence that the syndrome accurately identifies individuals who are impaired in a meaningful way, and who therefore should receive help if they seek it. Again, this evidence is quite supportive for ADHD, at least when the diagnosis is carefully and properly established by using full diagnostic criteria (Barkley, 2006; Hinshaw, 2002a).

Finally, there is the need for an established dysfunction or pathophysiological process that enables us to understand the syndrome and identify it accurately, based on a causal process. This last point—what I have been calling "etiological validity"—remains contentious for ADHD in today's research environment: What is the best characterization of the dysfunction? To which children does it pertain? Because scientific consensus is lacking on this point, it is the focus of the present book.

THE HARMFUL DYSFUNCTION ANALYSIS

Putting these ideas together, the "harmful dysfunction" analysis of disease proposed by Wakefield (1992, 1999) has influenced modern conceptions of psychopathology. The DSM-III, DSM-III-R, DSM-IV, and DSM-IV-TR reflect Wakefield's views to a large extent, since they have been influenced by writers in his tradition (see, e.g., Klein, 1978; Spitzer & Endicott, 1978). The DSM-IV-TR (APA, 2000) notes that "no definition adequately specifies precise boundaries for 'mental disorder' " p. xxx), but offers the following as a working definition: There must be a "clinically significant behavioral or psychological syndrome . . . with present distress . . . or disability . . . or with a significantly increased risk of suffering," and it must "be considered a manifestation of a behavioral, psychological, or biological dysfunction in the individual" (p. xxxi). Thus the working definition *assumes* an impaired function in the individual, following Wakefield's logic. Unfortunately, the nature of the impaired function is unknown for most forms of psychopathology. This book traces what is known in this regard for ADHD. Part of the challenge with ADHD from within this framework is to identify this dysfunction (or to determine that it does not exist), so as to enable the appropriate refinement of clinical practice. I therefore summarize Wakefield's approach and note some problems with it, before suggesting its adoption as one framework for this discussion.

Wakefield (1992) advanced the harmful dysfunction analysis. The essence of this analysis is that any disorder (whether it be a medical disease or a mental disorder; he applied the same criteria to both) must include two components to be called a disorder. The first is a "value" component: The condition must cause harm, in the judgment of society. The second component is that there must be a "dysfunction" in a physiological, psychological, neurological, or other functional system that can be scientifically described and identified. The dysfunction is defined by the failure of the mechanism to perform its natural or evolved function. For example, the fear response functions to protect us from danger. In the case of phobia, it no longer performs this function. The dysfunction element is intended to be the scientific or factual component of the definition of disorder. Thus Wakefield attempted to construct a hybrid model—one that recognizes both the value component and the scientific/factual component of disorder, properly conceptualized.

In its details and practical applications, Wakefield's argument faces problems (Lilienfeld & Marino, 1999; Richters & Hinshaw, 1999). For example, mismatches between evolutionarily designed functions and rapidly changing cultural demands seem difficult for the theory to accommodate; this issue, in fact, often enters into debates about the "validity" of the ADHD construct. Furthermore, as Wakefield (1999) himself acknowledges, scientists do not agree on the evolutionary function of many mental and emotional systems relevant to mental disorders. Relatedly, some medical dysfunctions seem relatively obvious (e.g., blindness), but others are graduated (e.g., high or low blood pressure). When is such a gradation in functioning to be called "dysfunction," without a "harm" value judgment? See Lilienfeld and Marino (1999) for an alternative perspective on mental disorders.

Despite these and other issues, the harmful dysfunction analysis is useful for our purposes (Klein, 1999). It suggests a framework for beginning to determine whether ADHD, or indeed any form of psychopathology, is validly conceived of as a disorder. First, harm must be present. In the case of ADHD, the evidence for this is extensive (Hinshaw, 2002a), if the following are judged to be harms: statistically increased chances of serious accidents, school failure, peer rejection, career underachievement, and so on.[1] In practice, a clinician must make a judgment as to whether a child is suffering impairment before diagnosing ADHD or some other mental disorder (APA, 2000). The focus herein, however, is on the factual or scientific component—that is, the nature of *dysfunction*—in ADHD. Using the criterion of a dysfunction in the child is one way to evaluate and justify the need for etiological validation of the syndrome.

Determining the nature of within-child dysfunction is therefore crucial to confirming the validity of ADHD as a disorder according to Wakefield's criteria. As this book will show, several potential dysfunctions are established in ADHD at the level of group analysis, with scientists now examining which domain is most important or primary. If the first protection against medicalization is to work from some definition of a disorder that includes a factual component, then the harmful dysfunction analysis, despite its limitations, gives us one framework (however imperfect) in which to begin to do so.

MULTIPLE LEVELS OF ANALYSIS, A TRANSACTIONAL SYSTEMS MODEL, AND THE DANGER OF REDUCTIONISM

It is helpful to recall briefly that referring to ADHD as a "disorder" is not intended to create an analogy to single-factor metabolic or infectious diseases, but instead to multifactorial, polygenic conditions. This may seem an obvious point, but it is one that many lay and professional reviewers overlook. To put it another way, even as we researchers and clinicians begin to clarify the neurobiology associated with ADHD, we ultimately will need to consider contextual moderators in development to fully understand the developmental pathways of this syndrome of behaviors. Several additional conceptual elements are needed to make clear the framework guiding this book's argument.

First, developmental psychopathology assumes a "transactional systems" model, in which genetic, biological, psychological, and psychosocial mechanisms are dynamically related via multidirectional causality. This is illustrated in Figure 2.1, which depicts several different levels of analysis, each interacting with the others over time and thus with development.

This perspective reminds us that the specific contexts of behavioral expression are crucial to a full appreciation of genetic and biological contributions, and vice versa. Addressing the specific interplay of different levels of analysis is an often neglected feature of research on child problems (see Cicchetti & Dawson, 2002, and several papers on this theme in the edited special issue of *Development and Psychopathology*, 2002, Vol. 14, No. 3). This "levels of analysis" perspective also helps protect against false reductionism.

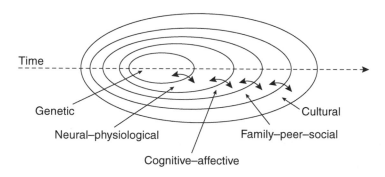

FIGURE 2.1. Multiple levels of analysis assumed in a systems perspective.

Second, a corollary of this transactional systems model is *multidirectional* rather than linear causality. For example, a very active, impulsive child may demoralize his or her parents, leading to less structure at home, which worsens the impulsivity. In another example, having a very oppositional, overactive child may lead to an overwhelmed mother's becoming depressed, or to arguments and couple conflict, which in turn affect the child's outcome. This principle is illustrated in Figure 2.1 by the small bidirectional arrows connecting each level of the system. Part II of this book, which is about one key domain of mediating causal processes, is integrated with Part III (about etiologies) via these types of causal loops.

Third, a developmental psychopathology perspective underscores the reciprocal importance to scientific advance of typical and atypical development, bolstering an emphasis on studying typical-range factors in temperament and personality in conjunction with psychopathology. This idea is illustrated in Figure 2.2, which depicts a hypothetical timeline of a child's development in relation to a predetermined threshold for labeling the child with ADHD; one might imagine various significant events along the timeline, enriching the story told. The child's behavior may reflect meaningful continuities in development in response to various changing contexts; however, attempting to summarize this by a dichotomous decision as to whether disorder is present or absent may not fully reflect these developmental dynamics. Therefore, when we consider extremes of inattention and overactivity in children, it is helpful to avoid *assuming* the existence of a static disease that accompanies the child throughout development. This assumption may be appropriate, especially if a chronic internal dysfunction is identifiable. On the other hand, the child's developmental pathway may in

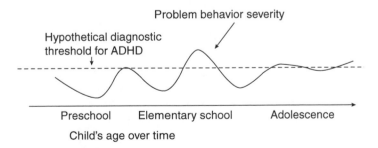

FIGURE 2.2. Hypothetical developmental pathway with varying adaptive and maladaptive responses to changing context.

some instances reflect characteristic vulnerability (or "liability") to exhibit a particular behavioral profile at certain times but not others.

Consistent with this concept, recent longitudinal data (albeit starting with preschoolers, for whom the clinical validation data for ADHD are still being gathered) suggest that even though children's rank orderings for activity level or inattention are quite stable over time during childhood, individual children meeting criteria for a particular ADHD subtype may not meet full criteria every year, or may meet criteria for a different subtype in different years. Lahey et al. (2005) followed 118 children initially diagnosed with ADHD, annually from ages 4–6 (wave 1) to ages 11–13 (wave 8). Over 20% failed to meet criteria for ADHD by the last two waves. A majority of children failed to meet full diagnostic criteria during at least one assessment wave; many of those children met criteria again at a later wave. A substantial number (37% of those with ADHD-C, 50% of those with ADHD-PI) met criteria for a different subtype at least twice during the eight annual assessments. Children initially identified with ADHD-PHI nearly all changed subtype or remitted in the ensuing years. Note that a similar pattern appears to hold for CD, with many children meeting criteria at one point in time, failing to meet them at another point in time, then again meeting the criteria at still another point (see Lahey et al., 1995).

If we can understand meaningful developmental pathways of children being studied under the rubric of ADHD (or some other significant behavior or emotional problem), we may better describe and thus better assist with their difficulties. It therefore is an important misconception to imagine that a syndrome must be explained by either extrinsic *or* intrinsic factors. In writings for the lay public, one sometimes gets the impression either that ADHD is caused by an inborn problem in the child (the classic disease model), or that it is not "real" but is "just a social construction." I hope that by this point, readers see the fallacy in these either–or views.

Fourth, a corollary to the third point is that most research, including genetic research, emphasizes determinants of individual differences in a trait (e.g., ADHD symptoms); however, these individual differences interact with effects on the entire population. When a population is subjected to risk factors for a multifactorial disorder (or, for that matter, for an infectious disease), *some* (not all) individuals will express symptoms of disorder. Which individuals? That in turn depends on which persons are vulnerable because of their genetic, biological, or social characteristics.

The extrinsic risks can move an entire population toward or away from risk for disorder, regardless of the determinants of individual variation in liability to disorder expression. This point is critical when we consider the possibilities for societywide prevention. For example, exposing the entire population of children in the United States to car exhaust containing lead in the mid-20th century increased the total population risk (and incidence) of mental retardation and developmental problems. Yet the individual children affected may have been those who were initially most vulnerable or liable to develop problems, due to their other constitutional or health characteristics. Without the lead pollution in their lives, many of these children would have been able to avoid developing a disorder. The lead pollution, doubtless combining with other risk factors, pushed more children over the hypothetical threshold line for developing a disorder. (I discuss lead's effects on development in Chapter 10, where citations and documentation are supplied.) Therefore, a complete picture of a disorder such as ADHD requires an understanding of the *extrinsic* risk context (including biological and social risk factors; see Chapters 10 and 11), as well as the *intrinsic* characteristics of children who are vulnerable to disorder and who have developed a disorder in that context (see Chapters 4–7).

Fifth, when problems develop, they are *mediated* via both intrinsic and extrinsic mechanisms or processes. In the case of ADHD, these could be difficulties in problem solving, attention, arousal, or other processes (as discussed extensively in later chapters). Therefore, to understand the overall trajectory of the argument in this book, readers must recognize that intrinsic risk factors are presumed to be mediated and moderated by extrinsic (context) conditions, and vice versa.

Sixth (and this point is crucial to the conclusions I highlight throughout this book), multiple pathways are likely. For example, both of the following may be true: (1) Some children with extreme hyperactivity and inattention, but no neuropsychological or other deficits, receive stimulant medication they might benefit from psychological services, but do not receive those services due to fiscal, societal, and educational forces. (2) In other children, the same surface behaviors entail marked neuropsychological and other impairments; they cannot be successful without medication as a support, and they suffer when this support is not made available. Grasping such distinct pathways or outcomes is essential to a complete understanding of ADHD.

So, to respect heterogeneity, this book aims to avoid blanket statements that attempt to account for the entire complex of phenomena captured under the rubric of "ADHD." I describe what has been learned by studying groups of children who meet the diagnostic criteria (or reasonable approximations of them), as well as by studying behavioral variation in the population without using the disorder concept. In discussions of the neuropsychological level of analysis—the putative dysfunction in the child—it is important to remember that this must be viewed as just one element of the total developmental picture for the child. Such a recollection is important for accurate theoretical formulation as well as sensible clinical practice.

Finally, an important caution is that many levels of analysis are available to us, but practical constraints permit us to consider only some of them in any depth. Part II of this book deals with just the neuropsychological level of analysis. This emphasis reflects a major focus in the scientific community; it is important in turn because of the need to understand within-child mechanisms. However, such effects are best understood within the context of the multilevel causal processes likely to be operating in development. Without that context, there is a danger of a false reductionism in our understanding of what the neural (and, for that matter, the genetic) correlates signify. Although scientific method relies upon a healthy reductionism in which we find explanatory mechanisms and isolate domains of inquiry, a less useful reductionism *assumes* that one level of analysis explains all other levels (see Miller, 1996; Turkheimer, 1998). This is an important distinction when we are examining the determinants of multifactorial behaviors over the course of development. Otherwise, mistaken assumptions will weaken scientific effectiveness (Horrobin, 2003). It would be a reductionistic mistake, for example, to assume that the answer will be found in neurobiology and thus to neglect family, school, or peer ecologies of behavior in ADHD. On the other hand, it would be an equal mistake to rely on an antibiological bias, to assume that the answer lies in societal factors, and thus to neglect potential breakthroughs on the neurobiological front.[2] In short, my intent is to analyze what is known at the neuropsychological level of analysis, without reducing all other levels to that one.

ADHD AND THE CONCEPT OF "DISORDER"

The currently prevailing operational definitions of ADHD, like those of other forms of psychopathology, are the descriptive symptom lists contained in DSM-IV-TR (APA, 2000) or ICD-10 (WHO, 1993). These operational definitions remain unsatisfying for nearly all disorders due to limited empirical support (Carson, 1991), lack of a developmental perspective, and absence of a biological or psychometric marker to establish diagnosis in relation to causal mechanisms. Moreover, the boundary between "nondisordered" and "disordered" is recognized as being fuzzy or approximate, and as relying in part on values particular to a sociocultural context (Wakefield, 1992; Lilienfeld & Marino, 1995), though this is not apparent in DSM-IV-TR.

Even so, to argue that ADHD does not seem much like a *classical* disease is to challenge a straw figure. ADHD resembles, if any disease, a multifactorial disease. All the same, the complexities in syndromes such as ADHD remind us not to expect the same sequence of break-throughs in ADHD as with classical diseases. Table 2.1 summarizes this state of affairs, showing where a disorder such as ADHD stands when evaluated through the inappropriate lens of classical disease versus the more appropriate lens of multifactorial disease.

Furthermore, some scientists question whether the disease or disorder metaphor is the appropriate guide to a science of ADHD at all. The developmental psychopathology perspective points to adaptation and maladaptation in varying contexts, to nondisordered and disordered developmental pathways, and to the plasticity of adaptation. Implementation of this perspective in terms of identifying and treating children with disordered behavior has not yet provided an alternative

TABLE 2.1. Is ADHD Valid as a Disease Entity?

	Implication for ADHD: Is it valid . . .	
Factual observation	as a multifactorial disease?	as a classical disease?
Statistical coherence	Yes	Yes
Familiality	Yes	Yes
External correlates	Yes	Yes
Lack of deterministic course	Yes	No
No single deterministic cause	Yes	No
Behavioral moderation of risk	Yes	Yes
Impairing with morbidity risk	Yes	Yes
Lack of robust biological marker	Maybe	No
Lack of laboratory test for diagnosis	Maybe	No
Characteristic treatment response	Yes	Maybe

to clinical research with children with extreme problems, but will aid conceptual integration later and enable us to suggest ways forward for the field. This perspective also reminds us that the criteria for a disorder such as ADHD are necessarily interim and not yet ready for reification. Rather, they should be revised as we better understand their statistical properties (Achenbach, 2000) and the causal and developmental pathways affecting extreme levels of these behavioral problems. Can we differentiate children whose behavior problems are properly classified as due to a within-child disorder from children whose problems are due to adaptation and context? The short answer is "Not well enough, yet." But I hope that a few chapters from now, readers will see that the field is approaching this point.

INTERIM SUMMARY

Few if any scientists today consider ADHD—or other psychopathologies—to fit the model of classic metabolic or infectious disease. ADHD, like other psychopathologies, better fits a multifactorial disease conception or metaphor. This view suggests that ADHD will have the following characteristics: (1) polygenetic contribution to susceptibility to disorder, but no single-gene cause in most cases; (2) varying course and probabilistic outcome; (3) biological changes that are small in magnitude relative to behavioral problems; and (4) genuine impairment.

In the sections that follow, I provide a brief editorial recap of the conceptual and controversial landscape in ADHD at the present time. In Chapter 3, I turn to the evidence with regard to the most likely neural systems to be involved in the syndrome, preparing for later integration across other levels of analysis.

* * *

A REVIEW OF THE MAIN ISSUES
DISCUSSED IN CHAPTERS 1 AND 2

We ultimately want to find out how ADHD works and where it comes from. To put it another way, what is the most important difference about these children, and what are the most important causes of that difference? As essential background, Chapter 1 has addressed why

ADHD is a source of controversies, and Chapter 2 to this point has discussed how we can define "disorder" so as to analyze the problem deeply. Both chapters have noted a set of healthy cautions as well as a workable framework for discussion. As a device to lay out my remaining goals in this book, I now review the status of selected issues in ADHD, indicating which ones will be discussed in this book and which will be left to others to address.

Conceptual Issues

Conceptual questions about ADHD can be roughly placed into three categories: (1) The data are sufficiently clear that the matters warrant little further discussion; (2) there are virtually no data, such that further discussion is premature; and (3) substantial data are in hand, but confusion continues. The third category is the one for which clarifying discussion may be most useful, and thus it is my focus.

Table 2.2 lists common questions sorted into these categories as I see them. The first section of the table, "Noncontroversies and their resolution," reflects issues that arise from mis-specification of questions and facts. These facts can be accepted. Readers should now recognize that ADHD has no laboratory test, that medication rates are indeed rising for unknown or multiple reasons, and that the "disease" metaphor indeed has a broad reach in our society. Nonetheless, the ADHD syndrome still carries substantial validity and utility, in that large numbers of children are seriously impaired, the syndrome has reasonable psychometric coherence and consistent external correlates, it confers an elevated risk of poor long-term outcomes, and standardized (if imperfect) assessment is available. At the same time, like most psychiatric classifications, "ADHD" is not ready to be reified in the same way as established classical diseases. The entity is still being defined, and dimensional or non-disease-related perspectives remain important to consider. To put this another way, application of the ADHD label offers no explanation in and of itself as to what has caused a child's problems. It simply identifies a set of phenomena requiring explanation. Because the issues in the first category are relatively non-controversial, little can be gained from additional discussion of them. They are therefore not considered further in this book.

The second section of Table 2.2 lists real public health questions that are important to resolve. Some of these issues are of critical public health and scientific importance, such as the possibility that severe behavior problems are increasing among children in Western society

TABLE 2.2. ADHD Questions and Controversies: Status of the Science

1. Noncontroversies and their resolution
   a. Is ADHD a "myth"? *No. Many children really are impaired as described by this syndrome.*
   b. Does the ADHD syndrome have statistical validity? *Yes.*
   c. Is ADHD a classical disease with a laboratory test for its diagnosis? *No.*
   d. Do genes play a role in liability to develop diagnosable ADHD? *Yes.*
   e. Does ADHD have a single cause, like a germ or a genetic defect, as in classical disease? *No.*
   f. Does the ADHD syndrome resemble other medical disorders in its characteristics? *Yes.*
   g. Does diagnosis depend in part on "subjective" perceptions of parents and teachers? *Yes.*
   h. Is diagnosis entirely subjective? *No. Standardized procedures provide some objectivity.*
   i. Is medication effective? *Yes. For most children, symptoms are suppressed.*
   j. Does medication provide a permanent cure? *No. Symptoms return when meds are discontinued.*
   k. Is ADHD being applied to wildly unrealistic percentages of children? *No, if 3–6% is realistic.*
   l. Is the cause of ADHD known in most cases? *No.*
   m. Are rates of medication treatment of ADHD rising rapidly in the United States? *Yes.*

2. Real public health and unknowns or controversies with insufficient data in hand
   a. What percentage of children may have adverse long-term reactions to chronic stimulant use?
   b. What is the nationwide prevalence of ADHD or HKD in the United States? In other nations?
   c. Why is there apparent variation in prevalence across cultures? Is it only due to methodology?
   d. Why do rates of medication prescription vary so widely across regions and nations?
   e. Are the right children receiving medication? How do we identify over- and undermedication?
   f. For which children might alternative treatments be as effective as medication?
   g. Is ADHD increasing in *true* incidence (apart from changing definitions/detection thresholds)?
   h. What are the obstacles to clinical use of best practices for assessment and treatment?
   i. Where are the natural boundaries to this syndrome, if any? Is it really an extreme point on a typical dimension of temperament?

(continued)

TABLE 2.2. *(continued)*

3. Key scientific questions with data available: Where have we arrived so far on these?

   a. What causes the extreme behavior and adjustment problems of most children with ADHD?

   b. What is the best characterization of the neurological, neuropsychological, psychological, or other "within-child" characteristics in groups of children with ADHD?

   c. How many children who can be classified as having the ADHD syndrome exhibit some type of psychological *dysfunction*, as required in formal models of disorder or psychopathology?

   d. What is the nature of genetic mechanisms in children with severe inattention and hyperactivity?

   e. What environmental or ecological causes or contributors warrant further study?

   f. Why is ADHD much more common in boys than in girls?

   g. What are the best scientific and clinical models for future understanding of this phenomenon?

   h. What is the appropriate boundary of the phenotype for study of etiology?

4. Important messages from critiques of ADHD

   a. Reification of the construct of ADHD is an important danger at this stage of knowledge.

   b. Reductionist thinking (e.g., relying solely on a genetic explanation) may limit understanding.

   c. Societal "medicalization" of behavior should be distinguished from scientific understanding.

5. Important messages from mainstream ADHD research literature

   a. The syndrome and the impairments are supported by extensive data.

   b. On average, children with an ADHD diagnosis are at high enough risk that help is warranted, if correct standards of care are applied to their diagnosis.

   c. Treatments can markedly improve quality of life for affected children.

and that appropriate treatments are not being provided in many cases. These issues should be placed on the national public health research and policy agendas. However, with virtually no data available to address them, it makes little sense to offer a book of speculations or polemics based on insufficient data. Therefore, I do not emphasize these questions, other than to briefly note best guesses at answers when these are relevant.

The third section lists scientific questions about the syndrome that have received extensive investigation; these are questions that we have come part of the way toward answering. This book focuses on these questions, in order to clarify where we are now, how far we have come, and where we need to go. The key focus here is the need to better understand the status of within-child mechanisms and to begin to integrate them with potential etiological (causal) mechanisms beyond the individual child. These disparate domains of investigation (mechanism and etiology) need to be more aggressively brought together in order for real breakthroughs to occur, and I hope that this book will spur movement in that direction.

Finally, the fourth and fifth sections of Table 2.2 summarize impressionistically some illustrative messages in the disconnection between the lay public and some academic critics on the one hand, and the mainstream scientific research community on the other. Legitimate concerns can be detected amid the distortions that inevitably accompany these controversies. Reification and reductionist thinking indeed are important dangers with a difficult set of phenomena such as ADHD. As society medicalizes these behaviors, scientific or clinical failure to recognize our own implicit assumptions can limit progress. Moreover, we are all well advised to remember that psychosocial context and developmental change may "explain" some of the phenomena. At the same time, the scientific community carries important take-home messages for the critics. Most central is that it is senseless to dismiss ADHD as "merely" a myth, in the face of massive evidence that this is a valid syndrome that severely impairs children who need assistance. Instead, we need to track our progress in understanding of the syndrome, as this book attests.

The Bottom Line

ADHD denotes a grouping of multifactorially determined syndromes without an established causal etiology and with fuzzy boundaries. Nonetheless, this grouping is useful and valid in aiding communication among researchers and clinicians and as a framework for identifying children who are impaired in meeting their developmental milestones. Important unresolved issues include clarification of developmental pathways, etiologies, mediating causal mechanisms, individuals to whom a given pathway might apply, and the appropriate boundaries of the phenotype (in other words, the best way to define the syndrome in order to capture true causally linked groups).

As scientific understanding improves, we should be able to better identify individual children with a "true disorder" (internal dysfunction, injury, or other abnormality that causes harm over time and across many contexts in their development), versus those with a problem in developmental adaptation. Currently, because the disorder is defined behaviorally, it is inevitable that both groups of children may be lumped together to some degree, despite the best empirically grounded efforts that went into creating the current criteria. Therefore, when we propose neuropsychological or biological models of ADHD, it is important that *heterogeneity* be considered. We must not assume that a given biological model will apply to all of the children currently falling under the diagnostic rubric. To put this another way, to how many diagnosed children does a neuropathological or etiological model pertain?

Expert readers will want to add other considerations to this discussion, such as mediating and moderating processes, recursive causal pathways, genotype–environment correlations, and more. I return to conceptual models later, taking into account some of these more sophisticated process issues (in particular, see Chapter 8). For now, the point is that we will need to consider both within-child mechanisms and contextual or extrinsic causal factors in order to have an accurate grasp of what ADHD may represent.

Clinical Implications

The essence of this background discussion for clinicians is in some ways another appeal to common sense. With regard to its validity as a disease, ADHD differs little from other psychiatric or behavioral syndromes. Its controversy centers on the urgency felt in society about the growing reliance on medications, rather than any unique status in terms of inherent validity. The simplistic argument that ADHD does not look like an infectious or metabolic disease is misguided, because most modern diseases do not fit that mold. The real question here is this: How well does ADHD fit the mold of a multifactorial disease? It is important for clinicians to recognize a child's developmental trajectory: The child may meet criteria for ADHD today, but may not meet them a year from now, perhaps despite ongoing impairment. Although the problem behaviors are often quite stable, they may not be stable in a given case if important changes in context occur. The bottom line here is that the wide individual differences among children with ADHD have to be recognized.

Recognizing that the medical model of multifactorial disease has much to recommend it, but that it also has key limitations (including the lack in DSM-IV-TR of any account of developmental course and process), will serve clinicians well. Thus a clinician can step outside of a narrow medical model without departing from a scientific understanding, if the clinician thinks deeply about a child's developmental needs, the child's accomplishment of developmental goals and milestones, and the developing pathways in which the child's temperament is both adapting to and molding the social context at home and school. Likewise, functional assessment is as important as diagnostic assessment. That is, it is important to evaluate not only whether the child meets criteria for ADHD, but in what way he or she is impaired and what is causing that impairment (Pelham, Wheeler, & Chronis, 1998; Pelham et al., 2005).

In all, it is advisable to be willing to think about the best "fit" for a child, and to be prepared to locate problems either within a child or within a context, as appropriate to the particulars of an assessment situation. Doing so will enable clinicians to take a sophisticated approach to the diagnostic and treatment challenges of these children.

How to Proceed: The Two Big Questions about ADHD

If we accept that as a descriptive syndrome ADHD has statistical validity as well as construct validity in relation to external correlates (including impairment), but that the various developmental pathways and causal mechanisms that lead to these problems are not fully understood, then we can begin to bring scientific investigation to our assistance. I suggest two broad questions to guide the discussion from here.

The first is "How does ADHD work?" This question concerns mechanisms: What is wrong? It is the main point of most scientific investigations today. Herein I am most concerned about within-child mechanisms, which can help us evaluate the extent to which there is a "dysfunction," as is necessary for an etiologically valid disorder. Here, to understand the status of the field, we must look at the neuropsychological or internal-process perspective on ADHD. Doing so can guide theory as well as inform assessment and treatment planning. Clarifying what we know on this front is the focus of Part II of this book.

The second question is "Why does ADHD occur?" To put it another way, "Where does ADHD come from?" or "Why does what goes wrong do so?" This is the question about causes (as opposed to within-child mechanisms). The question of endogenous (within-child) versus exogenous (contextual) contributions to ADHD becomes central. Understanding this causal level can inform prevention planning.

As we move to that level, the scientific data thin out—but do not disappear. Enough knowledge is in hand to enable us to begin taking preventive actions, as well as to inform high-risk/high-payoff research strategies (i.e., those that may have a less than 50% chance of success, but that if successful would result in major breakthroughs in understanding). Doing so requires integrated thinking about genetic factors (Chapter 9) and experiential factors (Chapters 10–11), including toxicological and other early risks. All of that is the focus of Part III. In Part IV, I consider integrated models and suggest research initiatives that warrant pursuit.

PART II

HOW DOES ADHD WORK?

CHAPTER 3

Neural Systems

Is something different about the brains of children with extreme forms of hyperactivity, impulsivity, and inattention—those who meet criteria for ADHD? What parts of the brain are potentially involved? What do those brain regions do? The neuropsychological and/or neurobiological level of analysis has received primary emphasis in much recent ADHD research. Reasons for this emphasis are many, including the dramatic effect of stimulant medications on the behaviors of children with ADHD, first reported by Bradley (1937). See Zametkin and Rapoport (1987), Castellanos and Tannock (2002), and the edited volume by Solanto, Arnsten, and Castellanos (2001b) for discussions of these effects and their implications for neural theories. But the overarching reason is the importance of the brain itself. Because it is the body's organ of thought, emotion, and behavioral organization, understanding how the brain works in ADHD is essential to a fuller understanding of the syndrome, and in turn to more effective remediation of it. Therefore it is worthwhile, even for clinicians doing psychotherapy, to gain some understanding of possible key brain functions in ADHD. Moreover, to follow the argument in this book, it will be necessary to grapple at least briefly with relevant neuroanatomy and neural circuitry. This chapter first provides an overview sufficient to enable readers to track the remainder of the argument in the book, and then furnishes more detail on the relevant circuitry for interested readers. Readers wishing to bypass the details can skip the "Detailed Description of Neurocircuitry . . . " section and still follow the remainder of this and the following chapters.

OVERVIEW OF KEY BRAIN REGIONS AND FINDINGS

Four Brain Regions Implicated in ADHD

Neuroimaging studies implicate four neural regions in ADHD: (1) the prefrontal cortices (especially the right prefrontal cortex); (2) the basal ganglia (in particular, the caudate); (3) the cerebellum (in particular, the cerebellar vermis lobules VIII–X); and (4) the corpus callosum (in particular, the genu) (Swanson & Castellanos, 2002). They are indicated in Figure 3.1, which also shows dopamine pathways (to be discussed later). I focus on these well-studied regions here, while recognizing that future studies may identify other regions as important, too.

Prefrontal Cortices

Why do children with ADHD fail to see the big picture? Why can't they keep simple instructions in mind for more than a moment? Why are they so impulsive? The answers may lie with difficulty in functions subserved by the prefrontal cortices.

The prefrontal cortices constitute a large region in the very front of the brain; they are distinct from the sensory and motor areas in the central region of the cortex. The prefrontal cortices include several subregions defined both cytoarchitecturally (i.e., by cell types) and

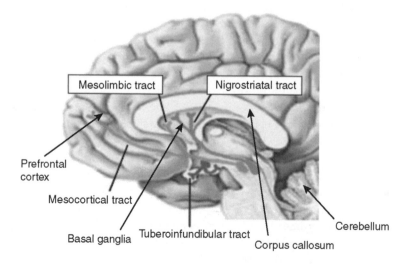

FIGURE 3.1. Key brain structures. Courtesy of www.thebrain.mcgill.ca, a project of Bruno Dubuc and the Institute of Neurosciences, Mental Health and Addiction of Canada.

functionally. Key areas relevant to ADHD are the dorsolateral prefrontal cortex (often associated with working memory or the ability to keep plans in mind), orbital prefrontal cortex (often associated with the ability to inhibit inappropriate actions), and anterior cingulate cortex (related both to emotional control and to cognitive control). These areas are heavily interconnected both with other cortical regions and with key subcortical structures in a series of neural circuits.

Via these circuits, prefrontal structures are involved in emotion regulation, executive functioning (working memory, controlling interference, interrupting inappropriate behavior), temporal organization of behavior, motivational responding (identifying potential reward), social judgment, and motor control (Fuster, 1997). They are thus obvious candidates for involvement in nearly all psychopathology, including ADHD. Patients with neural injury to various prefrontal regions exhibit an array of impulsive, unsocialized, emotionally unregulated, and amotivational syndromes, depending on the site of injury (Cummings, 1993; Fuster, 1997; Kolb & Whishaw, 1990).

Developmentally, the prefrontal cortices are among the last areas of the brain to mature fully. They continue to undergo synaptic pruning and myelination into adolescence and even into early adulthood (Benes, 2001). This late maturation makes these regions of keen interest to neurodevelopmental conceptions of ADHD, as well as of other psychopathologies. As Figure 3.1 illustrates, the prefrontal area is an important endpoint for long-fiber dopamine projections.

In children with ADHD, the best-replicated imaging findings involve the right inferior prefrontal cortex. Both structure and activity in this region appear to be related to difficulties with response inhibition and other cognitive control operations in children with ADHD (Casey, Castellanos, Giedd, & Marsh, 1997a; Rubia et al., 1999). In all, the apparent involvement of prefrontal cortices in ADHD is consistent with theories that the main difference in children with ADHD entails deficits in cognitive control (the ability to organize complex response sequences), especially working memory and response suppression (the ability to interrupt a response in a rapid decision context—e.g., the "checked swing" in baseball); alerting; or motivation (especially the extent to which a child cares about getting a reward).

Basal Ganglia

Why can't children with ADHD interrupt their behavior when warned? Why do they so often misjudge the consequences of their actions? These abilities depend on close coordination of prefrontal regions with subcortical structures subsumed under the term "basal ganglia." Located below and behind the prefrontal cortices (Figure 3.1), they include several specific structures. Most often mentioned in ADHD are the caudate and the putamen. These structures are closely interconnected with prefrontal regions, forming bidirectional "loops" of circuitry that work in concert to control unwanted response tendencies and to monitor whether current actions are moving toward the expected goal. As part of these circuits, these structures thus assist with motor control, with motivation and emotion (e.g., response to reward, anxiety about possible danger), and with executive and cognitive functions (including attention and suppression of a motor response). Several studies have shown abnormalities of the caudate, but the studies differ as to whether these are on the right or the left side. Data regarding the putamen and the globus pallidus remain preliminary and inconsistent.

Cerebellum

Why do 5 minutes seem like an hour to a child with ADHD? Why are so many children with ADHD uncoordinated or clumsy? Why do children with ADHD fail to learn from mistakes? Clues to these experiences may lie in abnormal development of the cerebellum. The cerebellum is a dense, complex structure with multiple projections to basal ganglia as well as to prefrontal cortices. It is a separate, differentiated subcortical structure located in the back of the brain (Figure 3.1). Understanding of its functions is still evolving. Researchers have recently been refining the historical idea that the cerebellum was primarily involved in complex, overlearned motor movement that required exquisite timing (e.g., ballet dancing). They now think that it is involved in a wide array of timing and temporal information-processing abilities, including detecting when expected consequences should occur (Ivry, 1997; Ivry & Keel, 1989). The cerebellum may be involved in other cognitive control operations as well, perhaps by detecting and coordinating the timing of their activation (Diamond, 2000). Several studies have found the cerebellar vermis to be smaller in children with ADHD than in control children (Swanson & Castellanos, 2002). This is a common finding in other disorders as well (notably autistic disorder and schizophrenia); however, the exact regions involved may be specific to ADHD—namely, lobules VIII–X (autism and schizophrenia may involve other lobules of the vermis). Although the functional importance of the vermis in ADHD is not fully clear,

Castellanos (2001) has suggested that the vermis modulates catecholamine functions. Therefore, these cerebellar regions are likely to
modulate the operations of the prefrontal–subcortical circuits. Overall,
involvement of the cerebellum introduces additional theoretical possibilities, including disturbances of motor timing or temporal information processing in general, as mechanisms contributing to ADHD.

Corpus Callosum

Finally, it is important to recall the lateral differentiation of the brain.
Although lateralization of functions remains incompletely understood
(and probably will not prove to be as neat as portrayed in early
popularizations of this concept), coordination of distinct functions
across the hemispheres appears to be important for effective cognition
and action selection. The corpus callosum is a thick bundle of fibers
that connects the two cortical hemispheres. It helps with interhemispheric communication and efficient information transfer, which are
necessary for complex cognitive and motor functions (Banich, 1998).

Despite imaging evidence that sections of the corpus callosum
may be smaller in children with ADHD than in control children, it has
sparked surprisingly little research. Behavioral probes of the corpus
callosum's integrity are available (Banich, Passarotti, & James, 2000a;
Banich, Passarotti, White, Nortz, & Steiner, 2000b; Passarotti, Banich,
Sood, & Wang, 2002) but are underutilized in efforts to develop assessment techniques for children with ADHD. Studies have also disagreed
as to which portion of the corpus callosum is reduced in size in samples with ADHD. However, findings of anterior abnormalities would be
broadly consistent with abnormal prefrontal cortical development in
ADHD, and would add the possibility of impaired interhemispheric
information transfer as a mechanism in the disorder.

Key Unknowns and Caveats

As will be apparent in the discussion to follow, many theories suggest
that other brain regions may also be involved in ADHD: the thalamus
(closely linked to the systems described above, in that the prefrontal–
basal ganglia circuits also include the thalamus); the amygdala (important in responding to unpleasant or potentially unpleasant situations);
the hippocampus (potentially important in motivation and effort); and
the hypothalamus. Some theories of ADHD suggest a role for arousal
processes, which involve neural loops between the brain stem reticular

activating system and the cortex. Brain stem structures have yet to be imaged in ADHD, in part because of limitations in the imaging technology. Moreover, imaging studies also show reductions in size of the temporal cortex, often ignored in discussions of neural involvement in ADHD (Swanson & Castellanos, 2002). Total brain volume is reduced in children with ADHD by 5% or more. Many imaging studies have failed to control adequately for total brain volume (Giedd, Blumenthal, Molloy, & Castellanos, 2001). However, this reduction in total brain volume is observed even with young, medication-naïve children and does not worsen over time, regardless of medication treatment (Castellanos et al., 2002).

Major Neuroimaging and Brain Wave Findings in ADHD

Both structural and functional neuroimaging studies have been reviewed by Giedd et al. (2001) and Swanson and Castellanos (2002), and more recently by Pliszka (2005). I follow these reviews closely here. Giedd et al. catalogued 6 computed tomography (CT) studies, 14 structural magnetic resonance imaging (MRI) studies, and 17 functional imaging studies (either positron emission tomography [PET] or functional MRI) of adults, adolescents, and in some cases children with ADHD. However, note that many of these studies were not independent of one another but emanated from the same lab, often with additional subjects (Swanson & Castellanos, 2002).

Structural Neuroimaging Findings

Table 3.1 summarizes the major structural neuroimaging findings in the ADHD literature, based on Giedd et al.'s (2001) review, a companion review by Castellanos (2001), and the summary from Swanson and Castellanos (2002).

A handful of studies in the last 3 years have not overturned these conclusions, but add some clarifications (Pliszka, 2005; Seidman et al., 2005). The magnitude of structural reduction in these key regions in ADHD is about $d \sim 0.5$–0.7 (see "Effect Size," below)—equivalent to a reduction of approximately 10–12% in volume, although slightly larger effects have emerged in the initial studies of the cerebellum (Swanson & Castellanos, 2002). Smaller caudate volumes were observed in a small sample (nine pairs) of identical twins discordant for ADHD (Castellanos et al., 2003), indicating that at least in some instances the source of these reductions in brain volume is not genetic, but environmental. As Castellanos et al. (2003) have noted, however, gener-

TABLE 3.1. Key Neuroanatomical Neuroimaging Findings in ADHD

Structure	Key ADHD findings
Prefrontal cortices	Reduced right > left asymmetry, with relatively smaller right side; underactivation of right medial prefrontal cortex during tasks
Basal ganglia	Abnormalities in caudate, but not putamen; reduced size of globus pallidus in preliminary studies; hypoactivation of caudate during executive task performance
Cerebellum	Reduced size of vermis, especially posterior–inferior lobules
Corpus callossum	Smaller rostrum (anterior and inferior region)
Caveats	Insufficient data on subregions of key structures; insufficient control of confounds; lack of data on thalamus and other relevant structures; danger of premature foreclosure on easiest-to-image regions

Note. Data from Giedd, Blumenthal, Molloy, and Castellanos (2001); Castellanos (2001); Swanson and Castellanos (2002); and Seidman, Valera, and Makris (2005).

alizing from twins to singletons on this point may be difficult, because twins may experience additional likelihood of perinatal traumas.

Castellanos et al. (2002) found that reductions in brain volume were apparent early in development and were nonprogressive. The fact that this reduction in volume emerges early in development could be consistent with a delay or deviation in neural development beginning prenatally.

Many imaging studies have lacked appropriate control for total brain volume (Giedd et al., 2001), although the findings in Table 3.1 have generally survived such control when it was instituted. The imaging literature itself suffers from several other imitations, including poor control of statistical artifact in most studies and difficulty imaging the specific subregions indicated by the parallel-loop model of prefrontal–subcortical circuits. Nonetheless, the imaging results are striking in suggesting potential internal mechanisms. They therefore can be kept in mind as we evaluate various mechanism-based claims about ADHD, and they lend credence to theories that implicate these key structures and their neural connections.

Neural Activation Patterns

Do the brains of children with ADHD operate differently from those of typical children? In addition to the work on brain structure, a growing literature on neural activation patterns in ADHD is emerging (see

Pliszka, 2005). Data using functional imaging (e.g., functional MRI, PET, and other methodologies) are still rather preliminary. However, key studies suggest atypical activation patterns in children with ADHD during cognitive control tasks (Bush et al., 1999, in a study of adults) and response inhibition tasks in prefrontal cortices (Rubia et al., 1999) and basal ganglia (Durston et al., 2003). Those imaging findings are convergent with the structural findings in suggesting that these regions not only are smaller, but are not activated in the same way in children or adults with ADHD as they are in controls.

Data using scalp electrical recordings (electroencephalography [EEG] and evoked response potentials [ERPs]) are much more substantial, although their precise meaning remains open to question. A large body of EEG wave form findings and a large body of early ERP studies suggest that ADHD is associated with (1) excess slow-wave activity (consistent with cortical underarousal), as well as (2) weaker evoked potentials to both stimuli and response cues (consistent with poor alerting as well as poor response mobilization). See Barry, Clarke, and Johnstone (2003a, 2003b) for review of these areas.

Neurochemical Pathways in ADHD

What does it mean when people say that ADHD is related to abnormal brain chemicals? This statement is, from a technical point of view, problematic. Nonetheless, a crucial complement to any discussion of neural structures is the possibility that neurochemical pathways may be relevant to ADHD. The candidates here include three of the biogenic amines: dopamine (although there is debate about which of the dopamine subsystems are most germane), norepinephrine (also called noradrenaline), and serotonin. Insufficiently examined to date are glutamate; gamma-aminobutyric acid (GABA); and various hormones and neuropeptides, including thyroid and gonadal hormones and the neuromodulators (e.g., vasopressin and others) that appear to be involved in impulsive and aggressive behavior in animals.

Given the incomplete state of our present knowledge about neurochemicals, it makes sense for now to focus on those chemicals and pathways that are fairly well studied and to evaluate progress in those areas first. I therefore discuss dopamine (a neuromodulator active in prefrontal regions and basal ganglia, important in reward responding and in cognitive control); norepinehprine (also found in prefrontal structures and cerebellum, and important in alerting); and GABA (throughout the brain, important in dampening unwanted neural activation).

In summary, neuroimaging studies indicate that ADHD is associated with (1) about a 5% reduction in total brain volume on average; (2) a 10–12% reduction in volume of key structures in the prefrontal cortices, basal ganglia, and cerebellum; (3) abnormal patterns of brain activation in these same regions on challenge tasks, although this imaging literature remains preliminary; and (4) increased "slow-wave" brain activity. Reductions in brain volume are present early in development (at least by preschool) and are nonprogressive, suggesting that they are due either to early insults or to genetic effects. One small imaging study of identical twins discordant for ADHD suggests that at least in some instances the etiology involves experiential causal factors.

DETAILED DESCRIPTION OF NEUROCIRCUITRY RELEVANT TO ADHD

This section provides more detail on neural circuitry for interested readers. Readers who wish to move directly to a discussion of functional implications should see "The 'Theoretical Brain' in ADHD," below. As I have noted in the preceding section, both cortical and subcortical brain structures are relevant to ADHD. The brain's cortical areas are connected to one another via frontal–posterior association loops and other cortical systems. Each is also part of neural circuits or loops connecting them to important subcortical regions. I focus only on the prefrontal–subcortical loops for now.

Most scientists now believe that at least five neural loops project from specific prefrontal regions to the basal ganglia and then to the thalamus.[1] The key structures in the basal ganglia are the striatum (composed of the caudate nucleus, of which the nucleus accumbens is part, and the putamen), the globus pallidus, the substantia nigra, and the subthalamic nucleus.[2] These structures are thought to be important in behavioral control as well as in emotional response and motivation. Three loops are of primary interest, consistent with the three most-discusssed prefrontal regions noted earlier. They are schematized in Figure 3.2.

Note that the structure of each circuit is similar, with projections from prefrontal regions to striatum and basal ganglia, and from the basal ganglia to the thalamus. The thalamus then projects back to prefrontal regions. Each loop projects to specific zones within the prefrontal cortices, basal ganglia, and thalamus, enabling the differentiation of the circuits and (hypothetically) of their functions as components of cognitive and behavioral control.

The circuits feature a "direct" path and an "indirect" path through the basal ganglia. The direct path, illustrated in detail in Figure 3.2, runs to the internal segment of the globus pallidus and substantia nigra pars reticulata (not shown), and then to the thalamus (Kandell, Schwartz, & Jessell, 1991). The indirect path, schematized on the left-hand side of Figure 3.2, projects from the striatum to the external segment of the globus pallidus, and then to the subthalamic nucleus. The subthalamic nucleus projects back to the globus pallidus (both internal and external segments) and the substantia nigra (again, not shown). The direct and indirect paths may have differential effects on activation versus suppression of behavior—a nuance not incorporated in most theories (for an exception, see Casey, Durston, & Fossella, 2001).

Three neurotransmitters are primarily involved in these circuits: dopamine, thought to serve a neuromodulatory function; glutamate

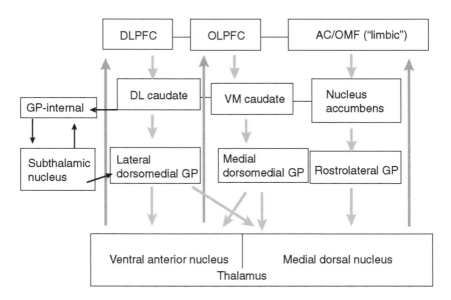

FIGURE 3.2. Three parallel prefrontal–subcortical neural pathways. DLPFC, dorsolateral prefrontal cortex; OLPFC, orbitolateral prefrontal cortex; AC, anterior cingulate; OMF, orbitomedial frontal; DL, dorsolateral; VM, ventromedial; GP, globus pallidus. Data from Cummings (1993) and Casey, Tottenham, and Fossella (2002).

(excitatory projections); and GABA, an inhibitory neurotransmitter (Casey et al., 2001; Kandell et al., 1991). Note that the net effect of glutamate or GABA projections on a person's responses can be excitatory or inhibitory, depending on the function of the neurons being modulated. In all, the distinct pathways probably differentially dampen or excite responsivity.

Consistent with the thumbnail sketch I have offered to open this chapter, scientists think that the three circuits depicted in the diagram influence different cognitive operations important to self-regulation. These partially distinct emphases are heuristic, even if qualified. The dorsolateral prefrontal circuit may support working memory, maintaining stimulus set, and thus planned or deliberate control of action. The orbitolateral prefrontal circuit may support behavioral set and may thus control behavioral output and behavioral inhibition. The anterior cingulate/orbitomedial frontal circuit may support emotion regulation and motivational response, as well as attentional control and conflict detection.[3]

These loops play an important role in rendering our theorizing more precise. ADHD probably involves not so much a discrete neural structure as one or more of these neural circuits. Involvement of these circuits nonetheless directs us again to working memory (holding a list, number, or name in mind for a few moments in order to complete a task), behavioral response suppression (interrupting an inappropriate response before it is completed), and related functions in neuropsychological models. They also provide a plausible neural basis for differentiating key regulatory functions at least partially from one another.

Other neural circuits are important to ADHD but are not described in Figure 3.2. First, loops among the cerebellum, basal ganglia, and frontal cortices (mediated in part by dopamine) are likely to be important in facilitating cognitive control and adaptation to context. These loops are increasingly believed to participate in sequencing, organizing, timing, and temporal organization of behavior, and thus also to be crucial to executive functioning (Diamond, 2000). They may be important in detecting violations in the expected nature and timing of events, with a cascade of effects on behavioral control and regulation (see Nigg & Casey, 2005).

The cortical–striatal loops work in concert with frontal–cerebellar circuits (which also link through the thalamus and receive morephinephrine and dopamine projections) to regulate complex behavior. The cerebellum, visible in the lower right corner of Figure 3.1, is a large and differentiated structure in the back of the brain implicated in temporal information processing, time perception and timing, motor control, and executive functions, as well as at least three psychiatric disorders (autism, schizophrenia, and ADHD). It also has extensive dopaminergic innervation (including expression of dopamine transporter) and noradrenergic innervation.

Furthermore, note that catecholamine circuits can be subdivided. To refer back to Figure 3.1, these can be schematized as three main circuits. The mesocortical dopamine circuit runs from the ventral tegmentum to the nucleus accumbens (sometimes referred to separately as a mesolimbic subroute) and on to the frontal cortex. It is involved in cognitive control operations, as well as (via the aforementioned limbic connections) motivation, reward response, and emotion. The nigral–striatal dopamine circuit runs from the substantia nigra to the striatum. It is involved in motor control; for example, its disruption is linked to Parkinson's disease. Third, neurons from the locus coeruleus and the ventral tegmental area carry norepinephrine projections, which innervate frontal cortex and other regions. These structures receive inputs from the cerebellar vermis as well. The ascending noradnerergic neurons are likely to be involved in attention, alertness, and signal detection (Posner & Petersen, 1990).

THE "THEORETICAL BRAIN" IN ADHD: WHAT FUNCTIONS ARE INVOLVED?

Overview

With these anatomical regions in mind, I now shift gears and talk about functional psychological, cognitive, or neuropsychological processes. These processes, which have been hinted at in the review of each brain region earlier, can also be organized into candidate systems related to the neural regions and their associated circuits. Although is is not possible to review all of the several hundred relevant studies, I identify the most compelling findings and direct readers when possible to comprehensive reviews of subdomains of these literatures. The relevant literature includes over 200 performance studies of cognitive function and several dozen physiological studies. It includes studies on clinically diagnosed samples and studies of correlates of behavior problems in community samples. To date, the neural regions involved in ADHD are still so broadly specified that many diverse functional interpretations remain possible. A goal of future research is to restrict these interpretations.

Some means of structuring the discussion of this vast literature is clearly needed. To do so, I suggest four functional domains as the prime candidates for dysfunctional neurocognitive mechanisms in ADHD. However, each of these domains includes subfunctions. Teasing the subsystems apart will prove to be important to clear thinking about neurocognitive mechanisms in ADHD. These domains, and for heuristic purposes the neural circuits with which they may be primarily identified, are listed in Table 3.2.

These four broad domains (1–4 in Table 3.2) are the topics of Chapters 4, 5, 6, and 7, respectively. The four domains include partially discrete functions within them (e.g., I list five attention functions and eight executive functions in this particular formulation), which are defined and explained in their respective chapters. As well, even this fairly comprehensive list of candidates is not exhaustive. For example, as colleagues and I have described elsewhere, language functions play a crucial role in the emergence of self-regulatory abilities (Nigg & Huang-Pollock, 2003; Nigg, Hinshaw, & Huang-Pollock, 2006). This point is important, because ADHD tends to co-occur with language-related problems (Baker & Cantwell, 1992; Tannock & Schachar, 1996). However, I do not emphasize it herein. Although I discuss temporal information processing in Chapter 7, it is not heavily emphasized here (see Toplak, Dockstader, & Tannock, in press). Basic memory functions remain of interest to some investigators. Nonetheless, the focus here is sufficiently broad to capture most of the neuropsychological features of ADHD.

I therefore review, in Chapters 4–7, the scientific status of 18 candidate neurocognitive dysfunctions in ADHD as listed in sections 1–4 of the table. Many writers have proposed much simpler organizations of self-control. However, at this stage the purpose in breaking these broad functional systems down into so many subfunctions is to strengthen our conclusions later. Thus, if we see that evidence on every putative function of a system points in the same direction, our conclusions will be surer than if evidence for a given system points in different ways for different subfunctions.

Attention

Is the core problem in ADHD truly "inattention"? To lead off Table 3.2, I have listed attention as an obvious candidate in an "attention deficit" disorder. Under this rubric, I list two low-level attention systems. The orienting system directs attention to a specific expected input ("Where

TABLE 3.2. Key Functional Neurocognitive Candidate Systems for ADHD

1. Attention (Chapter 4)

    A. Posterior attention system (parietal–thalamic attention network)
        i. Reflexive spatial orienting (where)
        ii. Perceptual selection (what)
        iii. Other bottom-up selection processes

    B. Vigilance system (right lateralized cortical–subcortical system)
        i. Alerting or arousal: Readiness for new or unexpected stimuli
        ii. Sustained attention (vigilance) to ongoing or expected stimuli

2. Cognitive control, effortful control, executive functioning (prefrontal-subcortical loops) (Chapter 5)

    A. Control of attention (selection and working memory) (anterior cingulate loop)
        i. Conflict detection
        ii. Control of interfering information/responses

    B. Control of motor response and behavior (orbital prefrontal loop)
        i. Suppressing or interrupting a prepared response
        ii. Delaying any and all response

    C. Working memory (dorsolateral prefrontal loop and associated cortical loops)
        i. Auditory working memory
        ii. Spatial working memory
        iii. Location working memory

    D. State regulation
        i. Activation (basal ganglia)

3. Motivation (Chapter 6)

    A. Reward system: Excitement/approach to incentive (cortical–limbic dopamine loop)

    B. Anxiety/behavioral inhibition system: Anxiety/retreat from *potential* threat (septal–hippocampal, amygdala loops)

    C. Fight–flight system: Panic/pain, emergency, or attack (imminent or actual)

4. Motor control and timing (Chapter 7)

    A. Motor coordination/execution (nigral–striatal pathways)

    B. Motor timing, and temporal information processing in general (cerebellar pathways)

5. Other areas

    A. Language

    B. Memory

is it going to happen?"). The alerting system gets the system ready for anything ("Something is going to happen, but I don't know what"). I group these all together because both systems operate somewhat outside voluntary control, although deliberate effort can override them to a limited extent. I argue that orienting has been largely disproven as a dysfunction in ADHD (at least in ADHD-C and at least in the visual modality), but that arousal (the ability to be alert) may well be involved in the disorder.

Cognitive Control or Executive Functioning

Is the core problem in ADHD inability to control or plan responses? To guide us in finding out, I have listed a high-level cognitive control or executive functioning system as the second system in Table 3.2. This system can be envisioned as having several subdomains. The nature and definition of these subdomains are hotly disputed topics in the literature today; therefore, any attempt to parse the executive domain is subject to dispute. I have tried to parse this domain in such a way as to make it easily convertible to other models. Overall, the executive system is involved in the deliberate or goal-oriented control of behavior. For example, when Tommy has to focus on his homework in order to be able to get playtime privileges this weekend, but really wants to leave his seat to talk to his friend at the pencil sharpener, he has to exert complex control: He has to remember the long-term goal, place value on it, and suppress the spontaneous urge to leave his seat. Failure in any of these abilities (holding in mind, suppressing irrelevant behavior) could lead to leaving his seat and losing his weekend privileges. Neuroscientists tend to prefer the term "cognitive control" to designate these functions, which require mental resources (i.e., they are harder to do if one is tired, or trying to do too many things at once). I argue that only some elements of this system are clearly dysfunctional in ADHD.

For simplicity, I have placed activation under the broad executive rubric. However, many theorists see this response system as outside of the executive domain and moderating it (Sergeant, Oosterlaan, & van der Meere, 1999); others see it as a component of very broadly defined executive operations (Berger & Posner 2000). Effort can also be seen as a distinct moderating process, or as part of executive functioning (Berger & Posner, 2000). However, because of its close relation with motivation (Scheres, Oosterlaan, & Sergeant, 2001; Sergeant, 2005), I omit discussion of it herein and instead focus on motivation.

Motivation

Is the main difference in children with ADHD that they aren't motivated? To structure an examination of this question, in Table 3.2 I also list three key motivation systems. An approach system (reward responsivity, or excitement) and a withdrawal system (punishment responsivity, or anxiety) are prominent subdomains in the motivational perspective on ADHD. I argue that dysfunction in a reward response system is more probable than dysfunction in a punishment response system in ADHD. Provocative but preliminary theories also note that the fight–flight system (fear, panic, rage) may be relevant in a subgroup of children with externalizing behavior problems; discussion of that potentially important suggestion is deferred until more data are in hand.

Motor Control and Timing

Is the problem in ADHD a more fundamental one of motor coordination or motor timing (or time perception in general)? To address this ancillary yet potentially crucial set of issues, in the fourth section of Table 3.2 I list motor control and timing, for which evidence remains sparse but hypotheses are resurgent. These systems are of obvious relevance and are receiving substantial empirical attention at this juncture. I check on the status of data about these systems, even though they constitute the most preliminary of the four areas under discussion. The possibility of a dysfunction in motor *execution* (as opposed to *preparation* for motor output) is directly related to the idea that some children with ADHD may have had neural injury, and so it is reminiscent of the earlier concept of "minimal brain dysfunction" with a modern twist. The cerebellum is important in motor timing, and in temporal information processing in general. Many theorists today prefer to emphasize temporal information processing. This is noted in Chapter 7, although I emphasize motor control here and in that chapter, due to its closer relation to clinical decision making and assessment concerns at present.

PLAN FOR THE REST OF PART II

In the remaining chapters of Part II, I scrutinize each of these four basic domains that may be crucial in terms of within-child dysfunction in ADHD. Overall, I argue that for two of these systems, involvement in at least a subgroup of children with ADHD may be considered to be established: executive response suppression (point 2Bi in Table 3.2) and alerting/arousal (1Bi in Table 3.2). For two others, a role appears quite probable, but the evidence needs to be improved: reward response (3A in Table 3.2) activation (2Di in Table 3.2). For other systems and functions, I clarify which are essentially ruled out and which require more examination. At the end of this book, I consider how to reconcile the involvement of multiple mechanisms in the syndrome via hybrid and multi-process theories.

Key Complexities and Remaining Issues

A few more words of caution are needed. First, numerous tasks are utilized in studies of neurocognitive operations in ADHD. Keeping these straight can be difficult for nonspecialists. No one task can provide a definitive answer to ADHD, because each task has its own particular limitations. Instead, we must look for convergent evidence from multiple types of information. As more putative measures of a domain converge, more confidence can be placed in its involvement. To enable readers to track these many measurement tasks, I include descriptive tables in each chapter to which readers can refer for more details about a particular method of measuring the abilities under discussion.

Second, the database for this literature remains limited in important ways. Most studies have been done with boys; minority groups are not well represented; and IQ and socioeconomic status (SES) effects are not consistently investigated as potential explanatory covariates. These are important limitations, to which I return in this book's concluding remarks. However, because they are pervasive issues, I do not belabor them when reviewing the literature in the main chapters of the book.

Third, the field still debates the construct validity of various task probes in challenging the intended psychological and neural systems. This question applies to physiological measures as well. Multilevel studies of neuroimaging, physiology, and performance remain important to "bootstrap" our understanding from one approach to another, as we look for convergence across techniques and methods. Readers are thus reminded to avoid premature reification of a given understanding of the disorder while new data are still emerging.

Fourth, we scientists have grown fairly accomplished at measuring and creating taxonomies of both behaviors and cognitive operations in children. Where we are less advanced is in describing a taxonomy of contexts for those behaviors and cognitive operations. Yet it will ultimately be crucial to identify and assess those contexts to understand fully how ADHD develops and is maintained. For example, the field has learned to differentiate "slow, careful" contexts (in which children with ADHD typically show hasty, careless, inaccurate behavior) from "fast, accurate" contexts (in which children with ADHD are typically slow and still inaccurate). As a second example, the field has learned to differentiate contexts in which both reward and punishment are possible outcomes from those in which one or neither of those consequences is cued. Yet we need far more differentiated accounts than these—accounts that capture developmental contexts at higher levels of analysis, including family conflict, peer relations, and other aspects of socialization that are likely to be important for ADHD (for more discussion, see Nigg et al., 2006). The effort to integrate cognitive difficulties with these developmental contexts will be important. Perhaps the most important thing will be to understand the early prenatal and postnatal context of neural development for children with varying behavioral and cognitive profiles.

Lastly, few of the findings to be reviewed are specific to ADHD (Sergeant et al., 2002); similar findings may also be seen in disorders that frequently overlap with ADHD, such as CD and reading disorder. Work in our lab has shown, however, various neuropsychological problems in ADHD are not explained by comorbid conditions. That is, when we statistically control for ODD symptoms, CD symptoms, or reading disorder or reading ability (as well as IQ), children with ADHD continue to have deficits in motor control, output speed, response suppression, and cognitive control in general (Nigg, Hinshaw, Carte, & Treuting, 1998; Nigg, 1999; see also Willcutt et al., 2001, and Schachar, Mota, Logan, Tannock, & Klim, 2000, for confirmatory findings). In other words, these group deficits are not "explained" by the frequent co-occurring psychiatric and learning problems of the children.

Yet studies that have checked the reverse—to see whether a particular executive or other deficit attributed to ADHD can be shown to be related to CD or reading disorder when ADHD symptoms are controlled for—are extremely rare. Pennington and Ozonoff (1996) could find no such studies, and therefore concluded that key executive deficits (notably response suppression) were specific to ADHD. Since that time, only a handful of studies have examined this important issue, with conflicting results. We (Nigg et al., 1998) failed to find control and motor problems linked with CD symptoms when ADHD symptoms were statistically controlled for in a regression model. But Seguin and colleagues (Seguin, Boulerice, Hardin, Tremblay, & Pihl, 1999; Seguin, Nagin, Assaad, & Tremblay, 2004) found that executive function deficits were associated with aggression after they partialed out ADHD symptoms. Those studies had very different samples; thus the degree of specificity of these deficits to particular behavioral syndrome clusters remains somewhat unclear. It is probably premature to conclude that such deficits are not specific to ADHD, as some reviewers have done. At the same time, more research on this issue is needed.

At a conceptual level, however, it is not clear that specificity is an important criterion for a causal mechanism in multifactorial disorders (Garber & Hollon, 1991). A deficit in, say, working memory may be present in two disorders, but may be causal in only one of them. Alternatively, such a deficit may be causal in both of them, but the exact form of the psychopathology may depend on moderating factors. The latter state of affairs is well recognized even in single-gene diseases, in which a single gene can cause multiple disease phenotypes (Worman & Courvalin, 2004). The diseases, however, share key features. Thus nonspecificity may be as much a clue to shared etiologies (relations among currently distinct disorders) as it may be evidence of any blind alley in the causal search.

That said, readers should be cautioned that the correlative studies to be reviewed in Chapters 4–7 are suggestive, but by themselves cannot demonstrate that these mechanisms, even if they are *dysfunctional* in ADHD, are part of the *causality* in ADHD. That will require some additional investigations and linkage to particular causal triggers, such as those discussed in Chapters 9–11.

Effect Size

Throughout the next several chapters, I often describe differences between children with ADHD and a control group (often, as just noted, a nondisordered control group). To enable direct comparison of the importance of effects in the different chapters, I make use of an effect size statistic, called d. The d statistic indicates how far apart two group means are, in standard deviation units. Thus $d = 0.5$ indicates that two group means are half of a standard deviation apart. Cohen (1988) provides cogent guidelines for interpreting the size of various values for d, and I follow his illustrative examples closely here. As explained by Cohen (1988), when $d = 0.8$, the effect may be considered "large" in the behavioral sciences; it is equivalent to a correlation of $r = .37$, or to about 14% of variance explained. As a frame of reference, $d = 0.8$ is equivalent to the difference in height between 13- and 18-year-old girls (about 1 inch), or to the difference in IQ between the average college freshman and the average holder of a PhD. When $d = 0.5$, the effect size is "medium" in size. This is an effect equivalent to a correlation of r = .25, or about 6% of variance accounted for in the outcome of interest (e.g., ADHD symptoms). It is equivalent to the IQ difference between clerical and semiskilled workers (about 8 IQ points). When $d = 0.2$, the effect is "small." This is equivalent to $r = .10$, or about 1% of variance explained. This is a small effect, but as we will see, such small effects can still be reliable and important in understanding ADHD. Although small, this effect would be equal to the difference in height between 15- and 16-year-old girls (half an inch).

SUMMARY AND CONCLUSIONS

Table 3.3 lists frequently asked questions that may come up for clinicians and other practitioners in relation to ADHD, and the best answers based on current knowledge as summarized in this chapter. Neuroimaging studies indicate that as a group, children with ADHD have about a 5% reduction in total brain volume and a 10–12% reduction in the size of key brain regions involved in higher-order control of behavior. The four main regions are the prefrontal cortices (crucial in coordinating complex, planned behavior, keeping things in mind, and overriding inappropriate responses), basal ganglia (a subcortical group of structures involved in controlling responses), cerebellum (important in processing timing of events and behaviors), and corpus callosum (involved in bringing different information together for optimal efficient response). These regions are closely interconnected in just a small number of key circuits, which are the probable loci for neurological involvement in ADHD. Structural abnormalities in these regions are apparent early in development, are nonprogressive, and at least in some instances are part of an environmental causal mechanism rather than a genetic mechanism (although they may reflect genetic influence in a majority of cases). Functional activity in prefrontal cortices and basal ganglia on challenge tasks is likewise different in groups of children or adults with ADHD than in nondisordered controls.

Because these circuits are so important in behavior, they support several core domains of functioning that remain as candidates for the

TABLE 3.3. Frequently Asked Questions about ADHD and the Brain

Question	Answer
Do brain imaging studies find anything in ADHD?	Yes, a 10% smaller size in key regions on MRI.
What brain regions are most important?	Prefrontal cortices, basal ganglia, cerebellum, corpus callosum.
What about brain waves and ADHD?	More slow waves (indicating low arousal) are observed on EEG scalp recordings in ADHD.
Are these findings reliable/replicated?	Yes
Are any of these indicative of brain damage?	The meaning of these data is still unclear.
So can brain scans be used to diagnose ADHD?	No.
Why not?	These are group effects; we cannot yet use scans to identify individual children who may have abnormal development in key brain circuits (although some clinicians are trying).
Do the brain scan findings "make sense"?	Yes. These regions are involved in the kinds of motivation, control, and attention abilities that seem to affect children with ADHD, and low brain arousal fits with poor self-control.

core area of psychological dysfunction in ADHD, or what I call "the most important difference" in children who meet criteria for this syndrome. These main candidates can be broadly described as (1) attention (including arousal), (2) cognitive control or executive functioning, (3) motivation, and (4) motor control and timing (or temporal information processing in general). Each has subdomains that will be important in adding sufficient nuance to our understanding of ADHD.

| C H A P T E R   4 |

Attention and Arousal

OVERVIEW AND DEFINITIONS

Basic Kinds of Attention

In evaluating candidate neurocognitive mechanisms in ADHD, I begin with the most obvious candidate: attention. The concept is obviously embedded in the very name "attention-deficit/hyperactivity disorder." Children with ADHD certainly seem to have problems paying attention and staying on task. Yet their inattentive behavior is often mysterious, puzzling, or baffling to parents, teachers, and even clinicians working with them. Why can Mary play video games for 2 hours without interruption, when she cannot focus on her homework for 5 minutes? Yet why can't Mike seem to pay attention even on the baseball field, a sport he really likes and wants to do well in? To understand how these different behaviors make sense, we need to identify more than one kind of "attention." Then we have to define it formally and measure it in the laboratory. Ever since seminal papers by Virginia Douglas and her colleagues in the early 1970s focused ADHD research on attention, the field has done these things, with striking progress (see Douglas, 1999, for additional perspective). Although attention is described here as a cognitive process, easily overlooked in a cognitive approach is the role of emotion and motivation in attention (Pennington, 2002). That is, emotions also govern attention (Derryberry & Tucker, 1994). If a child is angry, frightened, excited, the child's attention may be entirely focused on what excited him or her, to the exclusion of all else. However, the cognitive models are essential to beginning to evaluate attention in ADHD.

74

Selective Attention

For our purposes, "attention," broadly understood, refers to the ability to routinely filter the vast amount of information around us at all times. For instance, imagine that Mike is in a classroom with 25 other children (some of whom have interesting objects in their hands, and some with whom Mike has had recent memorable interactions); a teacher, Ms. Blake, calling for attention to material on the blackboard; a ticking clock; a pencil sharpener; two wastebaskets; a window with a big dump truck in full view; and more. Mike has to filter all of these details in order to focus on what is most important at that moment. Ideally, selective attention enables this to happen.

This ability, formally termed "perceptual selectivity" (Yantis, 1998), can take many forms. These include filtering on the basis of (1) spatial location (e.g., "If it is in front of me or close to me, I'll pay attention to it"; Erikson & Hoffman, 1972); (2) various object features, such as unusual shape or size (e.g., "Hey, look at that big truck out the window"; Triesman & Gelade, 1980; Wolf, 1998); (3) timing (i.e., "Something happened just now, or happened when I didn't expect it to"; Shapiro & Raymond, 1994); (4) movement; or (5) other object characteristics (Kahneman & Henik, 1981). Some models also emphasize a capacity pool for attention (Engle, 2002)—in other words, the idea that some of us can hold seven or eight things in mind while working, whereas others can only hold three or four things in mind while working. However, I cover the idea of capacity in Chapter 5 when I discuss "working memory."

Yet even if we define attention as perceptual selectivity (the filtering of the most relevant or important from a vast set of options, as just described), it still reflects multiple component abilities. Some of these are automatic, and some are deliberate. Operationally capturing these distinct abilities is a classic challenge in cognitive psychology, which has long debated whether attentional filtering occurs late or early in the processing of our environment. Recent work has integrated these views by suggesting that "perceptual load" determines whether an early or late selection process is involved in ADHD.

In some situations (e.g., high perceptual load), automatic, stimulus-driven processes guide selection. These are called "bottom-up" processes, because they are driven by lower brain centers. For example, we naturally notice someone moving fast to the side of us, or something loud (in Mike's case, Ms. Blake raising her voice over the classroom, or a Mary shrieking when Tommy pinches her), or something unexpected that happens near us (Ms. Blake suddenly rapping her knuckles on Mike's desk to get his attention—both loud and unexpected). These items are filtered into awareness automatically and attended to (at least briefly) without apparent effort, no matter how much else we may be trying to hold in mind. By the same token, events that are routine, familiar, or otherwise nonsalient are automatically filtered out. A theory that this ability is deficient in children with ADHD would suggest simplifying their environment, or shifting their activities or materials frequently, so as to activate this automatic filtering mechanism.

This ability can be formally measured with computerized reaction time tasks that carefully vary the types of distractors presented while a child completes a main task. When measured that way, the ability matures early in development and reaches near-adult levels by about third grade (Huang-Pollock, Carr, & Nigg, 2002). In the brain, it probably involves a posterior system that includes parietal cortical regions, as well as structures in the thalamus (recall from Chapter 3 that these are areas that have not been highlighted in neuroimaging findings in ADHD).[1]

In other situations, effortful, "top-down," goal-driven processes guide selection. These skills are strategic, relatively deliberate, and related to the concept of cognitive control. Thus, to return to Mike's dilemma of joining a friend for some clowning around at the pencil sharpener or ignoring his friend to focus on his spelling, the latter requires some deliberate filtering. Another example that illustrates strategy is a treasure hunt: A child is looking for clues that will help win the treasure hunt, so now attention is quickly focused on filtering possible clues (strange materials in the room) and ignoring information that is not a possible clue (the principal's beginning an announcement over the intercom). When assessed on computerized reaction time tasks, this ability is later-developing, still not fully mature even in junior high (Huang-Pollock et al., 2002). In the brain, it probably involves an anterior network that includes the anterior cingulate cortex as well as associated subcortical structures, as well as parietal cortex (see note 1).

These two types of processes interact continuously, each placing constraints on the other (Corbetta & Shulman, 2002; Schneider & Shiffrin, 1977). Sometimes automatic filtering can override strategic filtering, and vice versa. Research on ADHD (and typical development) attempts to isolate these two influences by using carefully constructed computerized reaction time tasks, as described later.

Attentional Orienting in Space

We can also think of attention as "orienting"—turning in space to where the relevant information is. A paradigmatic example is a quarterback dropping back to pass. He must locate relevant information by looking left, right, near, or far, on the basis of good automatic filtering (an unexpected player approaching from the left had better be noticed, or the quarterback will be sacked) as well as good strategic filtering (the quarterback must first look long, then look short, to maximize chances of a completion). Similarly, a child must be able to orient when playing sports, but also in the classroom, such as when picking up new words on the far end of the chalkboard. When attention is seen as an orienting response, it again has both a reflexive, automatic component, and a strategic or deliberate component. This ability is primary in the sense that it is difficult to filter the correct information if one is not oriented to it.

Arousal and Vigilance

A third kind of attention is the ability to stay alert ("arousal"). Thus in some situations, "I may not know what is going to happen, where it is going to happen, or exactly when it is going to happen, but I know if something happens, I better not miss it." This may be the state of a child waiting for the teacher to get to the main point of a lecture, or of a defensive cornerback on the football field waiting for the next play to begin. It is the state of a radar operator during wartime watching the coastal defenses for incoming aircraft or missiles, or of a meterologist during hurricane season watching for bad weather: Nothing important may happen for days on end, but the watcher must stay alert in case something happens. This ability to regulate arousal or alertness depends neurally on brain stem and other norepineprhine projections, culminating in the right frontal cortex, as well as other cortical–cortical circuits. Arousal is obviously low during sleep, and high during states of excitement or panic. Either very high or very low arousal can compromise self-control and goal-oriented behavior.

Assessing Different Kinds of Attention in ADHD

The complexity of these different kinds of attention and their component processes has led to a massive literature using a wide range of measurement paradigms in cognitive science. I do not survey all of the many approaches available (Triesman & Gelade, 1980; Theuwes, Atchley, & Kramer, 1998; Yantis, 1998; see Monsell & Driver, 1998), even though several have led to isolated but interesting studies of ADHD. Instead, I emphasize findings related to ADHD that rely on a small number of widely used approaches, which are relatively well studied and which allow some conclusions about the basic attention networks in the brain in ADHD. I focus in this chapter on (1) the posterior automatic system (both in filtering and in orienting) and (2) the right-lateralized alerting system. The strategic control of attention is covered in Chapter 5 in relation to executive functioning and effortful control mechanisms.

Theoretical Models of Attention

How are these basic systems reflected in formal models used in ADHD research? Studies of ADHD have generally relied on three broad concepts of attention: (1) visual orienting (how well a child notices where something happened or is about to happen); (2) visual or auditory selective attention (how well a child filters signal from noise); or (3) a neuropsychological component model. To enable easier integration of the literature on ADHD, then, I briefly difress to describe key models.

Orienting: The Posner–Petersen Model

Visual–spatial orienting is in some ways a privileged function because until a *location* is attended to, it is generally difficult to attend to *what* is at that location, regardless of how many object selection mechanisms are available (Yantis, 1998). With regard to spatial orienting of attention, Posner and Petersen's (1990) model posits (1) a posterior brain system that is responsible for relatively automatic cue response in visual orienting (focusing on a specific relevant location); and (2) an anterior system that is responsible for deliberate or strategic placement of visual attention, which is related to cognitive control. The automatic or posterior system orients visual attention almost reflexively to a sudden movement, appearance of a light, or other change. If ADHD is related to over- or underfunctioning of this system, as might be suggested by Mike's difficulty staying with Ms. Blake when she moves across the room or difficulty in picking up key information on the side of the board, then it should be detectable in formal probes of this system (i.e., computerized reaction time tasks). The anterior system moves attention deliberately (e.g., to achieve a strategy or a goal), and is considered in Chapter 5. A third system, which is variously referred to as an "alerting" or "vigilance" system (Posner & Petersen, 1990), enables establishing and maintaining an alert state ("ready for anything") as described earlier.

Selection: The Perceptual Load Model

With regard to describing object *selection* ("What is important from this busy classroom?"), a variety of models have traditionally been used. However, recent developments in understanding selection help us organize that literature. These developments suggest a way to think about this question: How do we know whether selection is "bottom-up" or reflexive versus "top-down" or strategic? Think of mental processing as involving a sequential set of steps, such as encoding, automatic filtering ("It's large or small, moving or not moving"), followed by strategic filtering ("Is it relevant to my goals?"), followed by action. Then we can think of "early" processes (the automatic filtering steps, necessary so as to save the limited-capacity strategic system for important or goal-relevant decisions), and of "late" processes (deliberate strategies, the limited-capacity strategic process). These stages are schematically illustrated in Figure 4.1. Using this approach, we can ask whether children with ADHD have problems in early or late selection mechanisms.

Lavie (1995) uses this approach to describe bottom-up or stimulus-driven versus strategic selection or filtering mechanisms. Our human capacity is finite, so we must preselect what we will attend to. How do we do so? Lavie distinguishes between early *perceptual* selection (relatively automatic) and later *cognitive* selection (which requires mental resources—the executive functioning system in Chapter 3, Table 3.2). This model is thus parallel to the aforementioned orienting model, in that it also specifies (1) stimulus-driven processes (probably guided by a posterior attention system) and (2) strategic processes (related to an anterior attention system in the brain).

Clinical Neuropsychological Models

Clinicians at this point have probably noticed that the Posner–Petersen and Lavie models have been little used in clinical assessment. How do these cognitive science models fit in with the assessment models used in clinical neuropsychology? One well-recognized neuropsychological model of attention, based on clinical measures, is that of Mirsky and colleagues (Mirsky, Anthony, Duncan, Ahern, & Kellham, 1991; Mirsky

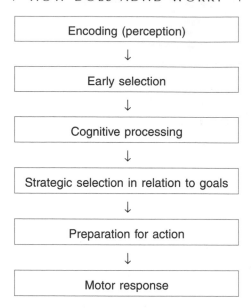

FIGURE 4.1. Hypothetical stages of information processing.

& Duncan, 2001). They posit five attentional functions. Two of these correspond to the two functions of the vigilance system: "sustain," measured by accuracy and reaction time on a continuous-performance test (CPT; see Table 4.1)—in other words, how quickly the child notices a rare target; and "stabilize," measured by variance of reaction time on a reaction time test or CPT—in other words, how consistent the response pattern is. Mirsky et al.'s "focus" function (illustrated in the Stroop color–word interference test) seems to me to fit within the anterior attention system, because it requires managing interference. However, I recognize that others (including Mirsky et al. in some writings) might link it with the posterior system. This may depend on how it is measured. The fourth ability is clearly an aspect of executive functioning, and also includes managing interfering information: "shift," measured by the Wisconsin Card Sort Test—in which the child must accurately sort the cards by abstract category (e.g., their color or shape), but then "shift set" when a new rule unexpectedly comes into play. The last ability pertains to short-term memory: "encode," measured by a digit span test—in which the child must remember a list of numbers and repeat them back. It is probably related to short-term memory, which I treat as distinct from these modules (short-term memory is discussed

TABLE 4.1. Key Laboratory Tasks Used to Measure Attentional Selection and Orienting in ADHD

Task	Brief description
Continuous-performance test (CPT)	There are several varieties of CPTs. Their common element concerns the ability to respond to a rare target over a period of extended time (e.g., 15 minutes in most studies of children, much longer in some studies of adult vigilance). For example, the computer may show a different letter every 2 seconds; however, when an X appears that was preceded by an A, the child is to press the response button. The target appears rarely (25% or fewer of trials). Successful detection of a rare target amid many nontargets is an index of vigilance. Signal detection theory can be used to computer a parameter called "d-prime" (d'), which combines hits and misses to calculate sensitivity to the signal. One can also look at the relative weighing of commissions and omissions and calculate a parameter called "beta," which signifies the response bias (e.g., tendency to overrespond or underrespond). Commission errors are responses to nontargets (in the present account, pressing the button for an N before for an A, or for an X not preceded by an A). The patterns of these errors have been extensively studied (Halperin, Wolf, Greenblatt, & Young, 1991; Nigg, Hinshaw, & Halperin, 1996), although many studies have failed to differentiate error types.
Spatial orienting task	The spatial orienting task is often called the "Posner orienting task" or the "covert orienting task." The child fixes his or her eyes on the center of the computer screen, with an instruction to press the key as quickly as possible when the child sees the target appear in either the left or the right periphery. The target is preceded by a warning cue that is either correct or incorrect in its spatial (left or right) visual field location. The task is illustrated later in this chapter (Figure 4.4).
Alerting task	The orienting task can have a condition in which a target appears with no cue—that is, an unwarned target appearing after a variable waiting period, so its time of appearance or location (left or right) cannot be predicted. Reaction time to respond to the unwarned cue indexes alerting, especially in the left visual field.
Perceptual load paradigm	In this computerized reaction time task, children (or adults) view a display with a target letter (say, X or L) embedded in a circle of nontarget letters. They must locate the target while ignoring the distractor. Outside the ring of letters is a very large distractor letter. The distractor letter can be a valid target (an L or X; difficult to ignore) or it can be an irrelevant distractor (easy to ignore). The ring of letters can be many (e.g., six letters; high load) or few (e.g., two letters; low load). The task is illustrated later in this chapter (Figure 4.5).
Dichotic listening task	A child is equipped with dual-channel headphones. One ear thus receives one stream of information, while the other ear can receive a competing stream of information. The task can then be manipulated to require filtering of information in one ear, to enable concentrating on information in the other ear.

in Chapter 5). Thus I discuss the first two of these functions in this chapter, and the last three in Chapter 5. Note, then, that clinical measures generally do not formally operationalize the automatic functions that are highlighted in the cognitive attention models.

Integrating Basic Models with Brain Networks of Attention

As I have mentioned, although these approaches at first seem quite different, they can be organized and grouped according to the component operation of three basic attentional networks in the brain. Thus the vigilance system handles alerting and sustained attention. The posterior attention system handles bottom-up or reflexive attention, including reflexive spatial orienting and perceptual (bottom-up) selection of information to filter. The anterior system handles strategic aspects of attention—that is, strategic orienting; filtering of information based on its meaning, importance, or goal relevance; and deliberate shifting of attention. In this chapter, I discuss the vigilance and posterior attentional systems in relation to ADHD. In the next chapter, I discuss the functions of the anterior system, along with other executive or cognitive control functions (see note 1 for additional comment).

THE VIGILANCE NETWORK IN ADHD

I begin with the vigilance network, because it serves to moderate the others. It depends on a network of neural structures that include the noradrenergic system originating in the locus coeruleus, the cholinergic system of the basal forebrain, the intralaminar thalamic nuclei, and the right prefrontal cortex (Parasuraman, Warm, & See, 1998; Posner & Petersen, 1990; Rothbart, Posner, & Rosicky, 1994). When it is linked to arousal, as I will do here, it may also involve the brain stem reticular activating system (involved in sleep–wake cycles and alertness state) and its cortical projections.

The Sustained Attention Function Is Intact in ADHD

Sustained attention is probably the most common, everyday idea about what is dysfunctional in ADHD. But what is "sustained attention," exactly? The concept has an extensive research history dating to at least the middle of the 20th century (Mirsky & Duncan, 2001). In the cognitive psychology literature, it means the ability to maintain a state of alertness and wakefulness during prolonged mental activity (Weinberg & Harper, 1993). A classic example (and the spur to research on this topic in World War II) is watching for enemy planes to appear on a radar screen. An example closer to home is driving a familiar route while watching for a new turn not usually taken. Two final examples, relevant to children, are paying attention throughout a class at school in order to pick up the day's homework assignment, and staying focused during a sports event waiting for the cue to action. Because of fatigue, everyone performs worse (slower and more variable responses, more errors) as minutes and hours go by with no variable signal. This is called the "vigilance decrement." The longer a person listens for key points in a monotonous lecture, or watches a radar screen with nothing happening, or strives to notice other rare events, the more mistakes the person will make, and the more slowly he or she will respond to what does happen (Parasuraman et al., 1998). Figure 4.2 shows a solid line representing a typical vigilance decrement, in which performance (let's assume that the *Y*-axis here is accuracy on a CPT— identifying rare letters; see Table 4.1) gradually drops off over time. The question has been whether children with ADHD have an *excessive* decrement, or, in other words, a specific sustained attention deficit. This is represented by the hypothetical dashed line in Figure 4.2, showing a steeper dropoff in performance over time. Superficial observation of children with ADHD seems to suggest that they do, because they appear to lose interest in tasks more quickly than other children do. However, this could be occurring for many reasons not relating to a formal measure of sustained attention.

In fact, when children with ADHD are assessed with computerized CPTs, this everyday observation of such children does not seem to be

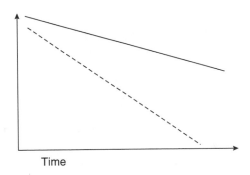

Time

FIGURE 4.2. Typical vigilance decrement.

attributable to a true sustained attention deficit. They generally do not show an excessive vigilance decrement except in very particular circumstances (especially those referred to as slow event rates). This suggests that the real problem is not sustained attention per se, but some other support process. We now know this because of the pioneering work of Douglas in the 1970s. Her theories (see, e.g., Douglas, 1972) stimulated the field to scrutinize attention more closely in the ensuing decade, with sustained attention being one key target of investigation.

Early computerized attention studies yielded inconsistent or negative findings for sustained attention (Sergeant & Scholten, 1985; Sergeant & van der Meere, 1990; Sergeant et al., 1999). Children with ADHD had a general tendency to show poor performance from the very beginning of a time course (Sergeant & van der Meere, 1990). This pattern was more consistent with an alerting dysfunction than with a vigilance or sustained attention dysfunction. When time-on-task effects are assessed in laboratory experiments, they typically fail to show deficits in ADHD-C(though most studies have relied on a DSM-III-R definition of ADHD; for reviews, see Sergeant et al., 1999; Huang-Pollock & Nigg, 2003). However, other data suggest that this general pattern depends on the event rate; at slow event rates (e.g., 8 seconds per trial rather than 1 or 2 seconds), a sustained attention deficit can be observed (van der Meere, 2002). This, however, seems better explained as a deficit in activation or another readiness process (discussed subsequently) than as a primary sustained attention deficit.

Overall, the most parsimonious conclusion is that the sustained attention function of the vigilance network is spared in most cases of ADHD-C. Further study of ADHD-PI may be useful, however, because the picture is less clear for that subtype. I now turn to the second function of the vigilance system: alerting or arousal.

The Alerting Function of the Vigilance System Is Impaired in ADHD-C

Many classic theories of ADHD emphasize a deficit in cortical arousal (Satterfield, Cantwell, & Satterfield, 1974; Zentall & Zentall, 1983) or, consistent with that idea, disruption in ascending noradrenergic neural systems that facilitate signal-to-noise detection (McCracken, 1991), which are pictured in Figure 4.3. Therefore, I consider data purportedly relevant to arousal as relating to the same neural network as the data on alerting. Alerting is viewed as a second function of the vigilance system by Posner and Petersen (1990); it can also be viewed as related to the ventral attention circuit described in note 1.

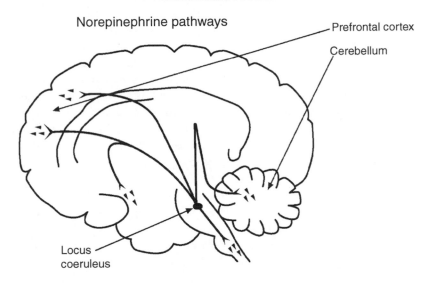

FIGURE 4.3. Noradrenergic projections. Courtesy of Dr. Timothy Wilens.

"Alerting" is the ability to prepare for what is about to happen when a warning is received, or to be ready to respond without warning. An example might be waiting during a short-answer test for the next question from the teacher, or waiting in a track meet for the starting gun to sound. An effective alerting system prepares for a rapid, accurate response. Although impulsive children make hasty responses in situations that call for waiting, they tend to make slow, inaccurate responses when time is of the essence—consistent with an alerting deficit. Failures in this system therefore could account for inability to regulate behavior or attention effectively in ADHD. Indeed, someone who is not alert (e.g., very tired) may also make hasty decisions when waiting is advisable.

In the laboratory, a deficit in alerting (or phasic arousal) is usually marked by either poor performance (slow, variable response times) on a series of single abrupt-onset trials (e.g., detecting a light the moment it appears and touching a key as quickly as possible; see Table 4.1), or poor (slow, inaccurate) performance from the very beginning of a reaction time task. On this type of reaction time task, responses must be very fast. So an average child might notice a light appear on the computer screen and press the key within 500 milliseconds (half a second). A child with ADHD might respond in 600 milliseconds. By the standards of fast measurement in computerized tasks, this is a large difference.

I have noted that alerting is related to the older concept of arousal. What is meant by "arousal"? This term is also used in different ways, but again we can draw a common theme from these different ideas. Traditionally, arousal was thought to be related to cortical–reticular loops in the brain that regulated states of wakefulness, sleep, and alertness (Mirsky & Duncan, 2001). One can talk about physiological arousal, cortical arousal, or arousal in any other bodily system; these may be distinct processes (Derryberry & Rothbart, 1988). When it comes to ADHD, generally we are referring to cortical arousal (Tucker & Williamson, 1984; Gray, 1982).

Arousal is modulated by one's emotional state. For example, anxiety or excitement (perhaps in response to a cue that something is about to happen, as when Mike hears the doorbell, which may indicate that he will get an expected letter with money in it for his birthday) lends subsequent behavior greater intensity and speed (Gray, 1982). For our purposes, arousal as a right-brain-lateralized process of activation by noradrenergic neurons (again, see Figure 4.3). This system responds to stimulus input and prepares to take advantage of new information by enhance the signal-to-noise ratio for novelty detection. This classical conception fits rather well with the formulation by Posner and Petersen (1990). A closely related idea was offered by Sergeant et al. (1999), who based their idea on a theory by Pribram and McGuinness (1975) about arousal. In this theory, again, arousal is a right-brain-lateralized alerting function, but Sergeant and colleagues specified that it functions during the early (information-encoding) stage of information processing (see Figure 4.1, above). Thus they suggested that responses early in a task (such as in the first moments of a CPT), or early on a trial, are most relevant. This is broadly consistent with the idea of an alerting function indexed by response quality from the very beginning of a laboratory measurement.

Although we have reasonable consensus on this *definition* of the relevant function, controversy attends the appropriate *measurement* of this alerting or phasic arousal function of the vigilance system. I therefore confine my remarks here to four laboratory measures for which there is reasonably widespread agreement (and little argument) that certain responses are reasonable indicators of problems with this functional system. These four types of test responses are as follows: (1) slow and variable responses from the very beginning of a time course in a fast reaction time experiment (accompanied by typical decline over time—in other words, typical slope, but atypical intercept, in a response profile); (2) slow responses on a series of unwarned, abrupt-onset events in a fast reaction time experiment; (3) low scores on the *d*-prime (signal detection) parameter on CPTs (see Table 4.1); and (4) certain patterns of slow-wave activity on scalp electrical recordings of brain electrical activity (EEGs) or of electrical response to stimulus onset (ERPs) on such recordings.

Reaction Time Speed and Variability

Reaction time studies generally support an arousal or alerting deficit. Because dozens of studies have used some type of rapid reaction time measure with children with ADHD, and have yielded a fairly clear story despite variability in their reporting, I do not exhaustively review data on reaction time findings in ADHD. Children with ADHD tend to be slow and variable *from the beginning* of a variety of fast-response laboratory tasks, as indicated by a detailed review of the early literature (Sergeant & Scholten, 1985); by a meta-analysis of this function in eight studies using the stop task (described in Chapter 5; Oosterlaan, Logan, & Sergeant, 1998); and by a meta-analysis of 14 studies using an orienting paradigm (Huang-Pollock & Nigg, 2003). We (Nigg, Blaskey, Huang-Pollock, & Rappley, 2002b) found that on a series of common clinical neuropsychological measures calling for rapid response—including Trail Making B, Stroop color and word naming, and rapid response on "go" trials on the Logan stop task—both ADHD-C and ADHD-PI were associated with slower response speed.

In a study of adults with ADHD, we (Nigg et al., 2005a) created two latent variables (essentially, composites of several tests) from a battery of neuropsychological measures. The tasks are described in detail in Chapter 5. The first latent variable was output speed, indexed by Trail Making A (rapidly connecting numbers in order), color- and word-naming speed on the Stroop (rapidly naming colors of rows of X's, rapidly reading color words printed in the same color of ink), and "go" reaction time on the "go" trials of the Logan stop task (rapidly pressing the X or the O key when the corresponding letter appeared on the computer screen). Slower scores on this composite "speed" score were strongly correlated with ADHD symptoms and the ADHD diagnosis. (The second latent variable, executive functioning, was also related to ADHD independently of slow speed.) Overall, the reaction time or speed data support a deficit in state regulation, consistent with an alerting or arousal dysfunction. However, as pointed out by Sergeant et al. (1999), many of these effects could also be consistent with an *activation* deficit, as discussed in Chapter 5. Therefore, other indicators must be considered to evaluate an arousal/alerting problem in ADHD.

Speed of Responding to Unwarned Targets

The second type of evidence is speed of responding to unwarned targets on the computer screen, particularly in the left visual field, versus warned targets. The few studies of unwarned targets provide some support, though it is mixed, for an arousal/alerting dysfunction in ADHD. This is measured fairly simply on a computer task, by instructing a child to respond as quickly as possible to a light that may appear at any time or in any location (see Table 4.1). Speed of key pressing after onset is an index of alerting. Because alerting is a right-brain-lateralized function, deficits are expected to be especially apparent to targets that appear in the left visual field. Despite the elegance of this measure of alerting, few studies have systematically examined results for unwarned, abrupt-onset events. Three studies used tests of reaction time to latereralized, unwarned targets in a lateralized (left vs. right) cue detection orienting paradigm (described in Table 4.1), with mixed results.

Our study of boys with DSM-III-R ADHD found a substantial effect (effect sizes[2] of $d > 0.8$, $p < .05$; Nigg, Swanson, & Hinshaw, 1997) in children and their biological (but not adoptive) parents for speed of response to fast, unwarned targets in the left visual field, consistent with a genetically influenced alerting dysfunction. Øie, Rund, and Sundet (1998), in a study of adolescents, reported an effect size of $d = 0.50$ for the group with ADHD on a similar task, but it was shy of significance with their small sample. Swanson et al. (1991), also looking at boys diagnosed with DSM-III-R ADHD, reported null effects for this condition, but effect size could not be computed from the data reported. More recently, a group at Cornell Medical Center has reported promising findings on a similar measure of alerting (Berger & Posner, 2000). Overall, the abrupt-onset alerting data tend to support an alerting dysfunction in ADHD; however, these data are surprisingly few, and this claim could be overturned with additional studies.

CPT Signal Detection d-Prime Parameter

In signal detection theory, d-prime is a measure of sensitivity to the difference between a target and a nontarget (Lachman, Lachman, & Butterfield, 1979). It is computed by examining how many targets were missed and how many were detected, and by looking at both omission and commission errors (in essence, determining the ability to discriminate a target [say, an X] from a nontarget [say, a T]). It is inversely related to the error rate, so a low d-prime score indicates poor performance. This index is widely accepted as an indicator of arousal (Sergeant et al., 1999). In ADHD research, it is usually assessed by administering a CPT (Table 4.1). The task requires staying alert, avoiding false-positive errors (responding to all letters), and avoiding omissions (missing the rare target letter). Although several dozen studies have used versions of the CPT to examine children with ADHD, not all included a control group or reported sufficient data to enable computation of the d-prime parameter. Losier, McGrath, and Klein (1996) conducted a meta-analysis of 11 CPT studies that reported ADHD versus control group effects in enough detail that d-prime could be calculated. They found clear evidence of an ADHD deficit on d-prime (ADHD group mean = 2.14, control group mean = 3.45, SE = .21, d = 0.74, p < .005)—a conclusion that has not been overturned, despite occasional negative findings. We (Willcutt, Doyle, Nigg, Faraone, & Pennington, 2005b) identified 30 CPT studies of ADHD and looked at simple omission errors; the aggregate effect size was d = 0.64 (23 of the studies 30 showed significant effects). The usual interpretation of this finding would be a deficit in the alerting/arousal function.

EEG Slow-Wave Findings

Despite variable findings and some interpretive issues, there is now fairly solid support for a low arousal/alerting dysfunction in ADHD, based on electrophysiological scalp recordings of brain electrical activity in ADHD. These EEG measures have been frequently investigated by researchers using various methodologies and definitions of ADHD over the past 60 years. Satterfield and colleagues (e.g., Satterfield et al., 1974) are often credited with the first work to use fairly contemporary definitions of ADHD and fairly contemporary methods. This group found higher rates of low-frequency ("slow-wave") brain activity on resting EEG (Satterfield & Dawson, 1971; Satterfield, Schell, Backs, & Hidaka, 1984), as well as ERPs (Satterfield & Schell, 1984) that they interpreted as consistent with low cortical arousal.

The idea of an arousal or alerting dysfunction continues to receive support in many (though not all) electrophysiological studies of ADHD (Brandeis et al., 1998; Monastra et al., 1999; Silberstein et al., 1998). Barry and colleagues conducted an extensive review of some 52 studies of EEG (Barry et al., 2003a) and over 60 studies of ERPs (Barry et al., 2003b) in ADHD and its historical precursors over the last half century; many of these studies were relevant to an arousal theory. They noted the recent emphasis on the elevated *ratio* of resting-state slow-wave EEG activity in ADHD, particularly the theta band or the theta-to-beta ratio. The predominant interpretation again has been under-arousal in groups of children with ADHD-C as well as ADHD-PI. ERP data are less clear, but seem to suggest abnormalities in a response known as the "contingent negative variation" and in an early marker called the "N1 component," both suggestive of abnormal early processing and consistent with an alerting problem in ADHD (Barry et al., 2003b; also see van der Meere, 2002).

Pertinent to our overarching theme of multiple causal pathways to ADHD, Barry et al. (2003a) also noted recent efforts to examine individual EEG/ERP differences in ADHD via cluster-analytic and related techniques. Preliminary but intriguing studies suggest that ADHD-C may be electrophysiologically heterogeneous. One subgroup had a high theta-to-beta ratio, interpreted as central nervous system (CNS) *hypo*arousal. Another, smaller subgroup had excess beta activity, interpreted as CNS *hyper*arousal (Chabot & Serfontein, 1996; Clarke, Barry, McCarthy, & Selikowitz, 2001b).

On balance, Barry et al. (2003a, 2003b) concluded that the EEG and ERP evidence is consistent with CNS hypoarousal in a substantial percentage of children with ADHD-C, as well as in at least a portion of children with ADHD-PI. CNS *hyper*arousal may be a feature in a subgroup, possibly those with high anxiety. The latter would be consistent with Newman and Wallace's (1993) observation that impulsivity can also occur under conditions of high anxiety, which they termed "anxious impulsivity." In view of the variation within ADHD samples on anxiety levels, it is likely that some have low anxiety (this group possibly overlaps with but is not identical with the cortical hypoarousal group), and that another group has excessive anxiety and hyperarousal.

Research on Alerting: Summary

Overall, a deficit in alerting or phasic arousal is important to consider in theories of ADHD-C. The data are fairly consistent across the four main laboratory probes of the health of this system. Although the data for ADHD-PI are less extensive, it appears that this subtype is also associated with this difficulty. It is unclear whether an alerting or arousal dysfunction can account for failures on other measures, such as executive tasks (Chapter 5). Brandeis et al. (1998) used ERP data to conclude that failures of stop inhibition on the stop task (described later) could be due to slow mobilization to a warning cue, consistent with an alerting dysfunction in the vigilance system. In all, an alerting or arousal problem is an important component of ADHD and a viable candidate for a within-child dysfunction in the syndrome, especially in ADHD-C.

THE POSTERIOR ATTENTION NETWORK IS INTACT IN ADHD-C

I now turn to the second attention system addressed in this chapter: the posterior or parietal attention system. As readers will recall, this system operates relatively automatically to orient attention in response to unexpected cues, and to filter perceptual information based on its superficial features (such as size, shape, and proximity).

The posterior attention network handles these functions. It receives extensive norepinephrine-rich projections from the locus coeruleus, and involves coordinated activation of the superior parietal cortex, the pulvinar in the thalamus, and the subcortical superior colliculus (Posner & Raichle, 1994; Rothbart et al., 1994). Specific components of the distributed neural network are specialized for rapidly engaging, disengaging, and shifting spatial attention (Posner & Raichle, 1994; Posner, Walker, Friederich, & Rafal, 1987; Rafal & Posner, 1987).

Several kinds of evidence are relevant to a claim about the posterior attention system in ADHD. These include (1) studies of automatic spatial orienting (referred to in the literature as "covert" or "endogenous" orienting; (2) studies of early perceptual selection in the visual modality; and (3) studies of early perceptual selection in the auditory modality. I consider these in turn.

Automatic Spatial Orienting

At least 14 studies have examined visual orienting in children or adults with ADHD. These used the spatial orienting task (Table 4.1), in which a child (or adult) waits in front of a computer screen for targets in the left or right visual field with various warning cues. The paradigm is illustrated in Figure 4.4. First, the child sees two empty boxes on the left and right sides of the computer screen (the figure is not to scale). Then one of the boxes brightens (this is illustrated by darkening of the

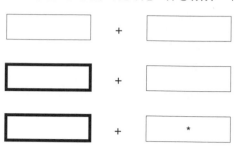

FIGURE 4.4. Typical spatial orienting paradigm. Each row represents one computer display sequence. Not to scale.

box lines in the figure). This cue naturally draws attention to that side. The target (the asterisk) can then appear on either side. In the figure, it is shown appearing on the opposite side, requiring the child to disengage from the cue and quickly move attention back to the other side to pick up the target and press the response key.

The reaction time to detect targets (and press the response key or button) after different kinds of warning is the outcome measure. These studies were comprehensively reviewed by Huang-Pollock (see Huang-Pollock & Nigg, 2003). Her meta-analytic review concluded that the posterior attention system is intact in ADHD-C. There was no evidence for any nontrivial deficit in the ability to move attention reflexively (the ability to move the spotlight of attention quickly across a computer screen, after a warning, to be ready to see what would happen there) or to engage (to stay put and detect a target after moving to the cued location).

One nuance was that occasional evidence popped up in some studies for a problem with disengaging. That is, once attention was locked on to a location, it was difficult for children with ADHD-C to let go of that location in order to pick up a target occurring someplace else in the field of vision. All studies that found group effects on these reflexive probes could be explained by a deficit in disengaging. Even so, most studies found no effect, and there was no effect when all studies were averaged together. Possibly a subgroup of children may exhibit this problem, but rather large samples (well over 100 children with ADHD-C, plus well over 100 controls) would be needed to chase down that fairly weak possibility. That study may never be done, due to the cost and the relatively small chance of meaningful payoff. However, it is important to note that only one study (Huang-Pollock, Nigg,

Henderson, & Carr, 2000; see Huang-Pollock & Nigg, 2003, for a reprinting of those data) looked at the ADHD-PI subtype. That study yielded negative results. However, many theorists continue to believe that the posterior orienting system may be disturbed in children with hypoactive, "spacey," inattentive behaviors. The hypoactive subgroup of children with ADHD-PI warrants further examination on this type of function, using more refined tests.

Early Perceptual Selection in the Visual Modality

What about the "early selection" function of this system? Several types of studies have looked at this type of filtering, using computerized tasks in which targets have to be picked out among distracting information (e.g., the letter L must be found amid an array of letters). This is analogous to what a child must do in picking up, relatively automatically, the important information in a busy classroom. Again, the evidence here was generally negative for an ADHD deficit: Children with ADHD tended to perform like nondisabled children. This was one of the first conclusions after the field turned its focus to attention in the 1970s (Berman, Douglas, & Barr, 1999; McIntyre, Blackwell, & Denton, 1978; Sergeant & van der Meere, 1988; Sharma, Halperin, Newcorn, & Wolf, 1991; Tarnowski, Prinz, & Nay, 1986; Taylor, Suohara, Khan, & Malone, 1997).

However, many of these studies did not control "perceptual load." If a child is alone in a room with one teacher, one desk, and no windows, there are very few distractions. The child does not need to use automatic filtering in order to focus on the teacher, because the perceptual load is low. All filtering can be done by central control or late-stage processing. On the other hand, if a child is in a very busy classroom with two dozen children (some moving to different work stations) and a teacher giving advice to one group, there is too much information to evaluate all of it fully. The child has to "prefilter" some of it out, in order to be able to use attention effectively for thinking.

This issue of the load, then, is crucial, because without the right level of perceptual load, one cannot be sure that the early selection mechanism was really challenged. In the laboratory, load is manipulated by varying the number or difficulty of items to be processed in an array of letters or symbols on the computer screen (some targets and some distractors). A computer display that has these various properties is illustrated in Figure 4.5 (see also Table 4.1). Imagine that the task is to pick out an X or an N in the circle of small letters, and to press the

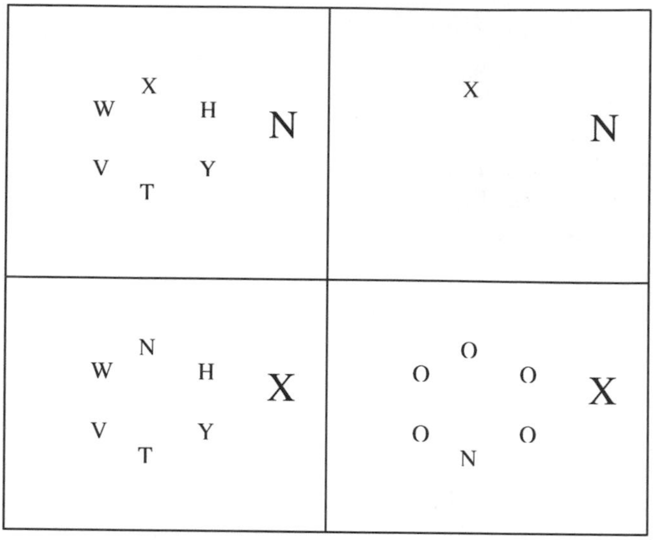

FIGURE 4.5. Varying perceptual load. Reprinted from Huang-Pollock, Carr, and Nigg (2002).

appropriate key indicating which target letter is there. One has to ignore the large distracting letter to the side, which will trigger an incorrect answer concerning the target letter. The upper two panels contrast a relatively high-load condition on the left (several letters in the circle) with a low-load condition on the right (only one letter in the circle). The bottom two panels illustrate how the same effect can be achieved by making the letters visually similar (all of the letters at bottom left are formed with straight lines) versus dissimilar. When load is low, early (automatic) selection is not needed for efficient processing. Instead, early selection "kicks in" when the load becomes too great (i.e., when necessary filtering must protect cognitive processing). Recent work by Huang-Pollock, in which perceptual load was carefully manipulated in this manner, seems to confirm the earlier reports: ADHD-C is not associated with any problem in early perceptual selection or filtering (Huang-Pollock, Nigg, & Carr, 2005). At the same time, there has been no evidence of an excessively *broad* filter in ADHD-C (i.e., letting in too much information). At present, there is thus little evidence to support an early selection deficit in ADHD-C, and the most parsimonious conclusion is that this operation is spared in the disorder.

What about early perceptual selection in ADHD-PI? A long-standing hypothesis in the field has been that ADHD-PI is associated with true posterior attentional deficits (Goodyear & Hynd, 1992; Milich et al., 2001). However, this has been scarcely investigated. We (Huang-Pollock & Nigg, 2003) reported no evidence of abnormal covert orienting in a small sample of children with DSM-IV ADHD-PI. This has been the only study to date to use the orienting paradigm with this ADHD type. In one of the few modern tests of early selection in ADHD-PI, we (Huang-Pollock et al., 2005) failed to find clear evidence for such a deficit, although a subgroup with "sluggish cognitive tempo" (i.e., the hypoactive, "spacey" behaviors mentioned earlier) gave some hint of a selective attention deficit. Thus the results were not particularly satisfying for the posterior attention model of ADHD-PI. However, the theory has received scant investigation. Overall, these types of data do not support a posterior attention deficit in ADHD-PI either, but clearly we must await further studies before drawing a firm conclusion for this group. In particular, a closer examination of the subgroup with sluggish cognitive tempo is warranted, since increasing data suggest that this subgroup may be etiologically distinct from either children with ADHD-C or other children with ADHD-PI (McBurnett et al., 2001).

A Complexity: Early Perceptual Selection in the Auditory Modality

In contrast to the fairly clear picture on visual tasks, the picture is much less clear in research using auditory tasks. In particular, the possibility of an auditory selective attention deficit in ADHD is supported by evidence that children with ADHD perform poorly in dichotic listening tasks, in which information fed to one ear must be ignored to concentrate on information fed to the other ear (see Table 4.1; Dalebout, Nelson, Hletko, & Frentheway, 1991; Davidson & Prior, 1978; Manassis, Tannock, & Barbosa, 2000; Satterfield, Schell, & Nicholas, 1994). Again, however, whether all of these studies tapped *early* selection (vs. strategic selection) is debatable.

Conclusions from this body of data are further complicated by confusion and controversy over another syndrome, called "central auditory processing disorder." This disorder is itself a somewhat controversial condition that is still undergoing examinations of its construct validity. However, the term is used to describe a condition in which nondisordered hearing is associated with disordered central (cognitive or perceptual) processing of sounds. Some investigators believe that the latter often co-occurs with ADHD but is missed in many studies (see discussion by Shapiro & Herod, 1994). Indeed, it has been difficult to establish the construct validity of central auditory processing disorder apart from ADHD, leading some observers to conclude that the syndromes are indistinguishable (see Shapiro & Herod, 1994, for an incisive discussion that remains relevant today). If samples of children with ADHD tend to include children with auditory processing problems, then one would expect findings on auditory perceptual attention tasks but not visual tasks. Because studies of ADHD rarely consider whether children may have central auditory processing problems (usually reports of "normal" hearing are enough), this remains an unclear area.

Shapiro and Herod (1994) found that auditory measures added to the discriminant validity of their neuropsychological battery. Overall, the role of auditory processing problems in samples of children with ADHD is unclear; if these are present in a substantial percentage of children, they could account for findings of apparent deficits in auditory selective attention in some studies.

AROUSAL AND SLEEP IN ADHD

I have noted that underarousal, poor alertness, and low vigilance are characteristic of samples of children with ADHD. One metaphor for understanding those difficulties is to imagine the behavior of someone who is very tired. Stress tolerance is reduced; alertness and vigilance are reduced; reaction times are slowed; and motivation to work or wait for delayed rewards is weakened.

This description may be more than a metaphor. We now know that there is a close relation between arousal and sleep. Indeed, the thalamic nuclei and thalamic–cortical projections that are involved in sleep–wake cycles are also involved in arousal (McCormick & Bal, 1997). More generally, the subcortical–cortical noradrenergic projections in the brain are important not only in vigilance and alertness, but also in typical waking and sleep (Berridge & Waterhouse, 2003).

Thus it might make sense that if arousal is impaired in samples of children with ADHD, sleep might be impaired as well. Base rates also suggest that this etiological possibility warrants investigation. Sleep disorders are relatively common among children in general (1–10%;

Gottlieb et al., 2003). Frequent and loud snoring occurs in about 10% of children under age 8; if evaluated on polysomnography, about 10% of this 10% will prove to have obstructive sleep apnea (O'Brien & Gozal, 2004; Ali, Pitson, & Stradling, 1993; Ferini-Strambi, Fantini, & Castronovo, 2004). An additional percentage of children have other sleep disorders, notably periodic limb movements. The pediatric literature indicates that impaired sleep can mimic ADHD, among other problems (Chan, Edman, & Koltai, 2004; Gottlieb et al., 2003; Kass, Wallace, & Vodanovich, 2003). Furthermore, it seems plausible that it could lead as well to the low-alertness findings that have been described in this chapter in relation to ADHD. Therefore, it is important to evaluate any evidence linking ADHD with undiagnosed sleep problems.

Sleep problems are so often reported by parents of children with ADHD that as late as 1980, the DSM-III presumed that excessive movement during sleep was a feature of the disorder. An absence of empirical research led to dropping this feature from DSM-III-R (APA, 1987), pending more study. Nonetheless, it continues to be clinically recognized that children with ADHD resist bedtime, may get less sleep, and may have more frequently interrupted sleep (Kirov et al., 2004). Whether this is a side effect of ADHD or contributes to their symptoms has been unclear, however. Ball and Koloian (1995) conducted a review of research from 1980 to 1994 about ADHD and sleep. They concluded that parents of children with ADHD reported more child sleep problems than parents of children without ADHD did, but polysomnographic studies yielded mixed results that did not clearly confirm elevated rates of formal sleep disorders in the children with ADHD. Yet to that time, only about 100 children with ADHD had been studied in sleep laboratories across all research

In the subsequent decade, sleep and ADHD have begun to receive far more intensive investigation, though results continue to be mixed. Corkum, Tannock, and Moldofsky (1998) found that although parents reported more sleep problems in their children with ADHD, objective measurement of sleep did not show a clear ADHD-related sleep abnormality. However, they did observe that children with ADHD were more active during sleep than were control children. Konofal, Lecendreux, Bouvard, and Mouren-Simeoni (2001) conducted polysomnography and video surveillance in an overnight sleep study of 30 children with ADHD and 19 control children. They also failed to find an increased incidence of sleep disorders in the group with ADHD, but again these children were more active during

sleep, exhibiting more arm and leg movements and a greater duration of movements. Kirov et al. (2004) conducted polysomnography
in 17 children with ADHD and 17 matched controls (as in the other
studies, children were on no medications). Once again, rates of
formal sleep disorders were not elevated; however, the pattern of
sleep was altered in ADHD, with shorter rapid-eye-movement (REM)
latency and more REM cycles in the ADHD group. It was unclear
whether this altered sleep pattern might account for the ADHD
symptoms, or whether it might simply be an additional correlate of
altered neurochemical activity in these children.

In contrast to these rather negative findings, Picchietti, England,
Walters, Willis, and Verrico (1998) administered a sleep interview to
screen a consecutive series of 69 children with ADHD, and followed
this up with overnight polysomnography in 27 children who passed
the screening questions for periodic limb movements. They identified periodic limb movement disorder (in which movements during
the night disrupt sleep continuously) in 26% of the children with
ADHD, but in only 5% of a matched control sample of children.
Crabtree, Ivanenko, and Gozal (2003) replicated this finding in their
series of 69 children; 43% of the children with ADHD showed
some sleep disorder (36% of the children showed periodic limb
movements, and the other 7% had obstructed breathing). Similar
replications were reported by Andreou, Karapetsas, Agapitou, and
Gourgoulianis (2003) using polysomnography. O'Brien et al. (2003)
concluded that children with ADHD referred to a sleep clinic and
children with ADHD in the community shared some sleep problems,
and that sleep disorders probably characterize a subgroup of children
with ADHD. LeBourgeois, Avis, Mixon, Olmi, and Harsh (2004)
found that by caregiver report, children with ADHD tended to be
sleepy during the day and to snore more often at night, but these
two features were not closely correlated.

In all, these more recent data provide mixed but intriguing evidence that a small subgroup of children with ADHD may have bona
fide sleep disturbances (particularly periodic leg movement disorder),
in addition to daytime sleepiness and frequent parental reports of sleep
problems (although such reports are not always indicative of sleep disorder) (Cohen-Zion & Ancoli-Israel, 2004). The percentage of children
who might be so affected remains unclear, due to varying results across
studies and a dearth of population-based studies with physiological validation of sleep status. Kirk and Bohn (2004) reviewed the charts of
nearly 600 children who had been referred to a sleep clinic and under-

gone a sleep evaluation. Periodic leg movements (defined as more than five per hour) were observed in 5.6% of the children, but 7.1% of the 28 children with ADHD. Two of the 13 children with periodic leg movements and no evidence of obstructive sleep apnea had ADHD. These data thus suggest only a mild relationship between ADHD and sleep problems in the population, at least when such problems pertain to periodic leg movements. However, additional population-based studies, as well as studies of clinic-referred series, are needed to clarify the conditions under which potential sleep disorders should be assessed fully.

The most parsimonious conclusion from this mixed literature is that multiple types of associations between sleep problems and ADHD may be occurring. Sleep problems may be a complicating side effect of ADHD in many cases; may be a second symptom of a neuropsychological dysfunction that is causing ADHD and sleep disorder together in other cases; and may be a contributing causal factor in still other cases (though probably only a small minority).

Studies are needed that evaluate representative population-based samples, and that link sleep disturbance with neuropsychological performance on measures of arousal and activation in children with and without ADHD. For example, Gruber and Sadeh (2004) assessed sleep for five nights via actigraph (a small wrist-watch-like movement detector worn on the arms or legs). They found that sleep disturbance was associated with worse performance on a neurocognitive battery for nondisordered control children, but not for children with ADHD. They concluded that sleep and ADHD are distinct pathways to neurocognitive impairment. Johnstone, Tardif, Barry, and Sands (2001) found that the excess EEG slow-wave activity typically seen in samples with ADHD was reversed (i.e., there was more "normalized" fast-wave activity) after sleep problems were treated. These were both small, preliminary studies, and they underscore the fact that research in this direction will not prove to be straightforward. Yet more evaluation of this type of linkage may well be quite informative.

In all, more systematic investigation of the role sleep may play in the neuropsychological findings of low alertness/arousal in ADHD appears warranted under a high-risk/high-payoff strategy. Too few studies have examined whether specific neuropsychological findings may be related to a subgroup of children with either poor sleep hygiene or a genuine sleep or movement disorder. Such studies might enable improved empirically sound clinical guidelines for routine screening of treatable sleep conditions in children with ADHD.

CLINICAL IMPLICATIONS

The apparent problems in paying attention that we see in children with ADHD are probably not "attention" problems per se (i.e., problems with automatical filtering and selection, or with automatic visual orientation to relevant information). Rather, they are related to a state of low alertness—of inability to mobilize mental resources quickly. In some children, this may reflect a state of low cortical arousal, which makes it difficult for the children to control or mobilize their resources. One way to think about this, which is sometimes helpful to parents and teachers, is to think about what it is like when we are very tired. At those times, our reaction time is slow; we are not very alert; it is difficult to pay attention to nonstimulating information; and we may speak impulsively. A child with ADHD may sometimes experience the world in the same way. In fact, sleep problems may be an important diagnostic rule-out in ADHD if other signs of poor sleep quality are noted during clinical evaluation.

A clinician can use findings of low alertness/arousal to help parents recognize that some of their child's difficulties may not be willful. Furthermore, this perspective is helpful in getting parents to understand that the child's ability to pay extended attention to a video game, television, or music concert does not counter an ADHD diagnosis in itself. In fact, being able to pay attention only when something really interesting, stimulating, or rapidly changing is going on would be consistent with a *less alert* child—and quite consistent with an ADHD diagnosis.

With regard to assessment, the differential findings in the auditory versus visual modalities in many studies with ADHD may indicate the value of assessing vigilance functions (e.g., via a CPT) in both the auditory and visual modalities. One instrument that makes it possible to do this is the Tests of Variables of Attention (TOVA; Greenberg & Waldman, 1993; see www.tovatest.com for more information), which provides CPTs in both auditory and visual modes lasting about 22 minutes apiece, plus instructions and practice. Although difficult for children to sit through, these tasks can yield clear information on vigilance performance. The TOVA includes normative data and provides a score for *d*-prime, as well as an "ADHD Index" (a combination of response speed and signal detection that has some degree of sensitivity and specificity for ADHD). Other commercial CPTs can also serve this function and yield similar scores. These include the Conners Continuous Performance Test II (for age 6 and above), which provides signal detection parameters (Conners & Jeff, 1999; see www.devdis.com/conners2.html), and the Gordon Diagnostic System (for ages 4–16), which is accompanied by its own machine to avoid potential problems with differential reaction times on different computer equipment (Gordon, 1991; for an overview of diagnostic and predictive validity of these tasks, see Nichols & Waschbusch, 2004).

Although these tasks and their suggested diagnostic cutoff points (such as the TOVA ADHD Index score) can contribute valuable empirical grounding to an evaluation, clinicians must take care not to place excessive reliance on such cutoff points in making a diagnosis of ADHD. For one thing, the sensitivity and specificity of these scores are far from perfect. In particular, many children with ADHD obtain average scores on these tests. For another thing, cutoff point accuracies will vary heavily with the base rate of ADHD in the setting in which the clinician is working. In other words, if the base rate of ADHD is low (e.g., one is screening a child in a school setting), positive predictive power will also be low. Tests can only improve partially on base rate or "chance" prediction of a disorder. On the other hand, in clinic settings where the base rate of ADHD may be 30% or higher, a positive score on a CPT may yield greater confidence that a child would meet consensus ADHD criteria. Yet in those settings, children with other forms of psychopathology (e.g., learning disorders) may also be expected to have an increased chance of problems on these tasks. In all, because performance of these instruments at varying base rates are not reported in their manuals, clinicians must use caution in weighing scores on these tests during diagnostic decision making.

A clinician can also consider assessing auditory and visual processing in relation to focused attention or working memory, using a test such as the Wide Range Assessment of Memory and Learning. If a problem is apparent only in the auditory modality, a fresh audiology examination or a referral for such an exam may be indicated, to make sure that hearing is unimpaired. Evaluation by a qualified audiologist for central auditory processing disorder may be of interest in designing ecological interventions (e.g., without distracting noise), despite significant concerns about the construct validity of this disorder.

When neuropsychological evaluation shows a low-arousal pattern (e.g., slow and variable reaction times, poor vigilance on a CPT, low alertness on interview and observation), additional scrutiny should be given to the possibility of a sleep problem. Referral for additional sleep evaluation or counseling for sleep hygiene may be important in some cases. In all cases, clinicians would be well advised to evaluate sleep hygiene and conduct routine screening for evidence of inadequate sleep (e.g., daytime sleepiness) that might warrant further evaluation (Marcotte et al., 1998). When a sleep disorder is found, its remediation may sometimes lead to improvement in the ADHD; however, the frequency of such improvement is unclear. In many cases, ADHD will coexist with a sleep problem, but the ADHD may persist even if the sleep problem is addressed. Nonetheless, identifying and treating sleep problems in children with ADHD are to the children's advantage. As for concerns that stimulant medications for ADHD disrupt sleep, data have not tended to support this concern (O'Brien et al., 2003) or have been inconclusive (for a review, see Kociancic, Reed, & Findling, 2004). Sleep disturbance that seems to be linked to medication use must be evaluated on a case-by-case basis, but the possibility of such disturbance is not necessarily a reason to avoid stimulant treatment.

The perspective that ADHD involves problems with vigilance can also be helpful with regard to intervention. For example, in cases for which medication appears to be an appropriate course of action, thinking of medication as "waking up" the underaroused cortical system—in much the same way as one might wake up a sleepy driver of a car (the "car" is the rest of the body and mind's control systems)—provides a simple heuristic by which a child and his or her parents can understand how the medication is supposed to help the child pay attention. Indeed, one reason why stimulant medication helps an apparently *over* stimulated child may be that the child's brain is actually *under*-stimulated. Waking it up with stimulant medication can help the child regain behavioral control.

Beyond that heuristic, designing behavioral interventions can be focused more usefully in some instances if one thinks not about the issue of *attention* (filtering), but the issue of *alertness*. How can the child be kept alert and engaged? This line of thinking gives rise to various ideas about interventions that involve relatively more frequent changes in activity, changes in materials, more brightly colored materials, and so on.

One of the paradoxical issues to emerge from this line of thinking concerns whether a child's environment should be *less* stimulating or *more* stimulating. For some children with ADHD, removing distractions may be important; for instance, they may do best taking an exam in the hallway instead of in the classroom. In other instances, more stimulation may be needed—turning up the lights, changing materials to those with engaging colors, or even having more background noise, such as music. Behavioral interventions may benefit from experimentation on the dimension of "degree of stimulation" in different environments and activities.

TABLE 4.2. Frequently Asked Questions about ADHD and Attention

Question	Answer
Why do *stimulants* calm my overactive child?	The underaroused control centers of the brain may benefit from the action of the stimulants.
Why isn't my child distracted during video games?	ADHD isn't due to problems filtering, but to problems with staying alert; video games are very stimulating, making it easy to stay alert.
Should a child with ADHD work in an isolated room?	In some instances this might help; some children benefit from more stimulation, others from less.
Why was my child given a boring computer test?	This is how we test for vigilance—one possible functional problem in ADHD.
Can a CPT diagnose ADHD?	No. It is just one indicator; accuracy depends on base rates of ADHD in the local setting.
Can ADHD be caused by a sleep disorder?	A sleep disorder can mimic ADHD. If sleep problems are suspected, the clinician needs to rule out a sleep disorder.

Moreover, less "mainstream" interventions come to mind readily from the viewpoint of a problem in alertness or vigilance. For example, the roles that a better diet, more exercise (for a review of exercise and ADHD, see Wigal et al., 2003), and sound sleep habits may play are all underscored. It is important for the clinician to ask about and evaluate "alertness hygiene" questions, and to advise parents and children accordingly. Occasionally, behavioral planning and therapeutic planning may have to emphasize restoring these important foundations of alert functioning. For example, a child who stays up after his or her parents are in bed, watching television until all hours, may benefit from adjustment of this daily lifestyle habit in addition to standard treatment.

Table 4.2 summarizes frequently asked questions about ADHD and attention that clinicians are sometimes obliged to try to answer.

NONEXECUTIVE ATTENTION IN ADHD: SUMMARY

Overall, the role of attention deficits in ADHD is one domain where we can say there has been substantial progress in our understanding. Of four distinct processes supported by two distinct neural networks, three are largely ruled out as major contributors to ADHD-C. With regard to the posterior attention network, there is very little evidence to suggest that either visual orienting or visual selection is involved in ADHD-C. The picture remains less clear for auditory selection, perhaps due to frequent inclusion of children with auditory processing problems in samples with ADHD. On the whole, support has failed to emerge for problems in the posterior component operations of engaging or moving; is minimal and probably not present for the disengaging process; and has not emerged for the early perceptual selection (high-load) process in the posterior attention network in ADHD-C.

Within the vigilance system, the sustained attention function appears to be largely intact (declines in focus over time are average in most situations for children with ADHD). Although deficits in sustained attention do appear at slow event rates (e.g., very understimulating situations), these appear to be best understood in relation to energetic factors (the ability to mobilize resources, discussed in Chapter 5 and by van der Meere, 2002), rather than to a primary attention problem. Thus, when attention is defined in these terms, there is no "attention deficit" in ADHD-C. Recent data, using newer models and better experimental probes of the selection system, have supported earlier studies on this point.

As for ADHD-PI, the suggestion that it may be associated with a posterior network dysfunction has not received sufficient investigation to allow firm conclusions. However, the data to this point do not appear to provide strong support for that hypothesis. Further investigation of children with sluggish cognitive tempo (a subset of those with ADHD-PI) may clarify matters here.

On the other hand, concerns that children with ADHD may fail to detect or process information from early in the processing stream

TABLE 4.3. Summary of Attention Functions in ADHD: Score Card to This Point

System/function	ADHD-C	ADHD-PI
Vigilance system		
Sustained attention	Intact	Intact?
Alerting/arousal	Affected	Affected
Posterior attention system		
Covert visual-orienting	Intact	Intact?
Early visual perceptual selection	Intact	Intact?
Early auditory selection	?	?

remain; those observations are probably explained by the substantial evidence supporting atypical functioning of the alerting process in the vigilance network in ADHD-C. This function may also be disturbed in ADHD-PI (Nigg et al., 2002b).

Table 4.3 summarizes the state of knowledge about these attentional systems in samples of children with ADHD. The bottom line is that only one of these functions appears to be involved in ADHD: alerting or (phasic, cortical) arousal. More research on auditory processing, and ADHD-PI, will clearly be helpful to the field.

| CHAPTER 5 |

Executive Functioning
or Cognitive Control

The functions to be discussed in this chapter are those that involve deliberate control of behavior, thought, or emotion. Such control is goal-directed and effortful, in that it requires mental resources. For adults, executive functions are invoked for situations and tasks that range from relatively routine (e.g., following a difficult recipe) to astonishingly complex (e.g., planning a company's growth strategy, organizing a NASA launch, or chairing a meeting of the local psychology or medical faculty). For children, depending on their age, common situations in which they must utilize executive functions include paying attention in class, even though other kids can be heard playing outside at recess; studying first and playing afterwards; playing their role on a team sport or acting in a play; waiting their turn for something to happen; keeping track of their homework on the way home from school; or forgoing an immediate treat for the sake of an impending dinner. Very young children may be observed to turn their eyes away from a forbidden candy or sing a song to keep their minds off a tempting but forbidden toy. These abilities thus emerge in rudimentary form in the toddler years, undergo significant development in the early school years (ages 4–7 or so), and then continue to develop throughout childhood and adolescence and into early adulthood.

When parents ask, "Why does my child with ADHD always lose his homework?", "Why does her desk look like a tornado hit it?", or "Why does he seem to approach homework at random?", they are asking whether the problem may be faulty executive functioning. Note that the term "executive functioning," though still used by clinicians, has begun to be replaced in the research literature by "cognitive control." I use the two terms interchangeably, despite slightly different connotations among specialists.

Whether viewed as "executive functioning" or as "cognitive control," this domain is not a single function, but entails multiple component functions. Indeed, without component functions we are left with a rather uninformative global concept, as if a miniature person inside each of us handles these abilities (the well-known philosophical problem of the "homunculus"). What are these component functions? There is no agreement on this point, and extensive discussions continue in the literature on the cognitive neuroscience of executive processes (Monsell & Driver, 1998), as well as in a rather distinct literature examining early development of these processes (Dempster, 1993; Harnishfeger, 1995; Rothbart & Bates, 1998; Zelazo, Muller, Frye, & Marcovitch, 2003; see Barkley, 1997, and Casey et al., 2002, for reviews).

Yet some structuring of possible components is needed in order to analyze the ADHD literature. Despite the intuitive nature of the concept and its venerable history of clinical utility in neuropsychology, it is widely agreed that the term "executive functioning" is insufficiently specified for formal analysis via neuroimaging or for the isolation of biological mechanisms that might be involved in the development of behavioral problems in children (Monsell & Driver, 1998; Pennington & Ozonoff, 1996; Zelazo et al., 2003). Factor analyses of batteries of executive function measures suggest that the domain is multicomponential (Barkley, Edwards, Laneri, Fletcher, & Metevia, 2001a; Robins & Rogers, 1998; Miyake, Friedman, Emerson, Witzki, & Howerter, 2000; Willcutt et al., 2005a).

A further difficulty has been related to conflating the idea of executive functions with that of "frontal" brain operations. As should be clear from earlier chapters, although prefrontal cortical regions are closely involved in many if not all executive operations, executive functions also depend heavily on structures in the basal ganglia, the thalamus, and (probably in at least some respects) the cerebellum. Indeed, some functions traditionally thought to rely on the prefrontal cortices, such as stopping a motor behavior (response inhibition), may instead be primarily supported by the subcortical ends of the neural loops (Kimberg & Farah, 1998).

Thus a contemporary conceptual neural basis for parsing cognitive control operations has been a series of parallel prefrontal–

subcortical neural loops, as described in Chapter 3. These loops, with modulation by cerebellar–cortical–basal ganglia loops, support the various component operations necessary for executive functioning. As outlined elsewhere (Nigg & Casey, 2005), one question at present concerns the exact nature of the interplay between (1) the cerebellar-frontal loops, which may detect violations in *when* something has occurred relative to expectations (as in a child's failing to gauge when the class will quiet down after the bell, thinking that a longer "grace period" will ensue, and clowning around beyond the time window of the teacher's tolerance); and (2) the thalamic–cortical loops, which may detect violations in *what* has occurred relative to expectations (as in the same child's failing to notice that children are not laughing at his or her joke as expected, thus again clowning excessively and disrupting the class). However, prefrontal regions are clearly important for some if not all of the component operations to be described next.

I adopt an organizational scheme for the components of executive functioning that borrows from (1) the neuropsychological account of Pennington (e.g., Pennington & Ozonoff, 1996); (2) the attentional account of Posner & Petersen (1990), noted in Chapter 4; and (3) the cognitive control model advocated by Casey et al. (2002) and others. The present scheme is designed to be "mapped onto" various approaches to executive functioning, so specialist readers can work from this account to their model of choice (for various models, see Barkley, 1997; Casey et al., 2002; Fuster, 1997; Lyon & Krasnegor, 1996; Monsell & Driver, 1998; Pennington & Ozonoff, 1996; Zelazo et al., 2003). Book-length treatments testify to the domain's complexity and the diversity of approaches available (Lyon & Krasnegor, 1996).

ORGANIZING THE COMPONENT FUNCTIONS OF COGNITIVE CONTROL

In parsing the executive domain, most experts agree on some initial generalizations. Most accounts include a role for "working memory" (variously defined, but emphasizing the ability to hold a goal or relevant information in mind, perhaps despite interference), which implies the converse ability to keep interfering information *out* of working memory and *out* of the set of response options (sometimes viewed as a distinct function). Most also include the ability to withhold or suppress prepared responses that become incompatible with the goal when the context changes dynamically, variously termed "response suppression" or "response inhibition." That function is emphasized in several theories of ADHD (Barkley, 1997; Schachar, Tannock, & Logan, 1993), although the terminology is in dispute as the inhibition metaphor's limits are realized.

Several theories of executive functioning (often presented as theories of frontal cortical functioning) exist. Norman and Shallice (1986) posit a supervisory attention system that presumably incorporates multiple operations. Others (Pennington, 1997; Willcutt et al., 2000b) provide a heuristic framework that includes working memory, inference control, set shifting/task switching, response inhibition, and planning. Fuster (1997) has argued that the hallmark of frontal cortical functioning is the temporal organization of complex behavior; as for components, he has emphasized working memory, "set" (motor attention), and inhibitory control (including suppression of competing information as well as no-longer-apt primary responses). In his influential theory of ADHD, Barkley (1997) has followed Fuster in emphasizing temporal organization, and for components offers very broad constructs that entail nearly all of self-regulation, including response inhibition, working memory, regulation of arousal–affect–motivation, internalization of speech, and reconstitution. Zelazo et al. (2003) emphasize a problem-solving model in which the key operations are problem representation followed by execution and evaluation.

Many of these theories attempt to specify primary functions and then subsidiary abilities that derive from these. Because those efforts remain speculative, I do not attempt a hierarchy of functions here. To organize findings about ADHD, it is useful to recognize further subcomponents within the working memory concept, as well as several commonly cited control operations. I therefore begin by dividing the executive domain into the two related but conceptually distinguishable areas of control and working memory (to which I later add activation). These can be simplified to enable correspondence to other models, such as the model of Pennington (1997) or Fuster (1997).

Control

Despite important differences, different theorists parse the area of control in roughly parallel ways. First, most theorists recognize a function that consists of filtering competing information to maintain task response. This function is for our purposes essentially equivalent to cognitive attentional selection, as described (though not discussed) in Chapter 4 (Lavie, 1995; Mirsky & Duncan, 2001). It is the ability to identify and resolve interfering information. Second, there are differing but related descriptions of the ability to suppress from working memory previously relevant information that is no longer relevant (Barkley, 1997; Harnishfeger, 1995; Casey et al., 2002). This can include the ability to put unwanted thoughts out of mind—an ability that seems to be impaired or overwhelmed in some anxiety disorders, such as obsessive–compulsive disorder and posttraumatic stress disorder (PTSD). Research to date on ADHD, however, has not effectively separated interference control from cognitive control or cognitive suppression (selective attention at the executive level). I therefore review these abilities together later for simplicity. Very little research has examined cognitive suppression (i.e., thought suppression) in ADHD.

Third, all theorists identify a function of suppressing, interrupting, or canceling a prepared motor response, either to accommodate new information coming online or to support a later goal. I have referred to this as "executive inhibition" (Nigg, 2001); Barkley (1997) has referred to it as "response inhibition." A more contemporary term might be "response suppression" or "response cancellation" (MacLeod, Dodd, Sheard, Wilson, & Bibo, 2003). However, there is broad agreement that the ability to stop a previously prepared response is a key component operation.

As an aside, it should be noted that the term "inhibition" has sparked controversy in academic circles of late. One issue is that whereas neural systems include inhibitory and excitatory connections, these are concrete, low-level electrochemical interchanges in the synapses of the brain and nervous system. At times, discussion of inhibitory processes in cognitive or behavioral terms seems to conflate the levels of analysis and to mix up neural inhibitory systems with inhibition of a behavior. Second, considerable discussion has ensued as to whether (1) cognitive interference control and (2) motor suppression truly entail inhibition or suppression of information, or simply the differential activation of competing streams of information (MacLeod et al., 2003). Computational models of many *cognitive* tasks indicate that human performance can be replicated by relying only on signal decay (withdrawal or cessation of the activation process that supports a response or a cognition). Thus whether "inhibition" is active, or simply passive decay, remains a key dispute for many but not all measurement tasks—in particular, those that emphasize cognitive processes (rather than motor output control). For other tasks that seek to assess the interruption of a prepotent motor response, this specific critique is less pertinent.

Crucially, some commentators have been less careful than MacLeod et al. (2003), resulting in misguided dismissal of a possible inhibition construct. In fact, important evidence supports the operation of such a mechanism. With regard to cognitive suppression, key performance paradigms supported by neural activation data (fMRI) provide powerful and so far unrefuted support for a distinct strategic suppression mechanism (Anderson, 2003; Anderson & Green, 2001; Anderson et al., 2004). With regard to response suppression, the existence of an inhibitory mechanism that suppresses a motor response is supported on at least two grounds. Animal neuroscience data show that (1) distinct brain regions are involved in executing versus withholding both attention and response (Baxter, Bucci, Holland, & Gallagher, 1999; Chiba, Bucci, Holland, & Gallagher, 1995); and (2) via single-electrode recording studies, specific inhibitory activity apparently functions centrally during a stop task (Hanes, Patterson, & Schall, 1998; Hanes & Schall, 1995). I therefore continue to refer to "response inhibition" or "response suppression" interchangeably, while recognizing that more data are needed to confirm whether a separate inhibitory mechanism is operating for many tasks used in human studies.

Poor response inhibition is often viewed as congruent with impulsivity and overactivity. Data as to the correctness of this assumption remain mixed (Logan, Schachar, & Tannock, 1997; Nigg et al., 2005a; Rodriguez-Fornells, Lorenzo-Seva, & Andres-Pueyo, 2002). It may be better viewed as a microprocess that helps keep behavior oriented toward the goal from moment to moment—and thus is at least as important for inattention/disorganization as for impulsivity per se. This ability is schematized in the baseball batter's "checked swing" when the ball suddenly breaks wide of the plate (Logan, 1994). Presumably, as real-world contexts evolve continually, we are continually "checking" behavior that might be cued by a given situation. Consider a teacher's control of impulsive responding in this classroom situation: One student walks into the classroom wearing a funny-colored sweater; another has an odd facial expression; a random joke pops into the teacher's mind; and in the meantime a rude student interrupts the conversation the instructor is having with still another pupil. In that 3-second interval, the instructor may have to suppress a handful of behaviors that "pop up" as potential responses, modifying actual responses in the process. Consider, alternatively, this situation in which a child must maintain organized, sequential (executive) behavioral control: In keeping her materials organized for school, Mary must allow some behaviors into action ("Put the pencil in the bag; make sure the homework is in there; throw in a fun comic book for the bus ride; zip the bag; remember to finish all this in time for my favorite TV show"), while controlling others ("Don't turn the TV on yet; don't put the bag in the closet where it may be forgotten in the morning; don't zip the bag up before checking its contents; don't answer the phone just now, because I don't want to miss my TV show"). Thus response suppression continually supports on-task, goal-directed behavior in dynamic fashion (Logan, 1994).

Note an important qualification here. Behavior can be suppressed for strategic reasons (I do not interrupt a speaker because I made a New Year's resolution to let people finish their sentences), or for reasons of anxiety (e.g., I do not interrupt a speaker because his or her angry tone makes me anxious, and I am afraid the person might turn on me). This second, *reactive* control of behavior is, in my formulation, crucially distinct from strategic control. Many research papers and theories of ADHD and inhibition fail to make this important distinction (Nigg, 2000, 2001), but it is crucial to making sense of pathways to ADHD. I therefore address reactive or motivated inhibition in the chapter on motivation (Chapter 6). In this chapter, I address strategic, "top-down" behavioral suppression.

Additional distinctions have been suggested in relation to control. Barkley (1997) has argued that the ability to delay a response is a key function that is distinct from interrupting a response. This distinction has some merit, as I note later, but for simplicity I cover delay (withholding all responses) along with interruption (suppressing a prepared response when new information appears).

Furthermore, the ability to shift response set, or to alternate response set, is often regarded as an ability distinct from response suppression (Mirsky & Duncan, 2001; Pennington, 1997). In suppression (inhibition), one merely has to stop a response. But in shifting, one has to activate another response simultaneously, so a total "stop" process may or may not be useful in a rapid-shift context. Distinguishing this ability is of value to our discussion, because shifting, especially in a rapid-shift context, likely involves additional demands on cerebellar circuitry in the brain (Berger et al., 2005).

Other components can also be suggested in a more detailed description of control operations from a neuroscience perspective (Monsell & Driver, 1998). However, the literature on ADHD is not sufficiently differentiated to render a more molecular model of these operations useful as yet. For our purposes, the basic heuristic set of abilities described here enables a meaningful organization of the ADHD literature. The basic breakdown of control is therefore as follows: (1) mental control, including interference control and cognitive suppression; (2) output control or response inhibition, including interrupting a prepotent response and withholding all responses; and (3) set shifting or response selection.

Working Memory

To keep something in mind while doing something else (e.g., remembering a phone number while searching for the phone, remembering a class assignment while talking to a friend) requires working memory. A problem in working memory could explain why children with ADHD so easily get thrown off track by new events, preventing them from completing their planned activities (e.g., abandoning homework in the middle because the phone rings, then forgetting to go back to it), because working memory involves protecting task information.

As is the case with control, several detailed conceptual models of working memory exist, and these differ in important ways (Baddeley & Hitch, 1994; Baddeley & Logie, 1999; Cowan, 1988, 1995, 1999; Engle, Kane, & Touholski, 1999; Hasher & Zacks, 1998; Kane & Engle, 2002). However, several themes are shared among these theories. Working memory is a limited-capacity ability closely related to executive attentional selection (which has been described in Chapter 4; Engle, 2002; Kane & Engle, 2002). Working memory, however, includes the ability to maintain an amount of information online and to activate some information or plans over others (it is thus closely related to mental control processes; Kimberg & Farah, 1998). This ability to maintain information in an active state differentiates working memory from interference control; even though working memory depends on interference control, it involves additional demands. This distinction is crucial for assessing the ADHD literature, as I show later.

Most models of working memory distinguish the ability to control or manipulate information (here, "working" memory) from passive storage (here, "short-term memory"; Baddeley & Hitch, 1994; Engle et al., 1999). Short-term memory is the ability to remember something passively and briefly. For example, in a digit span test, the child is asked to repeat a list of numbers right after hearing the list. Working memory, in contrast, includes storage and processing or manipulation of the information; it is the executive aspect of the system (Kane & Engle, 2002). For example, in a reading span test, the child reads a series of sentences while trying to remember the last word in each sentence. Mental arithmetic requires working memory; so does remembering a shopping list while talking with an acquaintance at the store. In these examples, information is either manipulated in the storage area, or held there while other information is entertained.

Many models also parse the storage area into distinct units, such as verbal and spatial. The central or control element may be nonunitary as well. For example, Baddeley and Hitch (1994) call the control element a "central executive," and identify two passive storage "scratch pads": one for verbal working memory (a "phonological loop") and one for visual–spatial working memory (the latter, in some renditions, is divided further into a module for object shape and a module for object location, as well as a module for events; Baddeley, 2001). These domain-specific storage modules or short-term memory modules, however, are integrated with the executive ability; this results in active working memory loops that are partially differentiated by content domain.

Neurally, the storage (short-term memory) modules are distributed in the brain depending on what type of information is being stored (e.g., whether it is something retrieved from long-term memory or new information just received, whether it is spatial or linguistic in form, etc.). Thus short-term storage may involve parietal cortical regions, as well as other cortical and subcortical regions (Baddeley & Logie, 1999; Cowan, 1999; Jonides, Lacey, & Nee, 2005; Smith & Jonides, 1997). In contrast, the ability to manipulate stored information and protect it from interference involves prefrontal cortical regions, especially the dorsolateral prefrontal cortex (Kane & Engle, 2002).

Figure 5.1 illustrates the cortical circuitry of working memory according to the Baddeley and Hitch model, for two major functions: (1) verbal working memory (the phonological loop, including left dorsolateral prefrontal cortex, Broca's area, and Wernicke's area) and (2) spatial working memory (left prefrontal and visual cortices).

Neuropsychologists often add another ability to the working memory domain, called "planning" (Pennington & Ozonoff, 1996). Planning is the ability to mentally organize a series of steps in temporal sequence in order to solve a complex problem. Playing high-level chess, for example, requires extensive planning. So does carrying out a complex recipe. Planning clearly requires working memory, but it probably involves functions such as reasoning and attentional and response selection as well, so the neural circuitry may be more diffuse. Because

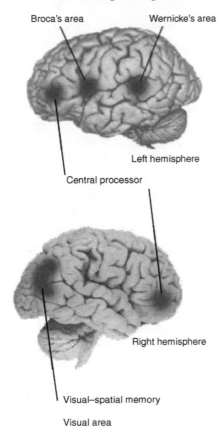

FIGURE 5.1. Brain regions in working memory. Courtesy of www.thebrain. mcgill.ca, a project of Bruno Dubuc and the Institute of Neurosciences, Mental Health and Addiction of Canada.

findings for studies of planning are somewhat different from those for working memory in ADHD, it is useful for us to make a distinction between these related abilities.

Activation

In order to respond effectively to a situation, a child must mobilize complex motor programs and hold this response readiness in an appropriate state of activation. For example, when Tommy is playing baseball and waiting at bat, he must be prepared to swing vigorously, but not until the right moment. Too much activation, and he will either swing too soon or too often; not enough activation, and he will swing too late or too seldom. According to Pribram and McGuinness (1975), activation is theorized to involve a neurally left-lateralized process supported by dopaminergic neurons, involving motor preparation for response output.[1] Consistent with the shared traditions in cognitive science, the activation system proposed by Pribram and McGuinness has also been related to attentional vigilance (e.g., Derryberry & Rothbart, 1997; Chapter 4). That similarity is readily apparent when we consider the example of Tommy at bat in a baseball game: He also has to be alert to every move of the pitcher, the catcher, and the ball.

But "activation" as defined by Tucker and Williamson (1984) places the specific emphasis on output preparation during a discrete response, rather than merely staying alert over a period of time during a task (Sergeant et al., 1999). They thus distinguish readiness to notice something (attention or vigilance) from readiness to respond (output or activation). In other words, this conception affords a broader consideration of relevant evidence, with an emphasis on motor preparation (output) rather than attention (input). Thus left-lateralized dopamine systems are theorized to be involved, rather than the right-lateralized noradrenergic system that is thought to support arousal and vigilance. For this reason, some view activation as an executive function (Berger & Posner, 2000), although others view it as subsidiary to executive functioning (Sergeant et al., 1999). I include it in this chapter for simplicity.

Synthesis

Although several components and subcomponents of cognitive control have been described above, sufficient data to enable evaluation of the state of knowledge about ADHD are not available for all of them. Thus I have shortened the list to conform to what data are available. Table 5.1 provides this simplified summary of the component operations that I consider in examining the reach of an executive functioning formulation of ADHD. In the table, I have reorganized the functions so that abilities related to mental control come first; abilities related to the intersection of mental and motor control come second (working memory); and abilities that control output response come last (response inhibition, set shifting, and activation). At an operational level, it is clear that we can measure the following operations. First, we can measure the ability to detect and prevent interference from goal-irrelevant information (interference control or late attentional selection); key neu-

TABLE 5.1. Useful Component Operations of Executive Functioning for ADHD Studies

Mental control: Attentional selection, interference control, thought suppression (anterior cingulate).

Working memory (holding information in mind and manipulating it; DLPFC).

  Verbal working memory: Short-term memory versus working memory (phonological loop).

  Visual–spatial working memory: Short-term memory versus working memory (visual–spatial loop).

  Planning.

Response suppression (suppression of a primary response on a cue; right inferior PFC, caudate).

Set shifting, response selection (PFC, possibly cerebellar loops in some tasks).

Activation (left-lateralized dopaminergic pathways).

Note. PFC, prefrontal cortex; DLPFC, dorsolateral prefrontal cortex; thought suppression is the same as cognitive inhibition; see text.

ral structures include the anterior cingulate for detecting response conflict, and the orbital prefrontal cortex and caudate for suppressing a response. Second, we can measure distinct elements of a working memory system, including a loop for holding and manipulating spatial information, and another loop for holding and manipulating verbal information. We can begin to ask to what extent ADHD is associated with deficits in specific short-term memory buffers versus deficits in the more truly executive working memory ability to manipulate information mentally.

Working memory is closely related to interference control and clearly depends on it. However, interference control may not require holding much information in mind. For example, on a Stroop task (see below), one must control interference but there is little need to manipulate information in mind, even though some working memory is probably likely involved (as pointed out by Kane & Engle, 2001). We can also measure the ability to put a thought out of mind that we do not want to think about (cognitive inhibition), in order to think about something else (Harnishfeger, 1995; Zacks & Hasher, 1994). This ability also supports working memory or is even inseparable from it (Zacks & Hasher, 1994).

To continue with control abilities, we can also measure the ability to suppress a primary response that we now do not want to make (the "checked swing"). This can include the ability to deliberately suppress all responding, or to delay or wait. This function appears to depend upon the right inferior frontal gyrus in the frontal cortex and upon the caudate in the basal ganglia, among other structures. It is disrupted by damage to either structure (Aron et al., 2003a; Casey et al. 2002). I have highlighted that this response is deliberate, strategic, and effortful, but not motivated by sudden or high anxiety or fear; otherwise, it falls into the reactive or motivational inhibition domain described in Chapter 6.

Finally, we can consider shifting of response set—the ability to alternate a response set in a dynamic environment (Mirsky & Duncan, 2001). This ability is related to response inhibition, but also requires rapid response initiation (Logan, 1994). Because it is often tested with tasks that require shifting while holding a rule in mind, it clearly requires the prefrontal regions. However, in some instances it also requires timing of the alternation, which may entail cerebellar operations.

MAIN FINDINGS
FOR EACH EXECUTIVE FUNCTION IN ADHD

Late Selection/Interference Control
Is Not Well Established as an ADHD Deficit

A basic skill with which children with ADHD appear to struggle is strategically filtering irrelevant information in order to concentrate on a task, such as ignoring other children's talk in order to work on an assignment. This ability is formally defined in attention studies as either "late selection" or "interference control." When formally measured, it is unclear that this ability is really impaired in ADHD-C.[2] This mechanism is part of an anterior attention system, involving the anterior cingulate (Posner & DiGirolamo, 1998). One can distinguish interference that is perceptual (too many basic stimuli) from that which is cognitive (meaningful stimuli) or motor (a response that is triggered by a cue) (Casey et al., 2002). Most studies of ADHD assess response interference; a handful have isolated cognitive selection.

Most ADHD research has focused on response interference, as operationalized on the Stroop task (Table 5.2); at least 14 studies have used this procedure to examine children or adolescents with ADHD. Note that considerable discussion continues as to the mechanisms involved in the Stroop task (MacLeod, 1991). One influential account notes that the Stroop involves both working memory (or goal maintenance) and conflict detection/control (Kane & Engle, 2001). Thus this task is not a pure measure of interference control independent of working memory. However, it isolates intereference control better than most

TABLE 5.2. Key Laboratory Tasks Used to Assess Interference Control or Late Selection in ADHD

Task	Brief description
Stroop task	This classic task has two or three conditions, depending on the design. The usual control condition is to name aloud as fast as possible the ink color of rows of X's (e.g., XXXX printed in red, green, and blue ink). Speed on this task is compared to speed on the interference task. In the latter, a child must name as fast as possible the ink color of a sequence of words, each of which is a color word different from the color of the ink (e.g., the word "red" printed in blue ink, the word "blue" printed in green ink). Because reading the word is a faster, more automatic process than naming the color, nondisabled children and adults are slower to name the words in the interference condition; the extent of this slowing versus the control condition is taken as an index of interference control. A range of related stimulus incompatibility tasks tap interference control without reading.
Flanker task	A flanker task is a type of selective attention task that can be designed to require perceptual or cognitive suppression of competing information. It is similar to the Stroop task, except that information is spatially distinct. For example, a child views a target area in the center of a computer screen, with an instruction to press the corresponding key depending on whether the X or N appears in the center. Immediately adjacent to the center letter are two "flanking" distractor letters that are to be ignored. The flankers can be incompatible (X or N) or neutral (e.g., F or D). It takes longer to respond to XNX than to FNF, because in the first instance, the flanker is a possible response that must be suppressed.
Directed-forgetting task	This task assesses the ability to deliberately suppress interfering thoughts. In a typical design, a child learns a list of words. The child is then instructed to forget that list so that he or she can learn a new list. After the second list is learned, recall and recognition are tested for the first list. If recall is reduced but recognition is not, it is viewed as suppression.

measures do, and as we will see, it yields quite different results for ADHD from those yielded by measures of working memory proper.

The classic Stroop effect entails attempting to name the ink color of color words printed in colored ink. No cognitive interference occurs when one must name the color red if the row of X's is printed in red. No interference occurs, either, if the simply reads the word "red" printed in black ink. Facilitation of reaction time (faster responding) occurs when one tries to rapidly name the ink color if the word "red" is printed in red ink. *Interference*, marked by sizable slowing in reaction times, is experienced when people try to rapidly name the ink color if the word "blue" is printed in red ink. The slower naming times to name the colors in the latter condition, as opposed to naming the colored X's or reading the color words in black ink, is referred to as the "Stroop effect." A large experimental literature over the past 50 years has examined how this effect works and debated whether a "suppression" mechanism is involved (MacLeod, 1991). Several functional brain imaging studies have established that, at least in adults, performing the Stroop and related tasks (e.g., the flanker task) activates the anterior cingulate cortex (Cabeza & Nyberg, 1997), a frontal region associated with the frontal executive networks described earlier (Posner & DiGirolamo, 1998).

Although some reviewers have concluded that children with ADHD show a deficit in Stroop interference, it is not clear that the majority of Stroop studies of ADHD have detected an interference control problem rather than simply an overall problem in slow responding. That is, slow response in, say, naming the colors of ink of *non*words (e.g., a series of X's in different colors) could be due to weak arousal or activation, rather than to poor late selection (Nigg, 2001). To isolate interference control on the color-word-naming condition, one has to correct for basic naming speed. Often this correction has been omitted from published reports; speed has simply been reported on color-word naming, uncorrected for color- or word-naming speed (e.g., Boucugnani & Jones, 1989; Das, Snyder, & Mishra, 1992; Houghton et al., 1999; Miller, Kavcic, & Leslie, 1996). Those researchers who made an effort to control for response speed have often failed to find a true interference effect (Gorenstein, Mammato, & Sandy, 1989; Grodzinsky & Diamond, 1992; Leung & Connolly, 1996).

On the other hand, Gorenstein et al. (1989) did find such an effect even with appropriate controls for naming speed. Furthermore, two studies of young adolescents used the Stroop interference score (corrected for reading and naming speed) and found an ADHD deficit (Lufi, Cohen, & Parish-Plass, 1990; MacLeod & Prior, 1996), although only the latter study controlled for IQ. Overall, evidence for an ADHD interference control deficit on the traditional paper-and-pencil Stroop task, apart from slow naming speed, is weak and rests primarily on studies of adolescents.

If all studies that examined the intereference effect are pooled, the results are not impressive for the Stroop task. van Mourik, Oosterlaan, and Sergeant (2005) conducted a meta-analysis of all such studies; that is, they pooled the results of all available data in the literature. They arrived at a composite ADHD versus control effect size of $d = 0.20$ (a very small effect; see the "Effect Size" section of Chapter 3), with a p value indicating that this effect was not reliably different from zero. This effect is sufficiently small that it might be difficult to "see" outside the laboratory, and so its clinical significance is doubtful at best. In all, it appears that Stroop interference is not a robust effect in ADHD.

Yet a stronger ADHD interference control effect may be seen with newer methodologies that rely on more precise timing of response, using computers. The paper-and-pencil Stroop task, in which a child simply names or reads a list on a page, is susceptible to various strategy effects. The alternative is to use a computer to give interference and noninterference trials one at a time, either in random order or in a prespecified sequence. These computerized tasks may create more effective interference and may challenge the attention system more effectively.

Using such an alternative method, Bush et al. (1999) failed to find an ADHD performance deficit (in adults), but they did reported differential neural activation in the ADHD group during the task. The interpretation of this activation difference as a deficit is problematic, however, when performance is typical. Carter, Krener, Chaderjian, Northcutt, and Wolfe (1995) matched children with ADHD and controls by age and sex, and excluded children with CD, ODD, or anxiety disorders. They found an ADHD interference control deficit. Jonkman et al (1999) administered a flanker task (Table 5.2); they too found more interference in the group with ADHD. Again, IQ was not covaried, although performance was uncorrelated with IQ in this small sample. They also obtained peripheral physiological and central EEG measures. The physiological data supported the conclusion that the deficit was not due to differences in speed of executing a peripheral response (effects were related to central, not peripheral, recordings).

However, we (Huang-Pollock et al., 2005) failed to find any ADHD effect on a flanker-like selective attention paradigm in a well-characterized group of children with ADHD-C or ADHD-PI. In our study, the group with ADHD-C showed almost perfectly average interference control (those same children had significant problems on other executive measures). The group with ADHD-PI also had average interference control, but secondary analyses of a subgroup with sluggish cognitive tempo (McBurnett et al., 2001), suggested that they may have had atypical attentional mechanisms. The sample size of children with sluggish cognitive tempo was too small to enable clear conclusions, however.

In short, newer computerized paradigms to date have yielded mixed and inconclusive findings of an ADHD interference control deficit. It may have been that task difficulty varied across these studies, accounting for some variation in results. In particular, variation in working memory demands (see the next section) could have been a factor in some studies. Unfortunately, the number of these computerized studies is still small, so meta-analytic or pooled effect sizes are not yet meaningful. If an ADHD deficit exists in the interference control domain, it is probably either small or highly dependent on exactly the right measurement conditions, suggesting that it is not the most robust area of executive functioning difficulty in the disorder.[3]

Overall, support for an ADHD interference control problem is rather inconclusive when working memory demand is minimized. Clarification of the extent of interference control deficit in ADHD awaits additional replication of recent computerized flanker and Stroop studies, and clearer demonstration that effects are independent of IQ.

Working Memory Is Impaired in ADHD

As noted earlier, working memory is closely related to the anterior attention network and interference control (Kane & Engle, 2002), except that it involves the additional requirement of maintaining a body of information online and working with it mentally. When this executive ability is linked with domain-specific short-term memory functions, distinct neural circuits are identifiable for visual or spatial working memory and verbal working memory (the phonological loop; Baddeley & Hitch, 1994). Pennington and Ozonoff (1996) provided an authoritative review of studies up to that time. They concluded that ADHD is not associated with a deficit in verbal working memory. However, they noted a significant ADHD deficit in planning, as assessed by various tower tasks (Table 5.3). Measures of spatial working memory, as defined herein, were largely unstudied in ADHD at that time.

More recently, two meta-analyses followed up that review with a review of studies published since 1996 (Martinussen, Hayden, Hogg-Johnson, & Tannock, 2005; Willcutt et al., 2005b). Both meta-analyses took care to evaluate the adequacy of control of comorbid disorders (especially learning disabilities) in studies of working memory, as well as to evaluate IQ effects. The findings reported below therefore survive those considerations, and I rely heavily on these two meta-analytic studies here. At least 20 experimental studies have looked at working

TABLE 5.3. Key Laboratory Tasks Used to Assess Working Memory, Short-Term Memory, and Planning in ADHD

Task	Brief description
Tower task	Several tower tasks exist, including the Tower of London, the Tower of Hanoi, the Stockings of Cambridge, and others. The idea in all of them is that discs or balls must be moved around on pegs (either manually or on a computer screen) according to certain rules, in order to arrive at a predetermined arrangement. A tower task requires visualizing the moves in advance and can be designed to place heavy loads on visual working memory and sequencing. It is considered a measure of planning.
Spatial span task	A spatial span task will typically ask a child to remember the sequence of a series of shapes or locations. For example, the Finger-Windows test asks the child to touch a pencil to a series of locations in the correct order on a paper after seeing the locations touched by the examiner. Many variations exist, either on the computer or with paper and pencil. When the span must be remembered backward, it is considered to tap working memory as opposed to short-term memory.
Digit span test	Several similar tasks exist on versions of the Wechsler Intelligence Scale for Children, the Children's Memory Scale, the Kaufman Assessment Battery for Children, and others. In all of these, a child must repeat a series of numbers (or numbers and letters). When they are repeated backward, the task provides a greater likelihood of tapping working memory.
n-back task	The child sees a series of letters (or numbers) appear one at a time on the screen. He or she must continually repeat aloud the number that was "n-back" (e.g., 2-back). For example, a sequence may be A, X, D (child says "A"), M (child says "X"), B (child says "D"). Difficulty is increased by increasing the number back to recall. The task can be modified to require remembering auditory or spatial information.
Paced serial addition test (PASAT)	The child hears a series of numbers and must continually provide the sum of the last two numbers—for example, 4, 3 (child says "7"), 1 (child says "4"), 5 (child says "6").
Porteus mazes	The Porteus mazes constitute a measure of planning. The child uses a pencil to trace a line through a complex maze to find the target point. Failure to anticipate future turns in the maze results in a failure on that trial, lowering the overall score.
Complex figure	There are several complex figure tasks (Lezak, Howieson, & Loring, 2004), but the Rey–Osterrieth complex figure is most often used in studies of ADHD. A child views a complex design and must copy it; later, the child is asked to reproduce the drawing from memory. Planning is involved, in that a better drawing and better recall are thought to follow from first viewing and analyzing the overall structure than from taking a piecemeal approach.

memory in ADHD in recent years, and additional studies have looked at short-term memory and planning.

Verbal Working Memory

In the domain of verbal working memory, pooled effect sizes are modest for both short-term memory tasks (passive storage) and working memory proper (manipulation) in ADHD. We (Willcutt et al., 2005b) reported that five of nine published studies showing significant effects, with an average effect size of d = 0.54. Martinussen et al. (2005), using different criteria for study inclusion, identified 16 studies with an average effect size of d = 0.47 for short-term memory and d = 0.43 for working memory. These effects were reliably different from zero (i.e., some type of ADHD effect was found), but medium in size. These data suggest that verbal working memory may be affected in ADHD, but that the effect is not as large as on some other neuropsychological functions. Moreover, these effects appear to depend somewhat on the particular measure of verbal working memory used, and do not appear to be robust to covarying the influence of comorbid symptoms (McInness, Humphries, Hogg-Johnson, & Tannock, 2003; Sonuga-Barke, Dalen, & Remington, 2003). Thus verbal working memory deficits are neither large nor necessarily specific to ADHD, although in mild form they appear to be one common feature of the disorder. In short, these recent reports tend to confirm Pennington and Ozonoff's (1996) conclusion that verbal working memory is not a robust deficit in ADHD.

Spatial Working Memory

In contrast to the state of affairs 10 years ago, spatial working memory is now better studied. This newer, albeit smaller, literature suggests quite a different story from that for verbal working memory (e.g., Karatekin & Asarnow, 1998; McInness et al., 2003). We (Willcutt et al., 2005b) noted that five of six studies found significant group differences, with an average effect size of d = 0.72. Martinussen et al. (2005), identifying nine relevant studies, found a larger effect of d = 0.85 for spatial short-term memory. They identified eight relevant studies of spatial working memory and a pooled effect size of d = 1.06 (the largest effect in the literature for an ADHD neuropsychological weakness). Thus spatial working memory is a robust deficit in ADHD, but this conclusion is qualified by the finding that spatial short-term memory (not an executive function per se) is also weak and may be accounting for a substantial portion of this effect. A further caution in this finding is the relatively small number of studies. As we (Willcutt et al., 2005b) found in comparing our findings to those of Pennington and Ozonoff (1996) on several executive tasks, effect sizes tend to shrink as the pool of studies grows. Nonetheless, these initial data are quite striking with regard to the potential importance of spatial short-term and working memory in ADHD.

Planning

With regard to planning, Pennington and Ozonoff (1996) noted that ADHD was associated with large aggregate deficits on tasks such as the Tower of Hanoi and Tower of London (Table 5.3), with a pooled effect size of $d = 1.00$, but the number of studies was small. More recent work (Klorman et al., 1999; Nigg et al., 2002b) supports an ADHD deficit on these types of tasks, but effect sizes are not as large when more studies are weighed in. We (Willcutt et al., 2005b) followed this up, with consideration of 26 studies. Results varied depending on the measure used. The strongest effects emerged for the Tower of Hanoi, with four of six studies showing significant group effects, and a pooled effect size of $d = 0.69$. In contrast, the Tower of London showed significant ADHD effects in three of six studies, with a pooled effect size of $d = 0.51$. The Porteus mazes (which also require paper-and-pencil skill) showed a significant weakness in four of five studies, with a pooled effect size of $d = 0.59$. The Rey–Osterrieth complex figure (copy trial) showed effects in five of nine studies, for a pooled effect size of $d = 0.43$. Pooling across all four measures yielded an unweighted average effect size of $d = 0.56$. Once again, this effect is notable, but not as large as some other effects. If ADHD is related to a deficit in the central executive function of spatial working memory, deficits should be large on the spatial planning tasks. However, unreliability is a concern with the tower types of tasks, and both the Rey–Osterrieth figure and the Porteus mazes have particular difficulties as measures of executive functioning. Thus planning effects may not have been well assessed with these measures.

Findings for Working Memory: Summary

It is striking that findings for spatial working memory are much larger than findings for verbal working memory in ADHD. Yet spatial *short-term* memory is a weakness in ADHD, perhaps accounting for many of the spatial *working* memory findings. If the central executive component of working memory is a unitary function (which is unclear), then if it is impaired, we should see a similar magnitude of deficits in verbal and spatial working memory tasks. Yet the data so far fail to show that pattern; instead, verbal working memory is only mildly affected. Therefore, the role of spatial short-term memory in ADHD is an important confound to be clarified in this literature. At least three possible explanations for this state of affairs can be suggested.

The first is that mathematics disabilities or nonverbal learning disabilities (which may preferentially impair spatial processing and spatial short-term memory; Rourke et al., 2002) have been inadequately controlled for in the initial studies of ADHD. Preferential control of verbal learning disabilities (e.g., reading disorder or dyslexia) would dampen findings on verbal working memory (effects are smaller in ADHD when such learning disabilities are controlled for) more than for spatial working memory or short-term memory. It may be that when mathematics and/or nonverbal learning disabilities are also controlled for, the working memory deficit in ADHD will appear modest in size.

The second possibility is that various forms of task impurity exist. For example, spatial short-term memory tasks may contain more working memory (executive) elements than verbal tasks (Kane et al., 2004). Along the same lines, verbal working memory tasks used in many studies (e.g., backward digit span) may not have been sufficiently difficult. Working memory is likely to be better tested with a more difficult dual-task design, such as asking a child to remember a word or number while completing an intervening task. Such tasks might show that the verbal working memory problem in ADHD is larger than it now appears, confirming a problem in a domain- general executive component of working memory.

The third possibility is that the central executive element in working memory is not unitary, but that there are significant differential operations for maintaining and updating spatial versus verbal information. If so, the ADHD findings could contribute to clarifying this issue of cognitive architecture. Then a specific weakness in spatial working memory could shed light on ADHD's etiology, particularly for theories that focus on right-lateralized neural weakness in the disorder. Findings of low vigilance (Chapter 5), poor response inhibition (this chapter), and poor spatial working memory (this chapter) are all consistent with a somewhat right-lateralized neurological weakness.

In all, the research reviewed here suggests a significant ADHD weakness in working memory, particularly in spatial working memory and perhaps in planning, though the magnitude of these effects remain in need of further scrutiny. These findings, however, are promising and have sparked renewed interest in working memory as a potentially important mechanism in ADHD (Castellanos & Tannock, 2002).

Response Suppression Is Impaired in ADHD-C

The basic control function of quickly interrupting a behavior as the context changes is critical to self-regulation and so is a logical focus for ADHD (Barkley, 1997). For example, imagine that Katie is trying to earn extra privileges for the weekend and so needs to avoid getting in trouble at school. She may be about to make a wisecrack to her peers when the bell sounds or the teacher begins talking. To progress toward her goal, she has to suppress that prepared wisecrack in a quick-decision situation. Doing so thus is important both in the moment, and in keeping behavior on task in an ongoing way. I refer to this ability as "executive response suppression" or "executive response inhibition," to distinguish it from anxious inhibition of behavior (discussed in Chapter 6 as "behavioral inhibition"). It relies on structures in the prefrontal cortices and in the basal ganglia.

Three main types of experimental evidence converge on this question in ADHD (Table 5.4). The first type of experimental data came from studies using the basic go/no-go task (Trommer, Hoeppner, & Zecker, 1991; Table 5.4). This task establishes a dominant response set by making most trials go trials (e.g., "Press the response key when you see any capital letter"). The response must be withheld on the relatively rare no-go trials (lowercase letters). Extensive neural imaging data support the preferential involvement of inferior regions of dorsolateral prefrontal cortex on the no-go versus the go trials (Casey et al., 1997b; Konishi et al., 1999; Vaidya et al., 1998). EEGs and magnetoencephalograms (MEGs) also reveal preferential frontal activation on the no-go versus the go trials (Yong et al., 2000). Taken together, all of these imaging data support the notion that a separate, putatively inhibitory process is involved on the behavioral suppression required by the no-go trials, and that success at inhibiting on those trials depends on specific activation of prefrontal regions.

Meta-analyses indicate an ADHD response inhibition deficit on this task; that is, children with ADHD make excessive go errors on no-go trials (Barkley, 1997; Pennington & Ozonoff, 1996; Sergeant et al., 1999). In a particularly careful study that featured case matching, paired matched trials, MRI measurement of brain volume, and statistical control of age and IQ effects, errors on the inhibition trials were

TABLE 5.4. Key Laboratory Tasks Used in Studies of Response Inhibition in ADHD

Task	Brief description
Go/no-go	One must withhold response on rare no-go trials. In a typical version of the task, randomly alternating stimuli are presented (e.g., an A and a B, or two different visual designs). The child is instructed to respond to the A but not to the B. The A is presented more often, in order to create a response set or prepotency toward responding. Errors in response to the B are taken as an index of failed inhibitory control.
Stop task	The stop task presents equally probable stimuli (e.g., an X and an O) with the instruction to press a corresponding key as quickly as possible, depending on which letter appears; this creates a prepotent tendency to respond on most trials. On a minority of trials (typically 25%), a signal (e.g., a tone) indicates that the child is not to respond. Timing of the tone is varied to estimate the speed of the inhibition process (essentially, how much warning the child needs to interrupt the response), independently of the speed of the response output process. Physiological data indicate that a central (cognitive) process and a peripheral motor process are involved; responses can be interrupted even after peripheral nerves (on arm and hand muscles) have begun to fire (see Logan, 1994). To measure inhibitory ability, older versions of the task calculated stop signal reaction time (SSRT) as the slope or dropoff in inhibitory success at successively shorter warning intervals. Newer versions estimate SSRT (or warning time needed) more directly, using a dynamic tracking algorithm. The go trials of the task provide a measure of rapid decision-response time, and variability of those response times can also be analyzed in relation to response variability.
Antisaccade task	This is an ocular–motor task in which eye movements are monitored. On each trial, a signal appears in the visual periphery, creating a reflex response to move the eyes toward that signal. The reflex is difficult to resist. On some blocks of trials, children are told not to move their eyes toward the signal. Instead, they may be instructed to delay their response or to move their eyes away from the signal. Errors toward the signal, as well as presignal anticipations, are taken as indices of inhibitory ability or ability to suppress motor response.

associated with smaller size of structures in right prefrontal cortex and basal ganglia for boys with ADHD but not for nondisabled boys (Casey, Castellanos, Giedd, & Marsh, 1997a), implying that abnormality in these structures was related to performance deficits in ADHD. Vaidya et al. (1998) found that children with ADHD made more commission errors than did controls in two versions of the go/no-go task. The children with ADHD showed different patterns of neural activation with functional MRI than did the control children, but patterns of activation on this type of task still await consistent replication. However, the go/

no-go task has been criticized as not functionally isolating inhibition. That is, the failure to withhold a response on a no-go trial could be due to strong prepotent go processes, not to disinhibition (Schachar et al., 1993). A further problem is that this task requires selective attention and decision making; this confound has made isolation of the inhibition function via neuroimaging problematic (Rubia, Smith, Brammer, & Taylor, 2003).

As a result, interest has shifted to the stop task (Logan, 1994), which attempts to separate response output and inhibitory processes by varying the timing of the no-go warning (Table 5.5). It then estimates how much warning is needed in a fast (milliseconds) response context to interrupt a response that was about to be made. Mathematical modeling (Logan & Cowan, 1984) and peripheral physiological data (reviewed by Logan, 1994) support the idea that stop and go processes are isolated by the task. Likewise, functional MRI data indicate that the stop response (as opposed to the go response) involves the mesial prefrontal and inferior prefrontal cortex and the caudate—regions similar to those identified with the no-go trials of the go/no-go task (Rubia et al., 1999). Children with ADHD consistently show weak neural activation on the inhibition portion of this task in imaging studies (Pliszka, 2005).

Recall that it is important to differentiate response suppression due to anxiety (*reactive* response, covered in Chapter 6) from executive response suppression, which is primarily strategic (low anxiety involvement). Extant data support the idea that this task activates controlled responding, but not reactive, anxiety-driven response interruption.[4]

At this writing, at least 27 different samples (controlled for multiple publications from the same data set) have been collected around the world to compare children with ADHD to controls on this task, making it perhaps the best-studied experimental task in ADHD. The key measure is the speed of the stop process, or how much warning is needed in order to interrupt a response. That is, children are rapidly pressing the computer key to designate an X or an O on the screen, and must withhold the response (often "midstride," as they are about to press the key) when a warning tone sounds. The length of time given by the warning is varied, so that the amount of warning time needed to be able to stop becomes the main outcome measure.

These studies have yielded a sample-size-weighted effect size of $d = 0.61$ for this measure of needed warning time (called stop signal reaction time or SSRT; Willcutt et al., 2005b). This effect resulted in 22 of 27 studies reporting significant group effects. An ADHD deficit on this ability is thus extremely well replicated. Only 12 of these studies used DSM-IV criteria to look at ADHD-C; 10 of these 12 found significant effects, with an average effect size of $d = 0.61$ again (unweighted average, $d = 0.70$).

The first studies of DSM-IV-defined ADHD-C also used a more recent version of the task, controlled for IQ, had samples that included boys and girls, and controlled statistically for comorbid ODD and CD symptoms, confirming an ADHD stop inhibition deficit (Nigg, 1999; Schachar et al., 2000) with similar effect size. Although the use of an auditory stop tone in combination with a visual go stimulus has been one confound to this task, Rubia, Oosterlaan, Sergeant, Brandeis, and Leeuwen (1998) used two different versions of the stop task with a *visual* stop signal; youngsters with ADHD again showed consistent inhibitory weakness.

However, questions remain about whether the slow "interrupt" function in ADHD on the stop task is a side effect of overall sluggish or low-arousal responding to all stimuli, as I have discussed in Chapter 4. For example, one study used ERP responses and found a weak neural response to the warning tone, suggesting that the need for more warning in order to suppress a response could be due to problems in alerting to the stop signal (Brandeis et al., 1998). However, frontal processing components were atypical in children with ADHD in another ERP study of the stop task (Pliszka, Liotti, & Woldorff, 2000), consistent with an inhibitory interpretation. Likewise, in their comprehensive review of ERP studies, Barry et al. (2003b) concluded that there was evidence of response inhibition failure in ADHD, based on ERP measures of response to go/no-go tasks.[5]

A third type of experimental evidence derives from the ocular–motor antisaccade and delayed-saccade paradigms (Table 5.4). The basic task design is schematically illustrated in Figure 5.2. The "boxes" in the periphery are far enough out that a child must move his or her eyes in order to identify the target arrow. The task is for the child to resist the box's brightening and to move his or her eyes in the opposite direction. These stimuli appear and disappear very quickly, so that if the child moves his or her eyes toward the onset (row 2 of Figure 5.2), the arrow briefly appearing on the other side will be missed. This paradigm therefore requires participants to control reflexive eye movements (saccades) when targets appear in the periphery of their vision. This task also differs from the stop and go/no-go tasks, in that it probably places unique demands on a frontal region known as the frontal eye fields.

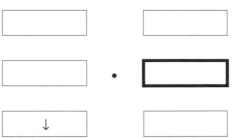

FIGURE 5.2. Schematic representation of the antisaccade task. Task instructions are to fixate eyes in center; ignore onset (row 2, right); identify arrow as pointing up or down.

However, support for the executive nature of this task comes from evidence that control is worsened by competing task demands, and that control on this task is impaired by anterior brain lesions, especially in orbital prefrontal cortex (Guitton, Buchtel, & Douglas, 1985). One might consider ability to suppress any response during a waiting period as a closely related mechanism, although it may show larger effects than seen for the ability to suppress response to the cue. Recall Barkley's (1997) suggestion that waiting or delaying a response may be an important, distinct ability.

Aman, Roberts, and Pennington (1998) found no differences between children with and without ADHD on an antisaccade task, but a floor effect was noted, in that even the control group had very high error rates on their difficult version of the task. Rothlind, Posner, and Schaughency (1991) also failed to find significant group differences on antisaccade errors. However, in a study of girls with ADHD, Castellanos et al. (2000) found deficits in ability to suppress the reflex response, but this effect was smaller than that observed for inability to suppress responses during the waiting period. The same pattern occurred in a study (Nigg, Butler, Huang-Pollock, & Henderson, 2002c) of an adult sample, the majority of which was female; the significant antisaccade error effect was nonsignificant after comorbid symptoms were covaried, but ability to suppress any response during a waiting period was deficient regardless of covariates.

Recent work in our lab (Carr, Nigg, & Henderson, 2005) replicates this last finding with a new, better-characterized, and much larger sample of adults with ADHD and control adults. Eye movements were monitored with an eye tracker. In this new sample, difficulty in suppressing the reflexive eye movement was apparent in the sample with

ADHD, consistent with a weakness in response inhibition. Again, response speed was slightly slower in the adults with ADHD, suggesting that they were exerting as much effort as the controls and were not adopting a "fast-guess" strategy.

Overall, evidence from the antisaccade task has been rather unequivocal with regard to ability to suppress all motor response during a delay period. All studies to date have found ADHD deficits in the ability to withhold all eye movements during the variable-delay waiting period between trials, and generally this effect has been more robust than that for antisaccade reflex errors (Munoz, Hampton, Moore, & Golding, 1999; Castellanos et al., 2000; Nigg et al., 2002c; Ross, Harris, Olincy, & Radant, 2000). Effects for suppressing reflexive eye movements have been less consistent, but nonetheless are generally supportive of a problem with response inhibition in ADHD-C.

Set Shifting Needs Further Study in ADHD

Although not featured in all cognitive neuroscience models, set shifting is regularly implicated in many neuropsychological tasks. Pennington and Ozonoff (1996) concluded that set shifting was impaired in ADHD, but the number of studies was relatively small. These findings have recently been updated (Willcutt et al., 2005b).

One classic neuropsychological measure of this concept is the Wisconsin Card Sort Test (WCST) perseverative errors score (Mirsky & Duncan, 2001; Miyake et al., 2000; see Table 5.5). The WCST requires children to adopt a response set (e.g., matching cards by color) and then to switch to a different response set (e.g., matching cards by shape). Perseverating on the initial response set is viewed as a weakness in set shifting. This measure, however, shows only modest and effects in ADHD. The recently reported meta-analytic effect size across 24 studies of ADHD was $d = 0.46$, with the majority of individual investigations failing to find a significant effect (Willcutt et al., 2005b). This effect was quite similar to that reported by Pennington and Ozonoff (1996). The largest WCST studies accordingly provide mixed results (Houghton et al., 1999; Klorman et al., 1999; Nigg et al., 2005a; Pineda, Ardelli, & Rosselli, 1999; Pineda et al., 1993; Willcutt et al., 2001).

However, as a measure of set shifting, the WCST is limited by heavy reliance on working memory (remembering which sets have been tried) and by a reliance on errors rather than reaction times (error scores are notoriously problematic in terms of psychometric properties; see Miller, Chapman, Chapman, & Collins, 1995). It thus

TABLE 5.5. Key Laboratory Tasks Used to Assess Set Shifting in ADHD

Task	Brief description
Trail Making Test	The Trail Making Test is from the Halstead–Reitan battery. In "Trails A," the child traces a line in order to a series of letters scattered randomly on the page (A, B, C, D, etc.). In "Trails B," the child must alternate letter–number–letter (thus tracing A, 1, B, 2, C, 3, etc.). The difference between B and A time is viewed as an index of set-shifting ability.
Wisconsin Card Sort Test (WCST) perseverative errors	The child must match a series of cards to a target card; cards include varying numbers of shapes, varying shapes, and varying colors. Thus the child must decide whether to sort by color, by number, or by shape. After 10 consecutive correct matches, the sorting rule changes, but the child is not told of the change. Thus the child must notice that the old rule is no longer working, determine the new rule, and again this continues for 10 correct matches, up to a total of six categories (in the full-length version). The test requires working memory, abstraction, and set shifting.
Switching task	Two sub tasks are learned, and a cue indicates which task is to be done on a given compute trial. For example, a blue screen may indicate that objects are to be counted; a red screen may indicate that they are to be named. Varying the proportion, speed, timing, and frequency of switches enables isolation of various component elements needed in the switch. However, inhibition may be required for switching.

lacks the precision of millisecond reaction time probes and may not be sufficiently reliable to assess this function. Alternative error measures of set-shifting ability may show an ADHD-related deficit (Koschack, Kunert, Derichs, Weniger, & Irle, 2003), but face the same psychometric limitations.

The Trail Making Test from the Halstead–Reitan battery (Table 5.5) is often cited as a speed-based measure of set shifting (Pennington & Ozonoff, 1996), although not all theorists agree. In any event, several studies of ADHD have used it. We (Willcutt et al., 2005b) reported that 8 out of 14 studies found a significant ADHD deficit; the composite effect size was $d = 0.55$. This medium-sized effect converged quite well with the conclusion from the studies of the WCST. However, conceptual and methodological problems with this task remain, including the demand for fine motor control.

Therefore, recent studies have begun to borrow methods from cognitive psychology that rely on reaction time measures of shifting. Although varying in detail, these designs all induce a response set and then measure reaction times when the primary response set must be changed; they can be established to monitor dual-task performance (performance cost of doing two things at once) or switching costs (see Altmann, 2004a, 2004b; Monsell, 2003; Pashler, 1998). Switching tasks seem to involve frontal cortical regions, as well as the cerebellum in some designs, but imaging work on these tasks is still not definitive (see the review by Monsell, 2003). Lesion studies suggest that the basal ganglia are also involved (Aron et al., 2003b).

These tasks have enabled more fine-grained investigations to clarify whether switching is a separate operation or is the culmination of processes such as task activation, working memory, or response suppression (Altmann, 2004a, 2004b; Mayr, 2002; Monsell, 2003). However, application of these more refined paradigms to ADHD has barely begun. Initial studies provide some evidence of ADHD deficits in rapid, controlled shifting (Cepeda, Cepeda, & Kramer, 2000; Hollingsworth, McAuliffe, & Knowlton, 2001; Perchet, Revol, Fourneret, Mauguiere, & Garcia-Larrea, 2001; Oosterlaan & Sergeant, 1998a, 1998b; Schachar, Tannock, Marriott, & Logan, 1995), but studies to date are too few and too variable in their methods to allow firm conclusions about the magnitude of the effect. For now, my conclusion is that performance on switching tasks is weak in ADHD, but it is unclear whether the effect is independent of more established problems with response suppression and working memory.

A key issue in the field, concerns the distinction between goal-directed switching of task set (an operation involving prefrontal cortex) and of attention within the same task (an operation involving parietal cortex and the dorsal attention network described in note 1 to Chapter 4; see also Shomstein & Yantis, 2006; Serenes et al., 2005). This distinction has not been well studied in ADHD.

Activation Processes Are Probably Disrupted in ADHD

Recall that activation is the ability to maintain readiness to respond. Dutch scientists have investigated this ability most heavily. They have relied on both time-on-task designs (does a child respond as quickly later in the task as early in the task?) and event rate designs (does a child with ADHD show better activation when events happen faster than when they happen more slowly?) (Table 5.6).

The event rate designs (Table 5.6) have provided the clearest evidence in support of an activation deficit in ADHD. Children with ADHD show average performance at medium event rates (e.g., a target every 4 seconds), but weaknesses at slow (e.g., every 10 seconds) and fast (e.g., every 1 second) event rates on both CPT (van der Meere,

TABLE 5.6. Tasks Used to Assess Activation in ADHD

Task	Brief description
Event rate go/ no-go	In the event rate version of the go/no-go task, the rate at which stimuli are presented is varied (e.g., every 1 second, every 4 seconds, every 8 seconds). The faster event rates are more activating for the child up to an optimum, then become too fast and lead to performance decline.
CPT beta	A CPT is administered (see Chapter 4). The child sees a series of foils (letters or shapes) and must respond when she sees a rare target (e.g., the letter X or a certain unusual shape). The beta parameter is calculated, which indicates the propensity to respond (impulsivity) or hold back (caution).

Shalev, Borger, & Gross-Tsur, 1995) and go/no-go tasks (Borger & van der Meere, 2000; van der Meere & Stermerdink, 1999; for a review, see van der Meere, 2002). Those researchers thus favor an underactivation explanation of cognitive and performance deficits in ADHD (Sergeant et al., 1999; van der Meere, 2002). In other words, varying the rate at which a computer presents stimuli can moderate response accuracy for children with ADHD.

Also supportive of a problem with activation are output response speed data—that is, the tendency of children with ADHD to respond slowly when asked to respond quickly on motor tasks (e.g., Carte, Nigg, & Hinshaw, 1996). Some physiological and late-component ERP data have been interpreted as further activation evidence (see van der Meere, 2002). Jennings, van der Molen, Pelham, Debski, and Hoza (1997) and Borger and van der Meere (2000) looked at cardiac response to the stop task and a standard go/no-go task, respectively. Both studies concluded that motor preparation and/or effort parameters are abnormal in ADHD. Dykman, Ackerman, and Oglesby (1992) found cardiac underresponse to warning stimuli in boys with ADHD; the effect was less clear in girls, but generally suggested a weakness in preparatory state.

On the other hand, some predictions about activation—most critically, predicted deficits on the CPT beta parameter (an index of risky vs. conservative response bias; Table 5.6)—have not been confirmed in ADHD (Losier et al., 1996), raising problems for the hypothesis of an activation dysfunction in ADHD. However, calculation of the beta parameter is vulnerable to ceiling effects, so additional data are needed.

In all, the limited experimental evidence available to this point favors continued consideration of an activation dysfunction in ADHD. Additional studies of event rate effects and other evidence for activation in ADHD will be important to clarify this effect and fix its magnitude.

As a final note, the regulatory model proposed by Pribram and McGuinness (1975), which has influenced European research on ADHD, included a module for effort. This concept, influential in cognitive psychology some decades ago, has suffered from lack of agreement on how to measure it and clarity as to whether it is really distinct from motivation (e.g., the reward response parameters discussed in Chapter 6). Sergeant et al. (1999) and van der Meere (2002) provide excellent summaries of the latest thinking on effort in ADHD, concluding that we lack compelling evidence of effort dysfunction in ADHD. However, if measurement issues are resolved, or if effort is equated with motivation as described in the next Chapter 6 (see Scheres et al., 2001), then the effort concept may be relevant, but still partially redundant with conceptions of motivation and reward response in ADHD. In view of its uncertain status and close relationship with motivation, I defer further consideration of effort here.

ADHD Subtypes and Executive Dysfunctions

Too few studies thus far have examined the DSM-IV(-TR) subtypes of ADHD to enable any firm conclusions about differences in executive dysfunctions among the subtypes. However, tentative comments are possible. Only three studies have included DSM-IV ADHD-PHI (Bedard et al., 2002; Chhabildas, Pennington, & Willcutt, 2001; Schmitz et al., 2002). We (Willcutt et al., 2005b) pooled all executive measures in these three studies and noted an average effect size of $d = 0.014$—in other words, a trivial effect. This finding adds to concerns that ADHD-PHI in childhood is less etiologically valid (and has less solid grounding with regard to syndromal validity) than the other two subtypes.

With regard to ADHD-PI, several studies have now looked at executive functioning in that subtype (Hinshaw et al., 2002; Klorman et al., 1999; Nigg et al., 2002b). These studies are too few to permit reliable estimates of effect sizes on any one measure; however, most studies have found executive function deficits in ADHD-PI. Indeed, it has been rare to find differences between ADHD-C and ADHD-PI (Klorman et al., 1999; Nigg et al., 2002b). Yet children with ADHD-C typically have somewhat larger deficits than those with ADHD-PI. This pattern of findings could be consistent with the idea that in a significant number of cases, ADHD-PI may be a milder variant of the condition seen in ADHD-C.

Future work to isolate a particular profile of executive function problems that may distinguish these ADHD subtypes remains of interest. For example, we (Nigg et al., 2002b) found that children with ADHD-C had a larger deficit on response inhibition (measured with the stop task) than those with ADHD-PI, but that this was only true for boys. Working memory problems may prove to be more apparent in children with ADHD-PI than in those with ADHD-C (or vice versa), but this question has not been much studied.

CLINICAL IMPLICATIONS

Children with ADHD can have marked problems in working memory (inability to maintain crucial information in mind while doing something else) and response inhibition (inability to suppress irrelevant behaviors as the context changes). They may also have difficulty with rapid set shifting (reorganizing responses), with preparing a rapid response, and with planning (sequencing). Altogether, these difficulties in executive functioning may be clinically very significant; they may contribute to problems with disorganization and inattention (Nigg et al., 2005a), to problems with impulsivity, and to impairments in academic achievement and other important life areas (Biederman et al., 2004).

As part of assessing a child presenting with possible ADHD, it can be valuable (or even essential) to assess the degree of cognitive and functional difficulty the child is experiencing with regard to control of interfering information, working memory, and response control. Identifying problems in these areas can help caregivers understand a child's difficulties in learning, studying, and participating successfully in extracurricular activities. Particularly valuable may be assessment of working memory in both auditory and visual modalities, as well as of the child's ability to remember complex versus simple information and abstract versus well-contextualized information.

It is important to remember that executive functioning problems are not necessary for a diagnosis of ADHD under DSM-IV-TR; the diagnosis is based on clinical history and behavioral assessment. However, ancillary assessment of executive functioning may be important to case planning. If a child has weaknesses in executive functioning, behavioral interventions can be developed to address them. For example, if the child has problems in working memory or planning, then in the short term teachers and parents can give the child smaller units of information when providing instructions. Over the long term, the child

can be given exercises (e.g., mnemonic tools) to strengthen these abilities. Although such interventions are still awaiting empirical validation
in ADHD, they have had some empirical validation in rehabilitation
studies of persons with head injuries (Sohlberg & Mateer, 2001;
Wasserstein & Lynn, 2001). Indeed, the possibility of applying interventions from rehabilitation psychology that are successful with head
injury to executive function weaknesses in ADHD is of growing interest, especially for ADHD in adults.

Attentional or other cognitive control training interventions for
children with ADHD are also being developed (Klinberg, Forssberg, &
Westerberg, 2002). The results of studies that evaluate and further
develop such interventions will be of interest in the field. Also of interest will be efforts to develop interventions with young children to
enable them to practice response interruption ("Stop, look, listen"), as
well as to focus and shift attention. Clinicians can consider these interventions as behavioral programs for children, but should keep in mind
that their efficacy has not yet been well established. A key obstacle to
establishing the efficacy of such interventions has been that intervention studies typically have not differentiated children who have ADHD
into those with unimpaired versus impaired executive functioning
(Biederman et al., 2004; Nigg, Blaskey, Stawicki, & Sachek, 2004a; see
Chapter 8). In all, such training interventions are worth investigating,
but remain as yet incompletely tested in formal trials with ADHD.

At the same time, it is important to keep in mind that a child with
ADHD and executive impairment should perform poorly on more than
just one isolated test. Even typical children will often have difficulty
with one particular subtest (Nigg, Willcutt, Doyle, & Sonuga-Barke,
2005b). Along the same lines, it is unfortunate but true that many clinical tests of executive functioning have limited reliability and normative
data. This state of affairs has begun to be remedied.

For example, two major new batteries have recently been published: the NEPSY (Korkman, Kirk, & Kemp, 1998; Kemp, Kirk, &
Korkman, 2001) and the Delis–Kaplan Executive Function Battery
(Delis, Kaplan, & Kramer, 2001). Both batteries have now been normed
on a stratified, nationally representative sample in the United States,
and test–retest reliability data have been provided. The NEPSY is a battery designed for children ages 3–12. Based on Luria's model, it
includes tests of focused attention (the Auditory Attention/Response
Set Task), of planning (the Tower Task—similar to the Tower of London), and of memory and learning. The scale internal and test–retest
reliabilities of these measures are generally respectable and even excel-

lent for executive function measures. Even so, subtest reliabilities typically range from .70 to .90, which are on the low end of ordinary acceptability for tests in which major decisions about a child are at stake. In addition, recent experimental work continues to focus on deriving better, well-validated, and reliable measures of other key components, such as vigilance and response inhibition (e.g., Dougherty, Mathias, Marsh, & Jager, 2005).

As for the other recently published test battery, the Delis–Kaplan battery (Delis et al., 2001) is entirely focused on executive function measures and covers the age range from 8 to 89. It thus cannot be used validly with younger children. A particularly useful feature is the inclusion of "control tasks," in which the same tasks are carried out minus the relevant executive components. This allows the clinician to draw some inferences about whether task performance is impaired because of cognitive control problems or because of more fundamental problems in task execution. The battery enables assessment of set shifting (with a task similar to the Trail Making Test), as well as response inhibition and working memory. Again, reliabilities are respectable (and are better than those for many past measures of executive functioning), but even so they vary into the inadequate range for some subtests. Thus scrutiny of the technical manual is advised even for this strongest battery of executive measures. Case formulation and treatment planning require identification of a convergence of data across multiple tests and sources of information.

Overall, even when using these new, state-of-the-art executive measures, clinicians must still be careful to avoid drawing strong conclusions from weakness on just one subtest, and must consider the broad pattern of both test results and behavioral descriptors to evaluate whether various components of executive functioning are problematic. Target behavioral interventions in the focal areas that are identified may be considered, but must be monitored in light of limited efficacy data.

The possibility of specific weaknesses in the spatial domain is noteworthy. It may be that a subset of children with ADHD has specific spatial or spatial reasoning problems, or even a full nonverbal learning disability syndrome. Evaluation to rule out this syndrome is warranted if a strong pattern of spatial or math weaknesses is noted, or if motor delays are apparent (Chapter 7).

Table 5.7 presents common frequently asked questions about ADHD and executive functioning that clinicians may face, and that this chapter has addressed.

TABLE 5.7. Frequently Asked Questions about ADHD and Executive Functioning

Question	Answer
Are children with ADHD just not trying?	No. They often have neuropsychological problems with response suppression and working memory.
Why doesn't my child with ADHD learn from mistakes?	The child may have problems with working memory or response inhibition, even when he or she "knows" the correct behavior.
Do some children attend better to visual information?	Yes. Assessing visual versus verbal learning and working memory may be very useful.
Do neuropsychological problems "fit" brain imaging findings?	Yes.

EXECUTIVE FUNCTIONING IN ADHD: SUMMARY

Executive functioning (also known as cognitive control) has been heavily studied in relation to ADHD, and a number of deficits ranging from medium to large in magnitude are apparent. Although control of comorbid and confounding disorders (such as learning disabilities and CD) has been lacking in many studies, a consistent literature has now emerged indicating that these main executive weaknesses are not accounted for by comorbid conditions (Barkley et al., 2001a; Nigg et al., 1998; Rucklidge & Tannock, 2002; Willcutt et al., 2001).

Executive functioning is not unitary; it reflects distinct operations that may differentially recruit distinct aspects of the prefrontal–subcortical neural loops involved in behavior regulation, working memory, and attention. Measures intended to probe executive interruption of a motor response have been the most extensively replicated with ADHD; however, large effects also have been noted in studies using measures of spatial working memory, although fewer studies have yet been published. It is unclear whether those effects are accounted for by difficulties in executive control or by difficulties in the visual–spatial scratch pad (short-term memory), perhaps due to uncontrolled nonverbal learning disabilities. On the other hand, verbal working memory effects may not yet have been fully probed in ADHD. In all, working memory deficits appear likely and will be a key focus of future studies.

At the same time, ADHD is not associated with clear problems in attentional control per se (selection and interference control) when working memory demands are low. Clever experimental designs that can isolate these components and clarify their functioning in well-characterized samples of children with ADHD should produce further advances in this area.

Finally, activation as a state regulation process appears promising as an element in the ADHD profile, at least for ADHD-C. Further independent replications of these effects are needed. Even so, these findings, along with findings on response suppression (however the latter comes to be conceptualized in emerging neuroscience and computation models) may converge into a theory of motor control problems in ADHD, governed by problems in interrupting a response and/or problems in activation (control) of response output parameters. Notably, most executive functioning research to this point has been confined to ADHD-C; however, a few studies of ADHD-PI have been completed, with inconsistent results. Key questions concern the actual mechanism involved in stopping a behavior (is it working memory or inhibition? is it frontal or is it subcortical?); the developmental sequence of the problems that have been described; and the integration of activation with executive functioning in new theoretical formulations.

Table 5.8 summarizes the state of knowledge on executive functioning problems in ADHD-C and ADHD-PI. Essentially no information is available about ADHD-PHI, so it is omitted. Because this area is so well studied that meta-analyses have been published, we can gauge apparent effect sizes for ADHD-C versus unaffected control children.

TABLE 5.8. Score Card on Status of Executive Functioning Deficits in ADHD

Executive Function	ADHD-C		ADHD-PI: Conclusion
	Conclusion	Effect size (*d*)	
Interference control	Unclear	0.20	Unclear
Working memory verbal	Weakly affected	0.43	?
Working memory spatial	Affected	01.0	?
Response suppression	Affected	0.61	Intact
Set shifting	Affected	0.50	Affected
Activation	Affected	Unknown	?

| C H A P T E R 6 |

Motivation

A common question about children with ADHD is "Are they trying?" That is, are they motivated? Parents and teachers often have extensive concerns on this front: "What should we expect of these children? What is their best effort? How can we get them motivated?" At the lay level, such questions seem simple enough. Yet, like the other concepts discussed in this volume, motivation involves several levels of both cognitive and neural representation. One level of motivation consists of values, long-term goals, and so on (Little, 1999). This is an important concern to parents and teachers, because it pertains to such issues as vocational training and long-term ambitions of children with ADHD. However, because this meaning of motivation is so little studied in ADHD, I do not discuss it here. Rather, in this chapter, "motivation" refers to more immediate situations, or a child's interest in and response to immediate incentives (i.e., reminders of or cues for impending reward or punishment). Whereas the chapters on attention (Chapter 4) and executive functioning (Chapter 5) are most relevant to the inattentive and disorganized symptoms of ADHD, motivation is probably most relevant to the hyperactive–impulsive symptoms.

MOTIVATION IN MODELS OF TEMPERAMENT AND PERSONALITY

To organize motivational response from a neuropsychological perspective, many options are available in the literatures on the neuroscience of emotion, on temperament, and on personality (see Nigg, 2000, for an overview). Models of temperament and personality are extremely important to motivation, because they tend to address emotional response—which is key to incentive-motivational systems. As a result, part of the discussion in this chapter concerns whether ADHD may reflect an extreme temperament, as well as whether there are cognitive deficits related to reward or punishment responses. I address temperament again in Chapter 8, but provide a needed overview here (see Nigg, in press, for a more extended discussion).

Many different temperament and personality theories are relevant to defining basic incentive–response motivational systems, including a tradition of temperament-based psychobiological theories of personality (Eysenck, 1955, 1967; Gray, 1982, 1991; Depue & Spoont, 1986; Depue & Collins, 1989; Depue & Lenzenweger, 2005; Zuckerman, 1991, 2001); trait-based models of personality (John & Srivastava, 1999; Block & Block, 1980) and of adult temperament (Clark, Watson, & Mineka, 1994; Tellegen, 1985; Watson, Kotov, & Gamez, 2006); trait-based models of child temperament (Eisenberg et al., 2001, 2005; Eisenberg & Morris, 2002; Kochanska, Murray, & Harlan, 2000; Rothbart & Bates, 1998); and psychobiological models of child temperament (Kagan, Resnick, & Gibbons, 1989; Kagan & Snidman, 2004). Most of these models converge on a small number of basic incentive response systems that underlie major temperament and personality traits (Rothbart & Ahadi, 1994). For example, many models emphasize three factors of extraversion, neuroticism, and control or constraint. These can be alternatively named as positive affect, negative affect, and constraint, or as approach, withdrawal, and control. Gray's (1982, 1991) model has been particularly influential in ADHD research, because it specified experimental predications to particular incentive contexts. He called the approach system the behavioral activation system (or BAS), and the withdrawal system the behavioral inhibition system (or BIS). Because most of the ADHD literature to date has relied on this model, I adopt a synthesized model here that draws upon the several approaches cited above (see Nigg, in press, for a more detailed exposition) but is interpretable within Gray's framework.

The basic working model that will serve for my purposes here is summarized in schematic form in Table 6.1. The control dimension pertains mainly to strategic control processes that have been discussed in Chapter 5; the table specifies that these are physiologically related to cardiac vagal tone (Calkins & Fox, 2002; Beauchaine, 2001), but cardiac vagal tone, heavily studied in externalizing behavior, is insufficiently studied in ADHD per se to enable much review here or in the prior

TABLE 6.1. Basic Trait Model

	Approach	Withdraw	Control
Behavior	Reward incentive	Potential punishment	Strategic control
Neural system	Dopamine–reward system	Amygdala–limbic system	Prefrontal–striatal
Peripheral nervous system indices	Heart rate increase (reward)	Skin conductance	Cardiac vagal tone
Temperament	Approach/ surgency	Withdrawal/ negative emotion	Effortful control
Personality	Extraversion/ surgency	Neuroticism	Constraint
Major affect	Positive	Negative	Neutral
Gray's model	Behavioral activation (BAS)	Behavioral inhibition (BIS)	

chapter. I focus on the incentive systems in the remainder of this section.

Central to this simplified model, then, is the reactivity of two basic incentive systems: approach and withdrawal, which are related to reactivity of autonomic as well as neural systems (Beauchaine, 2001). They are viewed as the top of a hierarchical structural model from which crucial subtraits emerge in development (Nigg, in press). Although some models view these in terms of valence (positive and negative emotions or affect), they are viewed here in terms of motivation (approach and withdrawal) for several reasons. Labeling these here as approach and withdrawal, rather than positive and negative affect, facilitates linkages between infant, child, and adult research on the one hand and cross-species, evolutionary, and neurobiological learning models on the other hand (Zuckerman, 2001). Recent physiological evidence is also consistent with this perspective. For example, left frontal EEG activation appears to be related to motivation (approach) more clearly than to valence (positive emotions). That is, some types of anger generate the same left-sided activation pattern as happiness or excitement (Harmon-Jones, 2003, 2004). These data indicate that it will not do to consider anger as only related to negative affect.

Admittedly, irritable frustration/anger factors in with negative affect (anxiety, sadness) in temperament studies of infants and children (as well as adults) (Lemery, Goldsmith, Klinnert, & Mrazek, 1999;

Putnam, Ellis, & Rothbart, 2001). Yet in the child factor-analytic data, anger also shares a *positive* correlation with aspects of approach (e.g., activity level), whereas sadness has a *negative* association with activity level (Putnam et al., 2001). Either (1) anger in response to frustration reflects both "negative" and "positive" affect (i.e., both approach and stress systems), or (2) multiple functional forms of anger must be considered. I adopt the second hypothesis here, but this is an empirical question. Thus I suggest that angry affect sometimes reflects a potential to overcome obstacles in anticipation of reward or reinforcement, emanating from traits such as surgency and reward responsivity. In other instances, it reflects a propensity to resentful, angry, hostile affect that is responsive to fear or anticipated negative consequences, as well as to panic, alarm, and/or stress response.

The approach trait is therefore defined as willingness to approach possible incentive or reward/reinforcement (it can also include active pursuit of relief from possible punishment—i.e., active avoidance of punishment). It is associated with speed of reinforcement learning. It is related to the personality trait of extraversion and includes elements in children such as activity level (of obvious relevance to ADHD), as well as surgency (Rothbart & Bates, 1998; Putnam et al., 2001; Shiner & Caspi, 2003). Disagreement remains as to the neurobiological core element of this supertrait (see Depue & Collins, 1999, and accompanying commentaries). It is conceptualized here as related in the CNS to the appetitive, dopaminergic systems, including the nucleus accumbens and ascending limbic–frontal dopaminergic networks. At the level of the peripheral nervous system (PNS), it is related to sympathetic activation, with one index being heart rate acceleration with the application of effort or the possibility of reward incentive (Beauchaine, 2001; Fowles, 1983).

The withdrawal dimension is anchored by readiness of withdrawal-related behavior in potentially unrewarding or uncertain contexts, or passive avoidance of potential punishment, as well as with associated affective reactivity (i.e., fear, anxiety, and sadness). This dimension is related to the personality trait of neuroticism. The reactivity of these responses is related at the level of the CNS to limbic–frontal neural circuitry. Depue and Lenzenweger (2005) describe fear as an immediate threat response involving short-term activation in the central amygdala nucleus, whereas anxiety reflects long-term activation to low grade threat associated with activation in the bed nucleus of the stria terminalis in the extended amygdala. Thus the reactivity of stress response or danger alarm systems (the hypothalamic–pituitary–adrenal axis and associated autonomic and hormonal effects, as well as the lateral hypothalamus, reticular formation, and other structures at the CNS level) is a key feature. At the level of the PNS, reactivity of this set of response systems is hypothesized to emanate in sympathetic activation of autonomic systems—in particular, electrodermal skin response to anticipated loss of reward (Fowles, 1983; Beauchaine, 2001).

Note that "behavioral inhibition" here therefore can have two meanings. First, in the presence of uncertainty (e.g., entering a room of unfamiliar peers), a child will suppress both emotional expression and exploration, and instead will carefully examine the situation (Kagan & Snidman, 2004). Likewise, an animal (e.g., a deer entering a clearing or a mouse entering an unfamiliar cage) might proceed with caution, automatically pausing to scan for danger and assess the situation with heightened attention to possible danger, while suppressing other behaviors. Second, in the case of imminent threat (fear or even panic, as might be experienced by an adult or child facing immediate physical attack by a larger and stronger person, or an animal encountering a predator), then a "fight–flight" or a "freeze" response can occur. In this instance, all behavior is suppressed; there is an actual rather a potential threat. Both behaviors are sometimes referred to as "behavioral inhibition" (note that this is completely distinct from "response inhibition" as described in the preceding chapter). Nearly all research on ADHD is focused on potential punishment and so refers to the first response described here. I refer to this as "reactive behavioral inhibition" or "motivational inhibition" (Nigg, 2000).

With regard to neural imaging data, fMRI studies show greater activation in the ventral amygdala when approaching negative information (i.e., fearful faces; Hare, Tottenham, Davidson, Glover, & Casey, 2005), whereas happy expressions elicit greater activity in the nucleus accumbens, a region associated with reward and appetitive behavior (Schultz, Tremblay, & Hollerman, 2000; Nestler, 2004). Amygdala activation (associated with avoidance of potentially unpleasant events) and nucleus accumbens activation (related to approaching a potentially positive event) appear to be mutually inhibiting responses (Hare et al., 2005).

Therefore, these two systems are thought to modulate one another (Gray, 1991). That is, activation of approach (possible reward) may damp down fear or anxiety, and vice versa. As a result, many theories emphasize the relative weighting of these two systems, rather than viewing them in isolation (Gray, 1991; Newman & Wallace, 1993; Patterson & Newman, 1993). However, from an operational viewpoint, it has been difficult to differentiate measurement of dysfunction in one individual system from dysfunction in their relative weighting. For simplicity, therefore, this chapter covers separately both approach (typically operationalized in ADHD research as responding to potential reward) and withdrawal (typically operationalized as avoiding potential punishment). Near the end I briefly consider integrative approaches, such as those proposed by Newman and colleagues.

APPROACH OR REWARD RESPONSE APPEARS ABNORMAL IN ADHD

The idea of a reward response deficit has remained viable if historically underemphasized in the ADHD literature. It is regaining currency in modified form today, due to the growing importance of animal models in understanding the neurophysiology of stimulant response and ADHD behaviors. Work by Gray (1971, 1982, 1991) on the basis of animal studies outlined a behavioral activation or approach system that activates motor response to signals for reward ("conditioned appetitive stimuli") and active avoidance behavior in response to cues for nonreward or punishment. For example, when Ms. Blake turns her back, Mike leaves his seat without permission to escape expected routine teasing from peers at his table. Gray suggested neural mediation by the ascending dopaminergic fibers in the reward or appetitive system of the brain (i.e., the mesolimbic dopamine system). These fibers proceed from the substantia nigra and ventral tegmentum to the basal ganglia (especially the caudate nucleus), limbic system, lateral hypothalamus, and prefrontal cortices. Contemporary models continue to accept the broad outlines of this hypothesized neural system for reward response in ADHD (e.g., Sagvolden, Johansen, Aase, & Russell, 2005). See Figure 3.1 for schematic illustration of the outline of these circuits.

Reward response abnormalities had been long suspected in ADHD (Douglas, 1972). Gorenstein and Newman (1980) proposed that an overresponsive approach (reward cue response) system as defined by Gray (1971, 1982) leads to difficulty inhibiting response in the presence of strong reward cues in the case of ADHD (for related ideas, see Gray, 1991; Newman & Wallace, 1993; Quay, 1988, 1997). In the meantime, the literature on ADHD emphasized both over- and underresponse to reward (Haenlein & Caul, 1987). It was hypothesized that an overactive reward system leads to overresponding in the presence of reward cues, but not when reward cues are absent.

The main problem with this formulation was the difficulty of experimentally demonstrating that children with ADHD "overrespond," compared to other children, when reward cues are offered (Iaboni, Douglas, & Baker, 1995; Oosterlaan & Sergeant, 1998b). For example, Milich, Hartung, Martin, and Haigler (1994) correlated adolescents' ADHD and conduct symptoms with commission errors in a reward-only condition on the go/no-go task (see Chapter 5). ADHD symptoms were associated moderately with commission errors for girls ($r = .53$), but not for boys. Iaboni et al. (1995) found no significant difference in children's commission errors in various incentive conditions on a go/no-go task. Oosterlaan and Sergeant (1998b) administered incentives on a modified stop task (see Chapter 5); there was no association of reward with ADHD responding. These types of findings created problems for a reward-based theory of ADHD. A comprehensive review of reward responding in ADHD was recently completed by Luman, Oosterlaan, and Sergeant (2005). They reviewed 25 studies (involving over 1,100 subjects). They noted that this has continued to be a mixed literature; it does not consistently support any one formulation about the role of reward responding in ADHD. However, they have concluded that (1) ADHD is associated with increased weighting of immediate over delayed reward; (2) children with ADHD may respond to high-intensity reinforcement; and (3) the limited physiological literature suggests underresponse (low sensitivity) of physiological reactivity to reward. As noted above, comorbid disorders, particularly CD, have been inadequately controlled for in this literature.

Conceptually, one way forward may be in the refined recognition that children with ADHD are overresponsive to immediate reward, but underresponsive to time-distal reward (Douglas, 1988; Tripp & Alsop, 1999). Thus the temporal properties of the reward and cue are crucial to theorizing in ADHD; a failure to control for these properties might account for some of the inconsistent results in prior studies.

Underresponse to contingencies has been reinterpreted recently in light of animal data by researchers in Norway. These more recent conceptions emphasize the tendency to underrespond unless reward cues are immediate. The operative concept in these more recent models involves a dysfunction in the tonic or phasic properties of the modulatory dopaminergic response to reward cues in the mesolimbic/mesocortical dopamine systems (Johansen, Aase, Meyer, & Sagvolden, 2002). This dysfunction leads to an abnormally steep "delay–reward gradient," which means that rewards become abnormally low in reinforcing power as they become distant in time (Johansen et al., 2002;

Sagvolden, Aase, Zeiner, & Berger, 1998; Sagvolden et al., 2005). The delay–reward gradient argument rests heavily on basic work in animal cognition using an inbred rodent model (the "spontaneously hyperten-sive rat"). Although there are some important difficulties with this par-ticular animal model of ADHD (see Ferguson, 2001; Sagvolden, 2001), the Oslo group has presented data on learning and extinction in chil-dren with ADHD that support the model (reviewed by Sagvolden, 2001). However, Luman et al. (2005) have concluded that behavioral data in support of this model are inconsistent. Nonetheless, it is worth considering this model for a moment here.

Figure 6.1 illustrates the idea of the steepened delay–reward gradi-ent and its hypothesized effects on learning and extinction in ADHD. In short, under this hypothesis, abnormal relative weighting of delayed and immediate incentives leads to overactive and impulsive behavior. Sagvolden et al. (1998, 2005), have hypothesized that extinction follow-ing learning should be impaired if there is a reward dysfunction, because new learning will fail to replace the prior overlearned behav-ior. This may be another reason why children with ADHD appear to be unable to learn from their mistakes— a common complaint of parents and teachers. Preliminary studies of children appear to support this prediction (Johansen et al., 2002).

Difficulty in tolerating delay may be related to reward response dysfunction. Sonuga-Barke, Dalen, Daley, and Remington (2002) have shown that children with ADHD consistently choose immediate small rewards over delayed, larger rewards, but their choice to do so is

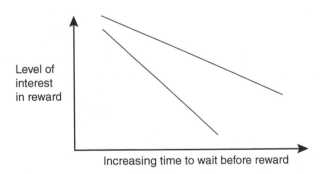

Level of
interest
in reward

Increasing time to wait before reward

FIGURE 6.1. Hypothesized steeper delay–reward gradient in children with ADHD (steep line) than in typical children (shallow line). Reward has more potency with a shorter wait time.

directly related to their wish to complete the current activity—in other words, to their intolerance of delays. Whether this is a "rational" choice to evade the experiment or a strong preference for immediate rewards remains in debate. Either way, this tendency to favor immediate over delayed (and larger) rewards is as strong as executive inhibition as a statistical correlate to ADHD symptoms (Solanto et al., 2001a).

A final note about this theory is that it suggests a role for social learning in the early development of ADHD. According to the theory, if children with ADHD fail to experience typical extinction of a behavior after it has been reinforced, parents may be left very little margin for error in helping these children to learn social rules and self-control. To put this another way, if these children have to "unlearn" misbehaviors by trial and error with parents, the "unlearning" process will be very slow. Any failure to sanction the misbehaviors immediately may make this process even more difficult. Many parents typically reward their toddlers' or preschoolers' appropriate behavior most of the time, but overlook some incidents. Most children still learn and internalize the parental expectations. This process will be much more difficult with a child with a steepened delay—reward gradient. The result may be that parents of these youngsters will require much more patience and persistence to get them to respond to parenting guidance and consequences. Data to evaluate this claim will be of interest.

In summary, reward and reinforcement response may be abnormal in children with ADHD, but consistent data to demonstrate this effect have been slow to emerge. Mixed findings across the literature make it difficult to draw firm conclusions. The basic idea of the delay—reward gradient dysfunction has recently been revived as a key ADHD marker. More careful consideration of reinforcement intensity and timing in future studies may clarify whether children with ADHD have an underresponsive or an overresponsive reward system, or whether there are two groups of children with ADHD (some under-, some overresponsive). Scientists therefore have begun to integrate reward response with temporal properties of actions and responses—that is, misjudging the timing of events, inability to tolerate waiting periods (perhaps due to difficulty with time processing), and poor time estimation (Castellanos & Tannock, 2002; Sonuga-Barke, 2002). The steepened delay—reward gradient may be related to problems in the "internal clock" in ADHD, as well as to problems in the basic dopaminergic reward circuitry in the brain. These theoretical ideas, while requiring more study, can potentially simplify the various competing regulation theories of ADHD.

WITHDRAWAL RESPONSE (REACTIVE INHIBITORY CONTROL) IS PROBABLY INTACT IN ADHD

If withdrawal responding was affected in ADHD, we would expect children with ADHD to have difficulty benefiting from warnings of possible punishment. In a sense, they would have insufficient anxiety or fear. Note that this circuitry is thought to be activated in response to impending (potential) punishment, not actual punishment; that is, it is very important to learning from mistakes. The logic here is that perhaps children misbehave because they lack typical response to cues for negative consequences. This insensitivity to impending punishment, or low anxiety, makes the process of socialization difficult for them and interferes with the development of self-control. As a result, these children move into later childhood and adolescence with impulsive, poorly regulated, and socially inappropriate behavior more typical of younger children. Hypotheses about this process in ADHD thus again primarily address hyperactive–impulsive symptoms rather than inattentive symptoms (Quay, 1997).

In Gray's (1982) model, the BIS is theorized to be anchored by the septal–hippocampal formation and to be mediated by the noradrenergic and serotonergic neurotransmitter systems. Quay (1988) suggested that ADHD might be due to a failure in avoidance learning, caused by a breakdown in the withdrawal system or BIS. Testing this concept has been difficult, however. One difficulty has been finding the appropriate probe of this withdrawal system or system in children. Gray's (1982) model relied heavily on animal research, in which animals received cues for extreme pain (e.g., electric shock) or potentially life-threatening punishment (e.g., a cat's scent for a mouse). Thus it may have often activated a *fear* circuit rather than an *anxiety* circuit. The analogue to human anxiety may thus be problematic. In any event, implementing probes of comparable strength in humans would be obviously unethical.

Nonetheless, in an effort to approximate a probe of an anxiety or fear system that would involve passive avoidance learning (in the face of impending punishment), two major measurement approaches have used incentive-based laboratory tasks and/or key psychophysiological probes (Table 6.2). Whereas a variety of other paradigms could be utilized, most research on ADHD to date has relied on either the modified go/no-go task or the card-playing/door-opening tasks, with a handful examining relevant psychophysiological responses to incentive cues.

TABLE 6.2. Key Laboratory Tasks used to assess avoidance learning in children

Task	Brief description
Motivated go/ no-go task	This task is similar to the basic go/no-go task described in Table 5.4, except that more stimuli are used (e.g., several letters or numbers)—some of which are paired with a reward ("If you press the key when you see an A, you win 25 cents") and some with a response cost or punishment ("If you press the key when you see a B, you lose 25 cents"). Various configurations of rewards and punishments are possible.
Card-playing task/door-opening task	In the card-playing task, each card played either wins or loses money. Early in the game, most cards win money, creating a reward-based response set to keep playing. As the game progresses, the probability that the cards will lose money increases. Typical respondents at some point realize this and stop playing before they have lost all their winnings. Impulsive participants play longer and lose more money. This is thought to demonstrate failure to suppress the reward-based response set when punishments appear. The door-opening task is the same, except that it involves opening doors instead of playing cards; thus it is more appropriate for younger children. Antisocial adults typically perseverate on these tasks (Newman & Wallace, 1993). O'Brian, Frick, and Lyman (1994) reported that response perseveration was observed only in externalizing children low in anxiety; this observation helped to validate the task as a probe of the passive avoidance system. In all, these tasks provide preliminary data on response regulation.
Physiological measures	Skin conductance to removal of reward in a motivated go/no-go task indicates activity of the reactive BIS. Heart rate response to reward indicates activity of the Approach System or BAS.
Observational methods	A young child enters a room of unfamiliar peers. The child may also be approached by an adult in a costume, or offered an object. Experimenter records time to approach, physical distance, and physiological responses.

Initial studies of psychopathy suggested a relationship to low anxiety (or low fear) and an underactive BIS (Fowles, 1980). Low heart rate was viewed as a prime marker (Raine, 1996, 2002). However, experimental incentive-based laboratory tasks yielded a less clear picture (see Newman & Wallace, 1993), leading Newman to modify his model of response regulation, which I comment on later in this chapter as an alternative to a "weak-BIS theory."[1]

Table 6.2 also lists a few examples of the numerous observational methods used in research on behaviorally inhibited (reactive) temperament (Kagan, 1997). These approaches represent a potentially very important but underutilized avenue for understanding the relation of ADHD to reactive inhibitory mechanisms mediated by either anxiety or fear. As conceived by Kagan and colleagues, behavioral inhibition is more heavily social in focus and related to innate anxiety to novel social situations. They assessed the construct via observations of young children interacting with unfamiliar and familiar peers, with the observers recording such behavioral variables as latency to interaction, physical distance maintained, and physiological variables (e.g., heart rate). Inhibited children are more socially withdrawn and more physiologically aroused in the face of an unfamiliar peer or social situation. Several longitudinal studies have linked this construct with later anxiety disorders (Biederman et al., 2001). Extremely low levels of inhibition (e.g., high exuberance) appear to be related to externalizing behavior problems (Biederman et al., 2001). However, these approaches have been little used to study ADHD per se as yet. In all, work on ADHD with this observational paradigms will be of keen interest and value in the field.

As noted above, most work on reactive behavioral inhibition in ADHD has used the card playing and go/no-go tasks, with a handful of relevant physiological studies. The go/no-go task with response contingencies can be criticized for not featuring a strong enough consequence to activate the anxiety system fully in humans. However, at least three physiological studies (looking at heart rate and/or skin conductance) have supported the validity of the task as a probe of reactive inhibition (Arnett & Newman, 2000; Iaboni, Douglas, & Ditto, 1997; Mezzacappa, Kindlon, Saul, & Earls, 1998).

Even so, the studies on ADHD remain few. In a careful study, Hartung, Milich, Lynam, and Martin (2002) recruited a sample of clinic-referred adolescents, including adolescent boys and girls who met diagnostic criteria for ADHD, CD, and ADHD + CD. Adolescent ADHD symptoms were unrelated to responses in the punishment-only condition on the go/no-go task, failing to support a weak-BIS formulation.

Iaboni et al. (1995), in a study cited earlier in this chapter, looked at children with ADHD and comparison children in four incentive conditions using the go/no-go task: reward only; punishment only; reward + punishment; and a fourth condition termed "response cost–reward," in which children earned money for inhibiting on a no-go signal and lost money for failing to respond to go signals. The boys with ADHD overresponded in all four conditions, contrary to the prediction of a weak-BIS model. However, in this repeated-measures design, it was possible that children with ADHD failed to distinguish between the conditions.

Yet Oosterlaan and Sergeant (1998a), using a modified stop task with reward and punishment conditions, also failed to find an association of response contingency with responding on the task in ADHD. Speed of the inhibition process was impaired in children with ADHD across all conditions, similar to the findings of Iaboni et al. (1995). In summary, the incentive-based experiments to date provide no clear support for a weak-BIS model of ADHD in childhood. As noted earlier, physiological studies may provide better evidence (Fowles, 1980, 1988). Fowles (1988) suggested that activity in the approach system could be indexed by heart rate response to cues for reward, and activity in the BIS by skin conductance response to removal of reward. The limited data using those methods in children with ADHD are thus quite important.

Lazzaro et al. (1999) observed reduced skin conductance level in ADHD, consistent with a weak-BIS effect, although response to punishment cues was not tested. In a better test of the weak-BIS model using Fowles's (1988) logic, Iaboni et al. (1997) found that, consistent with a weak-BIS hypothesis, boys with ADHD as defined by DSM-III-R exhibited abnormal skin conductance responses to removal of reward. However, a majority of this small sample with ADHD also had either CD or ODD (often a precursor to CD), and those symptoms were not covaried. If CD is associated in part with abnormal BIS activity (Fowles, 1980; Raine, 2002), then the result could be an effect of comorbidity rather than an ADHD-specific effect.

Nonsupportive results were obtained by Pliszka, Hatch, Bocherding, and Rogeness (1993), who looked at cardiac and skin conductance measures via a classical conditioning paradigm in boys with DSM-III-R ADHD with and without anxiety. They created a valid conditioned stimulus for punishment by pairing a computerized stimulus with an aversive white noise; they demonstrated that the conditioned stimulus generated a larger skin conductance response in all groups than a neutral stimulus. The subgroup with ADHD + anxiety showed nonsignificantly greater skin conductance responses (stronger BIS) than the other two groups, consistent with Gray's theory of anxiety. However, contrary to a weak-BIS theory of ADHD, the group with ADHD but no anxiety did not show any evidence of differing from the control group in skin conductance response. Heart rate parameters also did not differ across groups. Thus the weak-BIS model was not supported. ODD and CD symptoms were not controlled for.

In summary, the physiological studies of the weak-BIS model in ADHD have been inconsistent, and the performance studies have been largely negative. More such work is needed, including studies using observational paradigms and studies with better controls for comorbid conduct problems. Logically, the weak-BIS theory only pertains to the subset of children with ADHD who are low in anxiety (note that ADHD is associated with a higher-than-chance incidence of anxiety disorders). It may be possible to define and study a subset with very low anxiety and comorbid CD via weak reactive inhibition. Indeed, a substantial body of research now suggests that extreme low-fear or low-withdrawal reactions—including poor passive avoidance learning (Vitale et al., 2005), failure to recognize fearful emotions in others (Blair, 2001), lack of typical electrodermal skin reactions to potential punishment (Fung et al., 2005), low trait ratings of fearfulness (see Frick, Lilienfeld, Ellis, Loney, & Silverthorn, 1999), and lack of typical amygdala activation on imaging studies (in adults; Birbaumer et al., 2005)—all are associated with psychopathic tendencies in adolescence and adulthood, and therefore with a high risk of conduct problems, apparently distinctly from ADHD per se (Fung et al., 2005). These children may comprise a subset of children who have ADHD earlier in childhood, however (Lynam, 2002). In all, the most parsimonious conclusion at this point is that abnormalities of Withdrawal or punishment-related responding may characterize a subgroup of children with severe antisocial tendencies, but do not characterize the main group of children with ADHD per se.

RESPONSE MODULATION, ADHD, AND ANTISOCIAL BEHAVIOR

As noted earlier, Newman and colleagues (see Newman & Wallace, 1993; MacCoon et al., 2004) offered a modification of Gray's model. They suggested that "response modulation" is a relatively automatic process by which new information is regularly sampled from the environment to inform ongoing behavior. Thus the dominant response is continually integrated with feedback from the environment to enable its modulation. Deficient response modulation results in failure to modify a dominant response set (e.g., approach behavior in response to reward cues) once initiated. In short, a critical cognitive process can fail and disrupt motivational inhibition.[2] Because response modulation is portrayed as a broad cognitive process (MacCoon et al., 2004) that responds to affectively laden as well as affectively neutral stimuli, it could be related to failure to interrupt behavior for strategic or motivational reasons. Overall, Newman and Wallace (1993) suggested that in addition to the traditional weak-BIS conception of impulsivity, another major route to disinhibitory psychopathology arises from failure in interregulation of the BIS and the BAS. That is, the BIS fails to inhibit the approach system, so the dominant response set is excessively difficult to interrupt.

Newman and Wallace (1993) conjectured that response modulation is deficient in ADHD. In light of their findings for psychopathy, this idea is most readily applied to children with ADHD-C and comorbid CD—the group most at risk for antisocial and even psychopathic outcomes (Farrington, Loeber, & van Kammen, 1990; Lynam, 1997, 1998; Moffitt, 1990). However, Newman and Wallace (1993) suggested that the same response modulation deficit may underlie both ADHD and psychopathy, but may be expressed differently in those two syndromes because of other moderating factors in development.

The idea of a response modulation deficit has had only limited evaluation to date in ADHD. Of some relevance, however, may be data from the card-playing/door-opening tasks (see Table 6.2). Quay and colleagues pioneered use of the card-playing task with children and created the more child-friendly door-opening task as well; their early work confirmed that children with CD perseverated on these tasks (Daugherty & Quay, 1991; Shapiro, Quay, Hogan, & Schwartz, 1988). Two studies of children with ADHD yielded mixed results that failed to provide strong support for avoidance dysfunction in ADHD. Daugherty, Quay, and Ramos (1993) found that children with ADHD stopped prematurely on the task (the opposite of perseveration). Matthys, van Goozen, de Vries, Cohen-Kettenis, and van Engeland (1998) found that children with ADHD + CD perseverated more than other children, but failed to include a group pure ADHD group or covary severity of conduct disorder symptoms. However, Milich and colleagues (1994) found in psychiatrically-treated adolescents that levels of ADHD symptoms were correlated with perseveration on the card-playing task; yet conduct disorder symptoms were not controlled.

A mixed-incentive go/no-go task (i.e., one in which rewards and punishments are both possible on each trial) is the other tool that has been used to address this question. It is not a clean probe of response modulation, because excess commission errors could be due to an overactive approach system, a dysfunctional avoidance system, or poor response modulation. Nonetheless, these data are of interest.

Milich et al. (1994) used the go/no-go task in a "reward + punishment" condition (their reward-only condition was discussed earlier). Adolescent psychiatric inpatients received money for correct go responses, and lost money for incorrect go responses. Surprisingly, errors were not associated with CD symptoms. The sample may have included several youngsters with "adolescent-limited" antisocial behaviors, who, in contrast to those with persistent childhood-onset antisocial behaviors, are not expected to show psychological dysfunction (Moffitt, 1993). ADHD symptoms were associated with errors for boys but not for girls; however, correlations were nearly identical ($r = .33$ and $r = .32$, respectively). However, it was not clear whether this association would hold if conduct symptoms were statistically controlled for. Comorbid anxiety symptoms also were not controlled for.

Many of these issues were addressed in a careful follow-up study by the same group. Hartung et al. (2002, described earlier) recruited a fresh sample of clinic-referred adolescents, including adolescent boys and girls who met diagnostic criteria for ADHD, CD, and ADHD + CD. Both CD and ADHD symptoms were associated with errors in the mixed-incentive condition, consistent with a response modulation deficit. However, when CD and ADHD symptoms were examined simultaneously, for boys only CD symptoms were uniquely associated with errors, undercutting the finding related to ADHD. ADHD symptoms remained significant for girls. Results were independent of IQ, age, and reading ability, all of which were covaried. These data point to potential gender differences, but require further evaluation in light of the failure to show specificity with CD symptoms controlled for boys.

MOTIVATIONAL RESPONSES IN ADHD: SUMMARY

Overall, data on motivational problems in ADHD are mixed, and conclusions in this area are more tentative than in other areas of neuropsychology. The data provide tentative support for a modified reward dysfunction in ADHD-C, in which there is a steepened delay–reward gradient. Yet mixed findings continue to prevent firm conclusions about the core nature of this difficulty (Luman et al., 2005). Preliminary data are intriguing, but limited, regarding a possible response modulation problem in ADHD; this may be confined to ADHD + CD. An impaired avoidance system does not appear to characterize ADHD, although it may characterize a subgroup with ADHD + CD, and additional physiological studies are needed. This state of knowledge is sum-

TABLE 6.3. Score Card on Status of Motivational Effects in ADHD

Aspect of motivation	ADHD-C	ADHD-PI
Anxious inhibition of behavior	Intact	Probably intact
Reward response	Possibly affected	?
Response modulation	Insufficient data	?
Fear response	Intact?	?

marized in Table 6.3. Note that in the table I assume that most studies of children have examined anxiety rather than fear. This assumption may be debatable. In any event, it appears that as studied so far, low fear or low anxiety are not strong correlates of ADHD apart from CD.

CLINICAL IMPLICATIONS

The first crucial clinical implication from a motivational perspective is that during assessment, it is imperative to take note of whether the child's temperament is characterized by a fearful/high-anxiety style or a fearless/low-anxiety style. One straightforward evaluation approach here is to examine parent, teacher, and child self-report ratings of anxiety. The child self-report ratings can be obtained with the Multidimensional Anxiety Scale for Children (March, Parker, Sullivan, Stallings, & Conners, 1997), the State–Trait Anxiety Inventory for Children, or the Revised Children's Manifest Anxiety Scale (see Seligman, Ollendick, Langley, & Baldacci, 2004, for a comparative empirical analysis of these last two and other children's anxiety scales).

Note that a child can be both highly anxious and also impulsive or outgoing (these are two different temperament dimensions). The specific approach to behavioral intervention can be tailored for the child on the basis of an evaluation indicating whether the child has low or high anxiety. If the child has relatively low anxiety, then focusing on reward response may be especially useful. If the child has high anxiety, then focusing on behavioral consequences (response cost and mild punishment) may be effective and advisable. Work by Susan Crockenberg and her colleagues at the University of Vermont has provided fascinating empirical validation for this line of thinking. She finds that children with different temperament profiles, including high versus low anxiety, respond to distinct behavioral strategies differently (see Crockenberg & Leerkes, 2003, for a review). Likewise, the MTA (see Jensen et al., 2001) indicated that efficacy of treatment outcomes differed for children with ADHD plus anxiety without externalizing comorbidity (who responded equally well to behavioral or medication treatment) versus those with ADHD without anxiety (who responded best to medication intervention).

Thus the second obvious clinical implication of these insights concerns the structure of behavioral programming for the child when rewards are used. A common error is setting rewards or incentives too far into the future to motivate a child. For a child with ADHD at a given age, one may have to consider incentives closer in time to an event than otherwise, as one would with a somewhat younger child. For example, instead of rewards at the end of the week, some marker of reward may have to be provided immediately after behavior is successful (even if this is only a point or token for the weekly total). Parents may need to be guided to provide clear praise more frequently and immediately when a child is establishing appropriate behavior. Too often a behavioral program emphasizes costs or punishments, with insufficient attention to frequent reward. Also, the parents (or teachers) have too often neglected to maintain a positive and rewarding core relationship with the child. In the press of busy schedules and other demands, they may find that too many of their interactions are limit-setting and punishment/consequence-oriented. It may therefore be crucial to revise the behavioral program from the beginning, including instituting periods of unconditional positive interactions for a parent and child to build up their relationship. The latter, along with a reward-based behavioral plan for the child, may help boost the child's self-esteem as well, provided that care is taken to make the praise and reward authentic and not "pro forma."

The speculations about extinction learning are also fascinating in relation to potential clinical interventions and behavioral programming. For example, parents may have to persist in not reinforcing a maladaptive behavior—well beyond what they may consider a reasonable period of time or number of instances—before the child learns the implicit lesson that the behavior is not reinforced. Understanding the distinction between implicit associative learning and explicit information may be necessary in order for parents to recognize the need to persist in their response. To date, clinical studies have not deeply explored this concept, but it is an approach suggested by the theory that warrants more systematic behavioral and intervention testing.

Psychostimulant medication may work by enhancing the value of rewards (reinforcers) through dopamine release in the prefrontal corti-

TABLE 6.4. Frequently Asked Questions about ADHD and Motivation

Question	Answer
Why doesn't my child care about consequences?	Rewards may be too far away, or the child may have a weak response to potential punishment.
Why doesn't punishing my child work?	Some children respond more strongly to rewards than to punishments. Children vary temperamentally in their response to different types of discipline.
What does medication have to do with motivation?	Stimulants may strengthen the salience of rewards and make them seem more valuable to the child.

ces. With rewards now more salient, the child is better able to be motivated by less immediate considerations, and thus able to maintain appropriate behavior more easily.

In conclusion, consideration of the child's style (responding to rewards or responding to punishments), and of comorbid anxiety and conduct problems, may be most important for integrating the findings about motivational responses in ADHD. Frequently asked questions about ADHD and motivation are summarized in Table 6.4.

Motor Control and Timing

"Why is my son so clumsy? Is that part of his ADHD or something else?" "Why are some children with ADHD good athletes, while others appear to have motor delays?" In view of the historical importance of motor control problems to earlier conceptions of ADHD, notably the "minimal brain dysfunction" (MBD) concept (Clements & Peters, 1962), the underemphasis on motor control in recent ADHD assessment may seem surprising. Yet it may be seen as part of the field's reaction to the overinclusiveness of the old MBD concept. Indeed, highlighting motor control problems in ADHD could run the risk of returning us to an overinclusive understanding of the syndrome. At the same time, some analysis of this domain of impairment is vital to a complete account of different developmental pathways involved in ADHD.

In addition, problems with temporal information processing (e.g., "When my daughter is asked to wait an hour, why does she return in 10 minutes?"), long suspected in relation to impulsivity, appear relevant (Toplak et al., in press) and may be related to motor control problems in some children with ADHD (Piek et al., 2004). Although temporal information processing can be related to executive functioning (Chapter 5), it is also particularly relevant to the neural linkage in cerebellar–cortical loops in the brain. Therefore, this chapter considers both motor control and the processing of time, which (speculatively) may share a diathesis in the cerebellum's involvement in ADHD.

SEVERAL LINES OF RESEARCH ON MOTOR CONTROL/
TIMING PROBLEMS IN ADHD

I have noted earlier that rapid motor output is a problem in ADHD and may be related to response activation (Borger & van der Meere, 2000; Sergeant et al., 1999). I have also noted that the basal ganglia and the cerebellum—both structures classically associated with motor control—appear to be involved in ADHD. Sagvolden et al. (2005), in their dopamine theory of ADHD, posit that problems in the nigral–striatal dopamine pathway (important to motor control and involved in Parkinson's disease; see Chapter 3, Figure 3.1) may be a secondary feature of ADHD because the pervasive dopaminergic dysfunction affects all dopamine systems. These historical findings and recent theories raise the question of motor control as a factor in ADHD.

Clinicians, especially those trained in neuropsychology, may often note motor control problems in children with ADHD (Szatmari, Offord, & Boyle, 1989), even though they are no longer used as part of the diagnosis. Although major theories tend to underemphasize motor control, ADHD is often associated with a variety of motor control timing problems. These problems may be related to at least two central neuropsychological systems—the nigral–striatal dopamine pathways that are involved in fine and gross motor response *execution*, and the cerebellar–cortical pathways that are involved in temporal information processing and thus response *timing*.

Children with ADHD often have motor coordination problems (Piek, Pitcher, & Hay, 1999; Pitcher, Piek, & Hay, 2003) and have well-above chance rates of developmental coordination disorder as defined in the DSM (Gillberg, 2003). According to Gillberg's (2003) review, up to half of children with ADHD may have developmental coordination problems, depending on the sampling method used. This work also outlines a range of both gross and fine motor control problems, some of which may co-occur with particular ADHD subtypes. However, Karatekin, Markiewics, and Siegel (2003) noted that parents rated significantly more clumsiness and motor developmental delays in children with ADHD, even in a sample that failed to meet criteria for developmental coordination disorder; this finding suggests that subtle motor problems may be an issue even when the full criteria for the coordination disorder are not reached.

Earlier neurological thinking about minimal brain dysfunction included the idea that assessment of motor control (e.g., balance, overflow movements, and fine motor coordination) was a somewhat more objective indicator of a developmental condition than were behavior problems (Mostofsky, Newschaffer, & Denckla, 2003b). Following up on this earlier tradition, Denckla and Ruddell (1978) helped continue and develop thinking about motor control in ADHD. Their work emphasized overflow movements—either "mirror movements" (i.e., movement on the left side of the body while attempting to execute a difficult movement on the right side, or vice versa) or movement in the arms while attempting to execute a difficult foot movement. Recent work by Denckla and colleagues has been based on the idea that such movements may be related to failure of inhibitory mechanisms, including transcallosal mechanisms, which suppress excess movements during motor programming and execution (Mostofsky et al., 2003b). This line of work may reflect the role of the basal ganglia, sensory–motor cortex, and corpus callosum in ADHD.

This research group's assessment battery has been published as the Revised Neurological Examination for Subtle Signs (Denckla, 1985). It includes alternating movements and balancing tasks that are likely to probe cerebellar activity, as well as fine motor coordination tasks that probe activity of the prefrontal and premotor cortices and the basal ganglia. We (Carte et al., 1996) demonstrated that boys with ADHD had difficulty on both leg and arm movements, and that they also had difficulty on the alternating hand position task (a likely cerebellar probe); these effects were larger on more effortful than on less effortful versions of the tasks. We (Nigg et al., 1998) also showed that these effects were not explained by comorbid oppositional, conduct, or learning problems in this sample of boys diagnosed with DSM-III-R criteria. Thus these motor probes clearly tap a significant problem for typical samples with ADHD.

More generally, work emanating primarily from Sweden has focused heavily on developmental coordination disorder in its overlap with ADHD (Gillberg & Rasmussen, 1982; Gillberg, Rasmussen, Carstrom, Svenson, & Waldenstrom, 1982; Kadesjo & Gillberg, 1998). The assessment tools used in this work have included surveys relying on the DSM criteria for developmental coordination disorder (see APA, 2000, for the current version of these criteria), as well as a direct assessment battery. This battery also emphasizes alternation and balancing tasks that probably require intact cerebellar functioning (Gillberg, Carstrom, Rasmussen, & Waldenstrom, 1983). However, a wide range of potential movement problems are considered in their work. Pitcher et al. (2003) used the Movement Assessment Battery for Children (Henderson & Sugden, 1992) and found that boys with

ADHD-C and ADHD-PI (but not ADHD-PHI) subtypes had impaired fine motor ability. They concluded that fine motor problems in ADHD were apparent and were not due only to inattention or hyperactivity. Effects were not observed in balance or gross motor abilities, but the sample sizes were small. However, other work from the Swedish researchers indicates that children with ADHD have difficulty modulating grip force (Pereira, Eliasson, & Forssberg, 2000; Pereira, Landgren, Gillberg, & Forssberg, 2001; Steger et al., 2001), which may be more likely to reflect abnormality in striatal (basal ganglia) structures than in the cerebellum (Ivry, 2003). Moreover, difficulty in preparing and planning complete movements—examined in several studies of children with ADHD, using tasks that assess simple accuracy and velocity of arm and hand movements (Eliasson, Rosblad, & Forssberg, 2004; Yan & Thomas, 2002)—indicates problems that go beyond the cerebellum and involve basal ganglia and cortical motor control systems. In particular, it is possible that jerky movements on arm target tasks could reflect poor planning or poor control, implicating the basal ganglia or frontal regions.

Another program of work has emanated from Australia. Researchers there have also found a high degree of association between motor control problems and ADHD (Pitcher et al., 2003). A key question is whether this association is explained by problems in executive functioning or in timing. Piek et al. (2004) found that children with developmental coordination disorder and those with attention problems as measured by the Child Behavior Checklist (CBCL) shared deficits in response time and variability of response time, but not in measures of executive functioning. This suggests that the subcortical networks may be the most important for understanding the overlap of ADHD and developmental coordination problems. It also suggests the potential for discriminating children with attention problems into those with motor control or timing problems, and those with executive functioning problems—a speculative possibility that awaits further verification.

As alluded to already, yet another recent line of work has begun to explore the role of motor timing and temporal control of response directly (Barkley, Koplowitz, Anderson, & McMurray, 1997; Barkley et al., 2001a; Barkley, Murphy, & Bush, 2001b; Toplak et al., 2003; for a review, see Toplak et al., in press). This work has been influenced both by Barkley's (1997) theory emphasizing temporal organization of behavior as mediated by prefrontal areas, and by increasing interest in cerebellar involvement in ADHD in terms of disruption of an "internal clock" (temporal processing) as well as motor control. For example, Brown and Vickers (2004) found that a small group of adolescents with ADHD had more difficulty on timing tasks only when they required a motor response. Ben-Pazi, Gross-Tsur, Bergman, and Shalev (2003) found that children with ADHD failed to modulate their rate of tapping to a preset tempo, consistent with cerebellar problems. In a comprehensive review of a large number of methodologically varying studies emphasizing the role of the cerebellar network in temporal processing, Toplak et al. (in press) concluded that ADHD is related to problems in duration discrimination, duration reproduction, and finger tapping. Thus the temporal processing problems may be more fundamental than the motor control problems. Further, more refined analysis of temporal processing could therefore lead to increasing emphasis on it in understanding the etiology of ADHD, as well as the cognitive processing problems associated with ADHD.

CONSOLIDATION OF CEREBELLAR, STRIATAL, AND FRONTAL INVOLVEMENT IN ADHD AND MOTOR CONTROL/TIMING

As should be clear from the preceding discussion, ADHD often co-occurs with subtle difficulties in motor coordination of varying kinds. These appear to be diffuse and to involve a range of motor control problems, perhaps reflecting subgroups with different types of motor involvement. Motor control problems in ADHD are not surprising, but are underresearched; it is unclear whether they are nonspecific indicators of immature CNS development, reflect a specific causal pathway to ADHD, or characterize a particular subgroup with CNS insult (see Chapters 10–11). If they are exhibited by a subgroup with early CNS insult, then these difficulties may be extremely important in tracing etiological pathways. Thus, perhaps ironically in light of its much-maligned historical status and overinclusive nature, the old "minimal brain dysfunction" concept may have a kernel of truth in light of more recent research on development and more subtle probes of neural functioning.

Motor control/motor timing problems may reflect central processing problems with preparing and maintaining a ready response state (Sergeant et al., 1999). Alternatively or in addition, they may emerge from involvement of frontal and prefrontal (and perhaps premotor) regions in programming motor responses accurately. Finally, they may involve execution of motor responses involving either the basal ganglia (e.g., inappropriate force of response) or the cerebellum (e.g., improper timing and temporal integration of motor movements). Any of these routes could be consistent with dopaminergic dysfunction in ADHD. However, whereas the basal ganglia are clearly involved in ADHD, the structures that appear to be involved are the caudate and the globus pallidus—not the substantia nigra, the putamen, or other structures thought to lie primarily in the motor pathway. Nonetheless, the heavy dopaminergic moderation of this system has led to suggestions that it may be impaired in some aspects of ADHD (Johansen et al., 2002). Perhaps this pathway is involved for a subset of children with ADHD.

On the other hand, imaging studies consistently implicate the cerebellum in ADHD—in particular, hypoplasia of vermis lobules VIII–X (Swanson & Castellanos, 2002; Ivry, 2003), underscoring interest in temporal processing and timing. It is clear, however, that the motor control problems associated with the disorder extend beyond what would be expected to derive merely from cerebellar insult. Rather, a more diffuse and distributed involvement appears likely. Overall, from the viewpoint of theoretical as well as clinical conceptions of ADHD, it may be very important to recognize the potential for etiological subtyping with regard to clumsiness, developmental coordination disorder, and motor difficulties generally. Integration of this line of thinking with neuropsychological models continues to require refinement, but these problems may be closely related to the motor output (activation) problems identified in the cognitive–energetic model of Sergeant et al. (1999). As with other domains of difficulty in ADHD, identifying specificity vis-á-vis other conditions requires continued work. For example, autistic disorder is also associated with abnormal cerebellar functioning (albeit potentially in a distinct region of the vermis from that involved in ADHD), and learning disabilities appear to involve overlaps with clumsiness, coordination problems, and timing problems similar to those seen in ADHD.

Prefrontal involvement also seems likely when one considers findings such as motor overflow. As discussed cogently by Mostofsky et al. (2003b), the concept here is that bilateral overflow problems emerge from the relative immaturity of cortical systems—presumably in premotor regions and the supplemental motor area (Mostofsky et al., 2003a)—that inhibit spreading activation to motor regions (bilaterally) during unilateral motor movement. Whether these top-down cortical systems involved in suppressing unintended movement during effortful motor execution are the same as those needed to interrupt an intended movement upon new information remains to be seen; the latter may, for instance, entail greater bottom-up striatal activation (Casey et al., 2002), as well as prefrontal activation (Aron et al., 2003a; Mostofsky et al., 2003a). However, some evidence suggests that the motor suppression abilities discussed in Chapter 5 (response inhibition or response suppression generally) and in the present chapter are correlated (Mostofsky et al., 2003b).

Motor control is interesting from the viewpoint of dual-process theories of ADHD in relation to symptom domains. Many of the functions discussed in this book (e.g., executive functioning) are largely *cognitive* in nature and may be expected to be related to inattention and disorganization, and perhaps to impulsivity. However, how they relate to *motor* hyperactivity has been less obvious. It may be that a second system related to motor functioning must be included for a full understanding of ADHD. Yet the literature reflects quite distinct hypotheses about how motor control per se may relate to the two-factor structure of the ADHD clinical profile. As summarized in Figure 7.1, one approach links motor inhibition problems with executive functioning (Sonuga-Barke, 2002); this approach is supported by data from our laboratory at Michigan State indicating that deficits in motor inhibition as well as executive functioning generally are specifically correlated with symptoms of inattention and disorganization, rather than with symptoms of hyperactivity–impulsivity (Nigg et al., 2005a). On the other hand, motor control and motor inhibition might be linked to hyperactivity (Mostofsky et al., 2003b). Further empirical specification of these relations will ultimately be needed to clarify matters.

Model 1:

Motor disinhibition → Executive functioning (planning) problems → Inattention, disorganization, and motor control/overflow problems

Model 2:

Motor disinhibition and motor control problems → Hyperactivity and hyperkinesis

---

FIGURE 7.1. Two implicit models for how motor control per se relates to ADHD clinical profile.

CLINICAL IMPLICATIONS

Despite the excesses of an earlier era, in which all manner of "soft signs" were taken as diagnostic of minimal brain dysfunction, recognition of motor control problems in a subset of children with ADHD may be quite important. Some data suggest that long-term outcomes are more serious when ADHD is accompanied by motor coordination problems (Gillberg, 2003). It may thus be important to identify and intervene in motor control problems for children with ADHD. Two overarching issues are noteworthy.

The first major issue is that standardized methods for assessment of motor functioning are not well agreed upon. Ivry (2003) notes that in the neurology literature, basal ganglia problems are presumably involved in choreiform movements (spasmodic or small jerky movements like those associated with Huntington's disease) and athetoid movements (slow writhing such as flexion, extension, or pronation of fingers and hands), whereas cerebellar problems are associated with dysdiadochokinesis (difficulty with rapidly alternating movements, such as the alternating hand supination–pronation featured in Denckla's [1985] motor battery), intentional tremor, and dysmetria (inability to arrest a movement at the desired point). Often these are simple to observe in neurological illness. The more subtle difficulties associated with ADHD will not be as obvious as those seen in neurological illness, but may be detected in some cases by more formal challenges.

Therefore, clinical and educational psychologists and neuropsychologists may wish to assess motor control in some normative way. Several batteries have been developed and published for this purpose. The Test of Motor Impairment was an early measure, which was subsequently replaced with the Movement Assessment Battery for Children (Henderson & Sugden, 1992). The latter is normed for ages 4–12 and requires 20 minutes to administer; it includes both a parent rating scale and a battery of fine motor tasks (manual dexterity), tests of ball skills, and balance tasks.

The Bruininks–Oseretsky Test of Motor Proficiency, Second Edition (Bruininks & Bruininks, 2006) includes subtests designed to assess gross motor development (running speed and agility, balance, strength, and bilateral coordination), fine and gross motor skills (upper limb coordination), and fine motor skills (speed, visual–motor control, and dexterity). A short form requires 15 minutes for a total score; the full version requires 45–60 minutes.

A range of other tools may warrant consideration. The Denckla (1985) Revised Neurological Examination for Subtle Signs is excellent for spotting motor overflow and getting a clinical impression of cerebellar and frontal motor control functions. For example, the hand pronation–supination test (Carte et al., 1996; Nigg et al., 1998) and finger sequential movements used by Denckla (1985) may provide a rough index of integrity of cerebellar systems. This battery has also been productive in the research literature demonstrating ADHD motor control difficulties (Carte et al., 1996). However, it lacks standardization and the normative data that would be needed for proper psychometric assessment. The Purdue Pegboard (see Lezak et al., 2004) is widely used to assess fine motor dexterity. The Wide Range Assessment of Visual–Motor Abilities also includes a pegboard task, but without the manipulative demands of the Purdue Pegboard. However, neither of these two pegboard tasks probes the timing, cerebellar, balance, or overflow functions that may be crucial in identifying motor control problems in children with ADHD. The Finger Tapping Test (from the Halstead–Reitan battery) assesses output speed, but again does not get at the features of cerebellar and callosal functioning often cited in the literature. The NEPSY (Korkman et al., 1998; Kemp et al., 2001) also includes a finger-tapping test for fine motor assessment. Finally, developmental level of motor control may also be estimated in terms of real-world functioning by careful interview of parents and observation of the child, using such normative developmental ratings as the Scales of Independent Behavior.

Thus clinicians are advised not to overlook the gross and fine motor domains in their evaluation of children with possible ADHD. As Gillberg (2003) points out, it is diagnostically crucial to determine carefully whether motor problems and perceived clumsiness result from impulsivity and failure to pay attention (i.e., a child knocks things over because of overactivity and rambunctiousness), or whether there are also primary motor problems (e.g., the child cannot throw a ball well, cannot button clothes, has labored/poorly controlled handwriting, and/or hates physical education class because of difficulty with coordination).

The second major issue concerns how to design the intervention. Fortunately, many intervention programs are available, once a clinician overcomes the tendency to overlook motor functioning entirely in the ADHD evaluation. As a first step, if initial clinical assessment suggests that motor development and coordination may be contributing to a

child's functional or self-esteem problems, or if initial neuropsychological evaluation indicates motor problems, then it may be beneficial to
refer the child for an occupational therapy evaluation. Such an evaluation can address real-world limitations of motor control and may suggest exercises that can assist with pragmatic and even athletic skills,
muscle strength and balance, and coordination. Many different intervention programs along these lines are available. Gillberg (2003) notes
that informing the child's physical education teacher about the motor
difficulties may take some pressure off the child and help resolve problems with participation in sports. Muscle strength (hypotonia), posture,
body image, and fine motor control (pencil grip, writing) all may
require remediation, and remediation programs for all of these are
available in the occupational therapy literature. Of course, if the child
is very young, and/or if motor problems are marked and have not been
medically evaluated, then referral for neurological evaluation may be
appropriate. DSM-IV-TR (APA, 2000) makes it clear that cerebral palsy
or other primary neurological disorders supersede developmental
coordination disorder diagnostically.

    With regard to a handwriting problem, it is essential to evaluate
whether the problem is with difficulty in language and verbal production, or if the difficulty is in the effortfulness and laboriousness of fine
motor control (as identified on some of the tests just noted, as well as
on observation of writing attempts). If motor control is the problem,
Pennington (1991) suggests that the most important intervention is to
train the child in keyboarding. Contrary to what people who are not
touch typists may think, the motor control requirements for keyboarding are much less than for handwriting.

    Problems in time perception and temporal processing may be
important, of course, over and above motor control problems per se.
Such problems might affect the ability to learn and to organize behavior. They have not been emphasized in this clinical comment because,
with regard to assessment of problems in temporal information processing and time reproduction, standardized assessment tools are in
short supply. Various new assessment methods are still under development (Toplak et al., in press) that will provide a more refined analysis
of these mechanisms. Eventually, clinicians may have additional tools in
hand with which to evaluate temporal processing as well.

    Finally, in framing the pertinent issues for parents, children, and
educators, the clinician may be able to ease some frustration and provide a sense of direction by helping caregivers to understand that

TABLE 7.1. Frequently Asked Questions about Motor Control and Timing in ADHD

Question	Answer
Why is my child so clumsy?	The child may have motor development problems that need to be addressed specifically.
Is my child's clumsiness part of his or her ADHD?	It is not part of the diagnosis, but often goes with ADHD.
Does a minute seem like an hour to my child?	It may, much as it does with younger children.

motor control delays are distinct from motivational, cognitive, or other self-control problems with which the caregivers are concerned. Helping caregivers see these distinctions may be empowering for them, may help them focus their guidance of a child more effectively, and may enable them to generate additional ideas for helping the child. Table 7.1 provides some examples of frequently asked questions relevant to motor control and time perception in ADHD.

SUMMARY AND CONCLUSION

Motor control problems are often overlooked in the assessment of children with ADHD. Although they are not diagnostic of ADHD, and despite the fact that they have often been overlooked in a "post-MBD" clinical world, they remain frequent overlapping problems and contribute to social and academic impairments. Several assessment tools are available for initial screening in a neuropsychological evaluation; referral for an occupational or physical therapy assessment may be indicated in some instances. The presence of motor control problems should alert the clinician to the possibility of a right-hemisphere dysfunction or nonverbal learning disability syndrome (Rourke et al., 2002). Neuropsychological assessment of this possibility may provide needed information for complete academic, social, and occupational planning for the child. Moreover, in terms of our quest for the etiology of ADHD and a conceptual understanding of its development, the frequent presence of frank motor control problems in ADHD is a stark reminder both of the involvement of subcortical structures in the syndrome, and of the strong possibility that some children with ADHD have experienced early CNS insult. The latter point may prove a power-ful clue in considering particular etiological pathways in ADHD, as we will see in Part II of this book.

Finally, the role of timing, time perception, and temporal informa-tion processing (all abilities that involve cerebellum or cerebellar–frontal connections in the brain) in ADHD is only now beginning to be appreciated. It remains unclear how far the field can go in using time perception problems to account for ADHD, but it seems likely that future theories will have to include an account of cerebellar function and of temporal information processing in particular.

PART III

WHERE DOES ADHD COME FROM?

Multiple Pathways

ETIOLOGICAL HETEROGENEITY

Clinicians and educators will readily recognize that not all children diagnosed with ADHD are alike. ADHD seems to be a heterogeneous condition. Indeed, popular books on ADHD emphasize its multiplicity (Amen, 2001). Clinical or educational observation makes it apparent that some children with ADHD are anxious, whereas others are fearless; some have motor coordination problems, while others are good athletes; some are hostile, whereas others are friendly; some have high IQs and find schoolwork easy to understand, while others have learning disabilities or below-average language skills. Likewise, some have average psychological test scores on neuropsychological examination, but others have multiple impairments. Some of their families are cohesive and high-functioning; others are overwhelmed and disorganized.

This variety may even be so overarching that inattention or hyperactivity perhaps should be thought of simply as a final symptomatic pathway for numerous conditions—in much the same way as we now think of a fever. Alternatively (and less drastically), perhaps ADHD should be thought of as a valid syndromal entity, but one that describes a wide set of conditions—much as we now think of cancer. Still another option is to view these differences as unimportant ancillary features of a shared, core disorder. This third option, however, is difficult to defend, because these variations typically exceed chance levels of variation (defined as population base rates). Thus they are telling us something about the nature of the problem.

Therefore, a fourth option, which I follow, is to think of ADHD as a valid syndromal entity—but one that is arrived at via a relatively discrete set of causal pathways, which may lead to somewhat different manifestations of the disorder (including its associated neuropsychological profiles). In other words, ADHD may have etiological "types," although these are not yet recognized or agreed upon in the field.

Similar concepts of multiple pathways or multiple causal streams into ADHD have been noted by several theorists (e.g., Castellanos & Tannock, 2002; Nigg, 2001; Nigg, Goldsmith, & Sachek, 2004b; Sagvolden et al., 1998). The idea was given further impetus by Sonuga-Barke (2002), who developed a relatively formal theory of multiple pathways to ADHD that emphasized both excutive and reward-based processes. He subsequently elaborated on this view (Sonuga-Barke, 2003) and his most recent work on this subject (Sonuga-Barke, 2005) dovetails well with the perspective outlined here. Significantly, he urged a shift from searching for a single core dysfunction to identifying multiple developmental pathways in which the varying deficits might be considered complementary rather than competitive (Sonuga-Barke, 2005, p. 1235). This general idea has become of keen interest to the field and therefore receives detailed coverage and further extension here.

Why do I think that children with ADHD may be neuropsychologically heterogeneous? Two basic considerations guide this argument. The first is the evidence reviewed in Chapters 4–7 for the effects on several neuropsychological functions in ADHD. Although it is conceivable that all of these different findings will be reducible to a single core deficit, I judge this to be unlikely. We are more likely to find that these different neuropsychological deficits are each needed to best capture the problems of meaningful subgroups of children with ADHD. Work on the covariation of these different types of neuropsychological problems will clarify the extent to which this supposition holds.

The second consideration is the high distributional overlap of ADHD and nondisabled control children on individual neuropsychological measures. The effect sizes on the most sensitive neuropsychological instruments, taken from Chapters 4–7, are summarized in Table 8.1. These testify to both the importance of significant neuropsychological problems in ADHD at the group level (supporting its validity as a genuine disorder marked by internal dysfunction; see Chapter 2) and the overlap in score distributions. To explain this concept further, I recap the logic that several colleagues and I have presented (Nigg et al., 2005b) in a recent summary meant to spur discussion of this possibility.

Consider the distribution of scores on, say, executive function measures in a sample of children with ADHD versus a sample of nondisordered children. Established effect sizes are in the range of $d = 0.60$–0.80 (60–80% of a standard deviation; see Chapter 3; I assume that the large effect shown for spatial working memory in Table 8.1 will shrink with additional studies). A d of 0.80 is equivalent to approximately a 50% overlap in score distributions between samples (Cohen, 1988). As noted in Chapter 3, Cohen (1988) offers that this effect size on the one hand may be considered "large." It is equivalent to the difference in IQ between people with PhDs and average college freshmen, or between college graduates and those with only a 50–50 chance of graduating from high school, or the average height difference between 13- and 18-year-old girls. So it is not insubstantial, and might very well reflect a true difference between two homogeneous but distinct populations.

On the other hand, in the context of identifying the etiological mechanisms of a mental or behavioral disorder, a 50% overlap in scores raises some concerns with regard to the likelihood that we have identified a causal driver of *all* cases of the disorder. In effect, some

TABLE 8.1. Summary of Neuropsychological Findings in ADHD

Domain	Status	Meta-analytic effect size (d)
Attention		
Perceptual selection	4	NA
Reflexive orienting	4	0.20
Alerting/vigilance system	1	0.75
Cognitive control/executive functioning		
Interference control	4	0.20
Working memory verbal	2	0.45
Working memory spatial	1	1.00
Planning	2	0.55
Response inhibition	1	0.60
Set shifting	2	0.50
Activation	3	NA
Motivation		
Reactive (anxious) inhibition	4	NA
Reward response (approach)	2	NA
Motor control and timing		
Motor control	2	NA
Temporal processing	2	NA

Note. Ratings of status: 1, replicated deficit, substantial in size (reliably larger than 0.50, based on number of studies; confidence interval around pooled effect size); 2, deficit probably exists, but aggregate effects are modest in size (not reliably larger than 0.50) or consistent results rely on a small number of studies (so pooled effect size has wide confidence interval); 3, possible deficit, but findings are mixed across different indicators, and positive findings rest on a small number of studies; 4, spared, or effect is too trivial in size to be clinically meaningful. NA, not available or not applicable. Effect sizes are rounded-off estimates; see Chapters 4–7 for details.

children with ADHD may be "carrying" the group effect, and those children may thus be an important subgroup to understand.

Circumstantial support for this supposition comes from the observation that samples of children with ADHD invariably exhibit greater *sample* variance (not to be confused with *within-child* variability) in their scores than do control samples. In clinical measurement, this excess sample variance is almost always on the "poor performance" end of the distribution. Thus we can argue that (1) the ADHD and control performance distributions overlap to a substantial degree in all studies, and (2) some children with ADHD perform in the average range. Consistent with that picture, efforts to evaluate the clinical predictive power of executive function tests in relation to ADHD tend to show that these tests have worthwhile sensitivity, but poor specificity (Barkley, Grodzinsky, & DuPaul, 1992; Doyle, Biederman, Seidman, Weber, & Faraone, 2000; Grodzinsky & Barkley, 1999; Hinshaw et al., 2002). In other words, individuals with "bad scores" are likely to have ADHD, but only a minority of children with ADHD exhibit a deficit on any specific test. Therefore, the absence of a specific neurocognitive weakness cannot be used to rule out ADHD (Grodzinsky & Barkley, 1999).

Such clinical results are expected when (1) there is substantial distributional overlap, (2) sample variances are unequal, and (3) the ADHD sample tail is on the "bad" end of the distribution. In short, the group effects reported in the literature may well be carried by a *subset* of the children with ADHD.

Table 8.2 illustrates the degree of sample overlap and percentage affected (when a 90th-percentile cutoff was used) in three major centers studying ADHD in the United States. As it shows, even with robust p values and effect sizes, most children with ADHD fell within the "normal" range (less than 90th percentile) on each task. We (Nigg et al., 2005b) repeated this exercise with all neuropsychological tasks available at these three centers; none achieved better group separation. One might get slightly larger separation of groups with a measure of working memory or motor control, but it likely would not be substantially different from that shown here.

This can be outlined in more detail using data from the Michigan State ADHD Project (as Table 8.2 shows, very similar results have been found in other major projects studying ADHD; see Nigg et al., 2005b). If we designate the 90th percentile as the cutoff for "normal" versus "impaired" performance, we can classify children as "normal" or "impaired" on their neuropsychological scores. On the stop task (our best-performing measure on this exercise with $d \sim 0.9$ and $p < .001$),

TABLE 8.2. Illustrative Widely Used Neuropsychological Measures Comparing Children with ADHD-C to Controls: Group Differences and Percentage Classified as "Impaired" in Three Samples

Measure	Sample	Effect size			% with ADHD-C scoring beyond control 90th percentile
		d	η^2	p	
SSRT	MI (all)	0.88	0.133	< .001	51
	CO	0.79	0.101	< .001	45
RT variability	MI	0.75	0.123	< .001	48
	CO	0.77	0.125	< .001	44
Stroop color word	MI	0.50	0.045	< .05	25
	CO	0.84	0.132	< .001	44
	MGH	0.62	0.09	< .001	25
CPT	MI	0.91	0.11	< .001	37
	CO	0.54	0.053	< .001	35
	MGH	0.17	0.01	.11	16
Trail Making	MI	0.35	0.033	< .05	27
	CO	0.35	0.031	< .01	24

Note. CO, Colorado; MGH, Massachusetts General Hospital; MI, Michigan State; RT, reaction time; SSRT, stop signal reaction time; CPT, continuous-performance test commission errors; Trail Making, Trails B time. The MI data (Nigg et al., 2004a) were obtained through a multistage community recruitment and screening procedure using parent and teacher ratings, culminating in a structured diagnostic interview to confirm diagnoses. Sex was covaried in the MI analysis. The Colorado sample (Willcutt et al., 2005a) was a subset of participants from the Colorado Learning Disabilities Research Center twin study (DeFries et al., 1997). A school-based screening procedure was used to identify twin pairs in which at least one twin met symptom criteria for DSM-IV ADHD, and full DSM-IV diagnostic criteria were used to confirm diagnoses. One twin from each pair was randomly selected for these analyses. The MGH sample (Biederman et al., 1997) consisted of children consecutively referred to a pediatric psychopharmacology clinic (n = 405). Children were comprehensively evaluated with structured diagnostic interviews. Children in each sample also completed other measures, but none provided any result substantially different from what we illustrate with selected measures here. Data on ADHD-PI and ADHD-PHI are omitted (results for those groups were never better than for ADHD-C). Sample breakdowns: MGH, 231 controls (109 boys, 122 girls), 145 children with ADHD-C (59 boys, 86 girls); MI, 62 controls (37 boys, 25 girls), 79 children with ADHD-C (61 boys, 18 girls); CO, 307 controls (137 boys, 170 girls), 63 children with ADHD-C (45 boys, 18 girls). d, effect size statistic in standard deviation units; η^2, partial eta squared, or effect size in terms of proportion of variance explained (Cohen, 1988). Adapted from Nigg, Willcutt, Doyle, and Sonuga-Barke (2005b). Copyright 2005 by the Society of Biological Psychiatry. Adapted by permission.

that cutoff point classified 10% of control children and 50% of children with ADHD as "neuropsychologically impaired." In other words, if one attempted to define a group of children with ADHD and "impaired" response inhibition in a clinical situation, one would identify about half of the children with ADHD. The others would remain unexplained. These unexplained cases might have a dysfunction in vigilance, reward response, or working memory, or (in a few instances), no dysfunction at all.

This observation in no way disqualifies executive functioning (or response inhibition) as a potential causal contributor to ADHD. Were we to repeat the exercise with any other leading putative ADHD dysfunction, we would find a similar story. Of course, this observation may simply indicate that two different populations of children still overlap somewhat in their clinical profile. But another and more interesting possibility is that there may be multiple pathways to ADHD, with only one of those pathways involving impaired response inhibition.

How might we evaluate this second possibility? Several studies have now approached this question in different ways. One powerful approach is to attempt to validate a putative "neuropsychologically impaired" ADHD subtype by family data. That is, do the relatives of children with ADHD and neuropsychological problems have poor neuropsychological performance themselves? Our recent report from the Michigan State project (Nigg et al., 2004a) provided a first look at this question. We divided the sample of children with ADHD into those that were affected and unaffected by neuropsychological impairment (according to by the 90th percentile rule), and then looked at neuropsychological performance in their first-degree *relatives*. We repeated this analysis for several tasks, including measures of response inhibition (SSRT), set shifting (Trails B), and state regulation (response time variability).

A heterogeneity model would predict that the relatives of children with ADHD but without evident neuropsychological impairment would not differ from relatives of control children, and that both groups would do better than relatives of children with both ADHD and evident neuropsychological impairment. Most of the results supported that model. For SSRT and response time variability, for example, the relatives of "impaired" children with ADHD indeed performed worse than the relatives of "nonimpaired" ADHD and "normal" control children ($p < .01$), whereas the latter two did not differ. Note that this finding held despite the fact that the two groups with ADHD had similar levels of symptom severity. Related findings associating aspects of family history with neuropsychological impairments were reported by

Crosbie and Schachar (2001), Schachar et al. (2005), and Seidman et al. (1995).

In a similar effort, Biederman et al. (2004) looked at impairment as an external validator of a "neuropsychologically impaired" subtype. They defined the impaired group at 1.5 standard deviations from the "normal" mean on a composite executive functioning score (not very different from the 90th percentile); this led to 33% of children with ADHD being placed in the "neurocognitively impaired" subgroup. That group also showed more impairment than the other children with ADHD in academic achievement, even though they had no more comorbid psychiatric disorders than the other children with ADHD did.

A second approach is to put competing pathways to work in the same regression model, as we have recently described (Nigg et al., 2005b). Our first example built on a finding by Solanto et al. (2001a) that a delay aversion task (a measure of how heavily a child weights a delayed vs. immediate reward) and inhibitory deficit (SSRT on the stop task) independently predicted ADHD status when included in the same regression model. We revisited those data courtesy of Mary Solanto and Edmund Sonuga-Barke, using our standard 90th percentile single-task cutoff. We found poor inhibitory control in 46% and poor delay aversion in 39% of the group with ADHD; 15% had delay aversion only and 23% had "pure" inhibitory deficits; and 39% had neither.

Using the same logic with a different set of pathways in the Michigan State sample, my lab (Nigg, 2006) assessed child perception of parental couple conflict (a known contributor to child disruptive behaviors; Grych & Fincham, 1990), along with response inhibition (SSRT) as an executive measure. These two risk factors correlated only $r = .03$ (n.s.), and in a simultaneous multiple regression to predict number of parent- and teacher-rated symptoms of ADHD exhibited by the child, both content of couple conflict (beta = .34, $p < .001$) and SSRT (beta = .29, $p < .001$) contributed uniquely. Of the children with ADHD-C, 42% had impaired stop inhibition and 62% had experienced extreme parental couple conflict (more than the 90th percentile for the control group), including 30% with both impaired inhibitory control and extreme couple conflict; 13% had only inhibitory dyscontrol and 32% had experienced only couple conflict; finally, 25% of the children with ADHD had neither extreme problem.

These data are only preliminary, but they suggest that it is plausible that ADHD (here, ADHD-C) reflects the final common outcome of multiple specific pathways. One pathway may involve a breakdown in the ability to rapidly suppress prepotent responses, and perhaps other executive function problems as well. A partially independent pathway may involve breakdowns in reward/reinforcement response, perhaps rooted in a shortened delay–reward gradient due to abnormal dopamine firing in the frontal–limbic circuit. A third path, perhaps overlapping with the second, may involve family conflict and psychosocial distress.

Could these partially distinct pathways reflect distinct etiologies or causes? I believe that this possibility deserves exploration. The idea of etiological heterogeneity needs to be modeled and further evaluated, preferably in population-based samples, so that such etiological subtyping can begin to be identified if it really exists. As this book turns to different etiological possibilities for ADHD in the ensuing chapters, it is important to keep in mind the possibility of different etiological pathways, perhaps operating through different within-child neuropsychological mechanisms. It may be that one type of insult or cause leads to one pathway (executive and/or reward response dysfunction), whereas another leads to an alternate ADHD cognitive phenotype.

ONE WAY FORWARD: DEVELOPMENTAL PATHWAYS BUILT ON EARLY TEMPERAMENTAL PRECURSORS

Ultimately, a developmental account is needed here if we wish to describe pathways. In this section I consider the idea of multiple pathways in relation to the development of self regulation using a temperament perspective (as introduced in Chapter 6). As Chapters 5 and 6 have illustrated, the development of self-regulation involves both reactive (affective or motivational) processes and effortful or controlled (executive or strategic control) processes (Rothbart & Bates, 1998; Eisenberg & Morris, 2002).

Direct parallels can be drawn between the traits identified by research on temperament and personality, and the neuropsychological functions discussed in the prior chapters (Nigg, 2000; Posner & Rothbart, 2000). Theories of temperament and personality posit a number of major traits. Although themes of temperament do not all agree, many theories still converge on the idea that the first three major traits are the following (see Chapter 6, especially Table 6.1):

1. The first major trait is labeled "approach" and is related to "extraversion" (Eysenck & Eysenck, 1985; Digman, 1990) or "positive affect" (Tellegen, 1985; Clark et al., 1994; Rothbart, Ahadi, Hershey, & Fisher, 2001). Extraversion (or "surgency") connotes positive affect but

also connotes social dominance, social confidence or sociability, and a preference for social interaction. From the perspective of the neural systems outlined in the prior chapters, extraversion corresponds to approach or positive anticipation of reward (Rothbart et al., 2001; Zuckerman, Kuhlman, Joireman, Teta, & Kraft, 1993), and is thought to be mediated in part by dopamine systems (Depue & Lenzenweger, 2005). Thus its involvement in ADHD could be consistent with the idea of dysfunctional reward circuitry as outlined in Chapter 6.

2. The second major trait is labeled "withdrawal" and is related to "neuroticism" (Eysenck & Eysenck, 1985; Digman, 1990) or "negative affect" (Tellegen, 1985; Rothbart et al., 2001). It primarily connotes difficulty coping with stress and high anxiety; secondarily, it connotes a propensity to sadness and depressed affect, thought to be related to limbic reactivity to threat or stress (Rothbart & Bates, 1998). However, when present in a high degree, this trait seems to be a general marker for psychopathology and is elevated in range of psychiatric disorders, including ADHD (Nigg et al., 2002d). Recall that in the negative affect realm, it is important to distinguish "anxiety" (response to uncertainty or potential punishment) from "fear" (response to certain or actual pain or immediate threat), as outlined in Chapter 6. Fear results in either a freeze response or a panic/flight response. It has distinct neural concomitants from anxiety, as explained in Chapter 6 (Gray, 1971; Depue & Lenzenweger, 2005). Negative affectivity in this sense is therefore related to reactive inhibition. Absence of or weak reactive inhibition is associated with conduct problems and psychopathy, but I have argued that it is not a direct driver of ADHD. Whether low anxiety, low fear, or both are key affective elements in some forms of antisocial behavior is an important issue. In the case of ADHD, little research supports low anxiety as a core issue when CD is absent (Chapter 6), and very little work on fear has been done.

3. The third major trait is called "conscientiousness" (Digman, 1990) or "constraint" (Tellegen, 1985) in personality research. In the case of children's temperament, it is called "effortful control" (Rothbart & Bates, 1998). This temperament trait is assessed in children by observing their deliberate strategies for managing frustration, temptation, and required waiting. For example, a child may look away from a very tempting forbidden toy so that the time will pass more easily. This trait connotes planful and organized approaches to life, as well as the ability in early childhood to deliberately override emotional and immediate reactions. Because it reflects the effortful redeployment of attention in the service of coping, theorists view this trait as related to the neuropsychological concept of executive functioning or cognitive

control, as described in Chapter 5. It thus is also related to the functioning and development of the anterior cortical neural circuitry (the same circuitry involved in working memory and response inhibition; see Chapters 3 and 5).

To find converging evidence for involvement of these networks in ADHD, we looked at personality traits. The pattern of relations between these "Big Three" traits and ADHD symptoms is similar to what we have seen for neuropsychological measures. Thus we (Nigg, Blaskey, Huang-Pollock, & John, 2002a; Nigg et al., 2002b) studied self-ratings and spouse/peer ratings of personality in several samples of adults (including college students, middle-aged parents of children with ADHD, and young adults with ADHD and controls). Symptoms of inattention and disorganization (the first ADHD symptom domain) were strongly related to low conscientiousness ($r = -.47$). Extraversion was related to hyperactivity–impulsivity, although this relationship was relatively weak, depended on which symptom scale was used, and seemed clearer for men than for women. Neuroticism was related to all areas of psychopathology, including ADHD. When we controlled for antisocial behavior, we found that hostility (low agreeableness, another trait in the "Big Five" model) was related to antisociality, but that low conscientiousness continued to be related to symptoms of ADHD.

To confirm these relations in children, we (Martel & Nigg, in press) used partial correlations to identify unique relations of reactive control, effortful control, and negative affect with domains of ADHD and other antisocial behaviors in a well-characterized childhood sample of 173 children with ADHD and controls (ages 7–13). Overlapping items were identified and removed from the temperament and psychopathology scales, and partial correlations were used to isolate unique relations between psychopathological symptom domains and temperament domains. Parent and teacher reports were examined. We found that there was a reliable, unique relation between low reactive control and hyperactive–impulsive symptoms (and that the relation of reactive control to oppositional and conduct problems was nonsignificant when hyperactive–impulsive symptoms were partialed out). Conversely, high oppositional behaviors were related to negative affect; the relation of ADHD symptoms to negative affect was removed when oppositional behaviors were partialed out. Inattention symptoms appeared to be related to either low effortful control or low resiliency, though this effect was difficult to replicate with teacher ratings.

Goldsmith, Lemery, and Essex (2004) followed children from birth through first grade, assessing them with multisource temperament measures and parent and teacher ratings of ADHD symptoms. Both cross-sectional and longitudinal multisource data indicated that ADHD was associated with low inhibitory control (effortful control), high anger, and hostile/aggressive behavior. Observational data were most illuminating, linking both the inattentive and hyperactive–impulsive behavior domains with low effortful control and anger, and linking hyperactivity–impulsivity primarily with high approach, though magnitudes of these associations were modest (r's in the .20–.30 range). Then, exemplifying the type of work needed to evaluate etiological linkages, Goldsmith et al., reported biometric model fitting of longitudinal twin data (controlling for item overlap). Both genetic and environmental sources of variance in early effortful control were shared with later ADHD symptoms. All of the genetic variance in later ADHD symptoms was in common with the genetic variance from earlier effortful control. This finding dovetails nicely with our personality data in linking ADHD specifically to the control domain of temperament as well as personality.

These traits and associations are summarized again in Table 8.3 (see also Table 6.1). The potential to bridge the neuropsychological findings in this way back to the temperament constructs is important, because it enables us to begin to imagine how early development might look, prior to the full emergence of abilities such as executive functions. The latter depend on difficult laboratory tasks that very young children (toddlers) cannot readily participate in. However, toddlers' ability to resist an impulse, their positive affect, and their negative affect can be reliably and validly measured by laboratory observations.

TABLE 8.3. Key Temperament and Personality Traits, and Empirical Relations to ADHD

Basic behavior	Affective activation	Neurobiology	Relation to ADHD
Approach	Anticipation of reward	Dopamine pathways	Weak/inconsistent, theoretical relation with impulsivity, hyperactivity
Withdrawal (anxiety)	Anxiety in response to uncertainty or possible punishment	Amygdala network	Neuroticism, low reactive control, related to impulsivity
Withdrawal (fear)	Fear, panic	Amygdala network	Low fear related to psychopathy, not ADHD
Effortful control	Nonaffective	Debated; prefrontal network; serotonin regulation of systems	Low effortful control related to ADHD, esp. inattention

From such observations, temperament researchers, particularly Rothbart and colleagues at the University of Oregon, have developed a conception of how these early traits develop. I follow Rothbart and Bates (1998) as well as Posner and Rothbart (2000) in summarizing that viewpoint here; see also Barkley (1997) for another more detailed developmental amount. Very early in infancy, responses to the environment are largely reflexive (orienting to what is novel, withdrawing from what is unpleasant). These reflexive responses may be seen as precursors to later automatic or posterior orienting of attention. I have noted in Chapter 4 that such reflexive orienting is generally spared in ADHD.

By middle infancy (about the middle of the first year), babies can be observed to approach and withdraw from opportunities around them, based on the associations they have learned—that is, based on seeing or hearing cues for anticipated reward (e.g., the sound of a caregiver approaching at mealtime) or cues for anticipated withdrawal of reward (e.g., the sound of a ringing telephone during a meal, which means that the caregiver has to stop feeding now because the phone is ringing). Positive and negative affect are now expressed in response to these learned cues (rather than only to pain or pleasure directly). This ability may be thought of as the precursor to the reactive approach (and withdrawal) tendencies discussed in Chapter 6. As I have noted there, differences in the development of reward/approach tendencies may be related to ADHD.

Finally, in the toddler years, young children can be observed to begin to override these learned cue reactions in order to soothe themselves or to gain new information. For example, children who are distressed by seeing a reminder of difficulty (e.g., a toy they are forbidden to play with) can be observed to direct their attention away from that problem and thereby calm themselves. Likewise, they can begin to learn words for concepts that are not inherently rewarding (e.g., "This is the carpet") by effortfully directing their attention to what a caregiver is saying, even though the cookies on the table look appealing. This ability is viewed as dependent on the emergence of frontal circuitry neurally, and as a precursor to later cognitive control or executive functioning. Cognitive control then continues to develop throughout childhood (Williams et al., 1999).

As just hinted, language development plays an important role in emerging self-control. The use of language to mediate understanding of parental expectations and to remind oneself about the rules is a powerful tool for self-control in early childhood and beyond. Language learning begins to develop rapidly in the second year, at about the same time as effortful control first emerges. As in the example just given, effortful control can also support language learning (Hollich et al., 2000), so these two self-regulatory tools are yoked and synergistically support one another.

The final piece of our early developmental explanation concerns the mutually influential nature of these abilities or self-regulatory systems. In the examples just given, effortful control can override affective approach tendencies, thus helping modulate and attune the development of those affective reactions to what is adaptive in the child's context. However, one can postulate that if these affective approach reactions are extreme, a child may have difficulty consolidating effortful control abilities, because they will be frequently breached by strong affective or reactive response. Alternatively, if effortful control abilities are weakened in early development by early neural injury, extreme genotype, or their combination, then affective (reactive) responses may also become maladaptive. We may thus see alternate routes to similar outcomes. Figure 8.1 schematizes this general self-regulatory system and its component processes.

We can use these basic traits along with preliminary data from the literature to form hypotheses about developmental pathways, described first at the most obvious level of clinical presentation. Table 8.4 outlines one such set of different pathways to ADHD that might warrant exploration. This outline reflects recent speculation about the importance of comorbid groups in ADHD (Jensen, Martin, & Cantwell, 1997a). It also reflects interest in early temperament contributions to externalizing behavior and conduct problems (Lahey et al., 1998). Support also comes from treatment outcome research. Reports from the MTA indicate that the most important differentiation may be that among (1) ADHD plus anxiety disorder (pathway 5 in Table 8.4), (2) ADHD plus ODD or CD (but no anxiety; primarily pathway 4 in Table 8.4), and (3) ADHD plus both anxiety and ODD/ CD (possibly pathways 1 and 3 in Table 8.4). Table 8.4 also suggests that one group of children with ADHD has a late-emerging problem that manifests itself when anterior cortical structures begin to influence attention, and may have relatively mild comorbid problems (pathway 1). A second group has extreme approach, but no real cognitive problems and a relatively benign course (pathway 2). A third group may have earlier-emerging difficulties in affect regulation and secondary problems in effortful control; they may have a more severe comorbid problem (pathways 3, 4, 5, 6). In addition, the pathways here address the reality that children with ADHD include those with

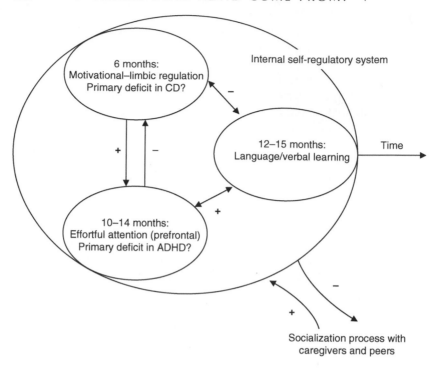

FIGURE 8.1. Schematic illustration of the processes that mutually depend on timing in development to support self-regulation, executive control, verbal learning, and socialization. Age ranges indicate the earliest point in which the emerging processes can be observed to control behavior. From Nigg and Huang-Pollock (2003). Copyright 2003 by The Guilford Press. Reprinted with permission.

high and low levels of anxiety, with implications for cognition and treatment response (Tannock et al., 1995).

A SECOND WAY FORWARD:
IDENTIFICATION OF DISTINCT EXTRINSIC ETIOLOGIES

The preceding formulation may have some promise in helping us to begin thinking about how children may arrive at ADHD via distinct developmental routes, exhibiting somewhat different behavioral profiles. A temperament perspective has the advantage of being able to accommodate the genetic findings of substantial heritability in ADHD (although temperament presumably can also be influenced by early

TABLE 8.4. Speculative Developmental Pathways to Different Clinical Presentations of ADHD, from a Temperament Perspective

ADHD pathway	Key developmental period	Developmental sequence and speculative temperamental precursors	Clinical presentation
1. Primary ADHD-C with secondary CD	Toddlerhood/ preschool age	Weak regulatory control at 1–2 years; secondary breakdown in ability to dampen negative affect, disrupted socialization a key moderator	Impaired executive functioning; mild deficits in affect regulation; secondary ODD or CD in some cases
2. Primary ADHD-C with little or no comorbidity	Infancy	Extreme positive approach at 6–18 months, with permissive socialization	"Normal" neuropsychological profile; little or no clinical comorbidity; altered delay–reward gradient
3. Secondary ADHD-C with primary socialized CD	Infancy	Extreme negative approach at 6–12 months disrupts later regulation development; thus secondary executive deficits	Mild executive function deficits; notable hostility and poor affect regulation; ODD, then CD
4. Secondary ADHD-C with primary unsocialized CD	Infancy	Extreme low anxiety (low negative withdrawal) disrupts later consolidation of regulation	Low arousal, low heart rate; aggressive conduct problems; risk for later psychopathy
5. Primary ADHD-C with anxiety	Infancy/ toddlerhood	Weak regulatory control at 1–2 years, with low hostility but high negative withdrawal (anxiety)	Executive deficits, with notable anxiety or anxiety disorder
6. Primary or secondary ADHD-PI	Infancy	Cognitive regulation is disrupted in relation to high anxiety/intrusive thoughts; high scores on anxiety	Inattentive on CPT but OK on executive tasks; high anxiety, maybe "anxious impulsivity"; overarousal

Note. Adapted from Nigg, Goldsmith, and Sachek (2004b). Copyright 2004 by Lawrence Erlbaum Associates. Adapted by permission.

189

experiential insults or benefits). To go beyond this, however, we can consider causal agents that may originate outside a child and affect the child. I consider extrinsic causal agents in the Chapters 10 and 11, with this multipathway structure as a context. Because this approach relies on the material covered in those chapters, I defer further description of it until Chapter 12.

CLINICAL IMPLICATIONS

The clinical implications of etiological heterogeneity are extensive—perhaps the most significant in this book. For many clinicians, the idea that children with ADHD are a heterogeneous lot is self-evident, but the problem is how to organize that variety meaningfully. Indeed, popular books on ADHD attempt to employ various subtyping schemes based on the various authors' clinical experience.

For example, one popular clinical book on ADHD (Amen, 2001) postulates six types based on hypothesized distinct single-photon emission computed tomography (SPECT) brain imaging profiles. These types may well map onto "mainstream" comorbid types (e.g., Amen's "overfocused ADD" resembles ADHD + anxiety disorders; his "ring of fire ADD" resembles ADHD + ODD; his "temporal lobe ADD" resembles ADHD + aggression; and his "inattentive ADD" resembles ADHD-PI with sluggish cognitive tempo).

This work has received only very limited exploration in the published, peer-reviewed scientific literature, and so cannot yet be formally evaluated. Related work has been done using EEG and quantitative EEG (Clarke, Barry, McCarthy, & Selikowitz, 2001a). This research has been reviewed by Barry et al. (2003a), who suggested that over- and underarousal might characterize two groups of children with ADHD-C, as noted in this book's Chapter 4. Efforts to apply this thinking to treatment and interventions will be of increasing interest. To date such efforts, including biofeedback and neurofeedback, are fascinating, but their efficacy is still insufficiently documented for general clinical use. Yet they illustrate the strong clinical interest in recognizing distinct etiological subtypes of ADHD, if etiology or mechanism-based subgroups can be independently identified and confirmed.

Attempts at subtyping ADHD based on EEG profiles are analogous to efforts at subtyping based on neuropsychological findings. Ultimately, the goal of all such work is to subtype the condition according to causal mechanisms—a point this entire book is highlighting. Yet all of these subtyping approaches remain in their infancy. They still lack systematic, controlled, independent trials in order to validate cut-off points, methods, linkages to treatment response, or outcomes. But they may in time become established as such studies begin to be done and their results begin to be reported. The focus here is on what is now relatively clear, and thus my intention is to ask these questions: (1) What is the core *functional* system? (2) What is the developmental course that would enable etiological subtypes to make sense?

Therefore, clinicians must strike a careful balance in thinking about the heterogeneity of ADHD. On the one hand, they must recognize that various subtyping schemes for ADHD remain preliminary and to a large extent speculative. The lack of consensus validation data on the ramifications of such speculative subtypes (e.g., on their courses, treatment responses, or long-term outcomes) requires that care be used in implementing such subtyping in clinical interventions or psychoeducation with parents and children. Furthermore, many interventions, including careful behavioral treatment and careful medication management—can lead to improvement for a majority of children with ADHD, regardless of their biological subtypes (Jensen et al., 2001; Swanson et al., 2001b).

On the other hand, the clinical reality is variety in children with ADHD. Intervention is most likely to be complied with and to address each child's unique needs if these various dimensions are recognized. Indeed, children with comorbid anxiety may respond differently to intervention than children without comorbid anxiety may (Jensen et al., 2001). Moreover, many parents are reluctant to accept medication treatment, obliging the clinician to include recommendations for alternative treatments. The chances of positive response and recovery for a child are highest with multimodal intervention, however (Swanson et al., 2001b).

On what dimensions should the clinician think about heterogeneity? Most obvious, and emanating from the prior chapters, are (1) the child's comorbid profile and temperamental style (aggression, anxiety) and (2) the child's cognitive and neuropsychological profile (learning disabilities, impaired executive functions, motor delays). Particular interventions with the appropriate validation data can then be tailored to the child's overall clinical profile. For instance, interventions to improve reading ability or motor control are well validated, as are interventions for anxiety or for ODD symptoms.

Once again, the bottom line—and a theme of this entire book with regard to clinical implications—is that a complete psychological and medical evaluation is essential to gain a full understanding of the appropriate intervention needs of each child with ADHD. Whether this becomes an advocacy issue for clinicians when parents do not have resources, or whether it becomes a matter of clinical best practices, will depend heavily on the type of population and setting at issue.

SUMMARY AND CONCLUSION

Neuropsychological models will not explain ADHD all by themselves. Various issues still remain to be resolved, despite the progress that has been made. However, a major insight in the field in the past decade has been recognition of the need to create formal models of causal heterogeneity. Multiple developmental pathways no doubt exist for children diagnosed with ADHD. I have suggested that the first step in identifying and understanding such pathways is to recognize that different elements of the regulatory system can be mapped (at least to some extent) onto distinct clinical and comorbid profiles. As a result, an initial set of hypotheses for longitudinal research on the development of ADHD pathways is to track the unfolding of these key regulatory domains.

These domains can be described from a neuropsychological perspective as involving vigilance, cognitive control or executive functioning, and reward response. They can be alternatively viewed from a temperament perspective as involving effortful control, reactive control, and approach tendencies emerging early in development. An integrated developmental perspective must consider the mutual influences of cognitive integrity, affective style or reactivity, and language development and facility in the development of self-regulation and of ADHD. Breakdowns in distinct elements of this mutually influential, dynamic developing system may lead to mechanism-based subtypes of ADHD that differ in important ways. For example, they may differ in their types of neuropsychological impairments. As such phenotypic distinctions come into focus, the next level of understanding will be to identify pathways in relation to specific etiologies.

CHAPTER 9

Genetic Effects

DISTINCTION BETWEEN ETIOLOGICAL AND MEDIATING MECHANISMS

Perhaps the most common question parents have for clinicians diagnosing ADHD is "What caused this?" Is it due to genetics? Is it due to poor diet? These are important questions. All of the neuropsychological theories reviewed in Part II address potential *mediating* processes (or perhaps additional syndrome features), not *originating* causes. They address what is wrong now, not what led to the problem. To put it another way, even if we were to agree on a definition of abnormal neural development (perhaps based on statistical risk of early death, injury, or criminality/substance abuse as outcomes), and if we establish that a neural system is abnormal in a child with ADHD, this does not tell us why it developed abnormally. The neural dysfunction may tell us about *how* the problem works, but not *why* the problem occurred. To address the latter issue, we must consider etiology proper.

The basic model guiding neuropsychological studies of ADHD is illustrated in Figure 9.1. The figure shows a single pathway for simplic-

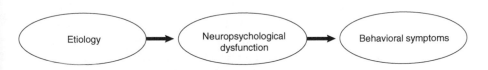

FIGURE 9.1. Simplified model of etiology.

193

ity, to illustrate the idea of a mediating process; however, note that I continue to consider multiple pathways later in the book. Neuropsychological impairment in this general model mediates the connection between the originating cause and the expression of behavioral and adjustment problems. Of course, there may be multiple originating causes even for one child, and there almost certainly are multiple causes across the whole population of children who could be diagnosed with ADHD, as I discuss later. Another qualification is that after the problematic course is underway, neuropsychological vulnerabilities may help maintain the behavior problems even if the originating cause is removed. Thus they may be causally contributing in a "maintaining" sense.

A final caveat is that the developmental process may not be as linear as depicted here; neuropsychological impairments, once underway, may influence the originating causes. For example, if the behavior problems are caused by a difficult home environment, leading to poor cognitive development, this problem in the child can now contribute to the environment (e.g., by causing poor peer relations, academic frustrations, or ongoing home conflict), maintaining the environmental cause of difficulty. This potential circular causality must be kept in mind in real-world and clinical thinking.

But for purposes of our understanding here, it is useful to think about the distinction between *originating* cause and *mediating* process. Why did the neural processes develop atypically? We need to understand the processes by which the disorder or behavior problem operates, and the context, risks, or agents that may have launched the cascade of processes leading to the behavioral maladjustment. This chapter begins our discussion of the latter set of issues. First to be addressed is the perennial topic of the role of genetics.

GENETIC INFLUENCES REQUIRED IN CAUSAL MODELS OF ADHD: BEHAVIORAL GENETIC FINDINGS

Our clients often tell us that a child with ADHD is similar to one of his or her parents. Family studies established long ago that ADHD "runs in families," with a two- to fourfold increased risk among first-degree relatives. How much of this familial similarity is due to genes, and how much to common family experiences? Does genetic influence mean that nothing will change the behavior? In Chapter 2, I have distinguished multifactorial, polygenic conditions from single-gene disorders. In a single-gene condition such as Hungtington's disease, an inherited genetic mutation determines the course of illness; in other words, that one gene has a very large effect. But in polygenic conditions (such as asthma, heart disease, and most psychopathology, including ADHD), many genes together exert probabilistic effects, amplified or dampened by experience. Each individual gene exerts only a small influence on the disorder. Cumulative effects of several genes are expected. In these polygenic conditions, it is meaningful to ask how much of the likelihood of the disorder may be attributable to genetic influence or genetic variation between individuals.

To answer the question about how much of the individual variation in liability[1] to ADHD is genetic, behavioral genetic studies use "experiments of nature" in the form of comparisons of (1) fraternal twins (who share, on average, 50% of their genes) and identical twins (who share 100% of their genes);[2], or (2) adopted offspring (no genetic similarity on average) and biological offspring (50% genetic similarity). These comparisons permit researchers to estimate the relative contribution made to a disorder by three basic components of variance that represent different types of etiologies:

1. *Shared environment effects.* These are effects that make twins more similar to one another than would be expected based on genetics alone (e.g., they are both raised by an alcoholic parent, or both attend a poor quality school).

2. *Nonshared environment effects.* These are effects that make twins less similar to one another than would be expected based on genetics alone, (e.g., they have different peer groups, or one chooses a positive extracurricular activity, or one is favored by a parent).

3. *Genetic effects or heritability.* Basic models estimate "heritability," which refers to additive genetic effects. Other genetic effects of course are possible, such as dominance effects, epistasis (gene–gene interactions), gene–environment correlations, and gene–environment co-action and interaction. Many of these are discussed later in this chapter.[3]

Each of these three basic statistics ranges from 0 to 1.00 (0% to 100%). Each is, technically speaking, a statistical component of variance partitioning; their sum therefore must equal 1.00 (100%). Each statistic reflects the degree to which differences between individuals in a given population are influenced by these three general classes of effects.

To see how these values are arrived at, consider the twin correlations for inattention in the Australian Twin Project (Levy & Hay, 2001; I am indebted to D. Hay, personal communication, November 2005, for this example). The correlation between scores for the identical (monozygotic, or MZ) twins (who share 100% of their genes) is .87, whereas the correlation between fraternal (dizygotic, or DZ) twins (who share 50% of their genes) is .42. Here the MZ correlation is almost exactly twice as big as the DZ correlation, consistent with a trait influenced primarily by differences in genes. In that same sample, the speech problems have a correlation of .91 for MZ twins and .65 for DZ twins. Here the difference between MZ and DZ correlations is not so large, and the DZ correlation is larger than .50 (i.e., larger than would be expected in a purely genetic model), suggesting shared environment effects. This particular shared environment effect makes sense when one considers that speech is developing in part through the behavioral interchanges of two young twins with one another. As another example, a compilation of twin data across several studies (described by McGuffin et al., 1994) indicated that extraversion had an MZ correlation of .51 and a DZ correlation of .21, suggesting substantial heritable effects but no effects of shared environment. In the same compilation, religious involvement had an MZ correlation of .60 and a DZ correlation of .58, consistent with trivial effects of heritability and large effects of shared environment. These intuitive examples can be modeled formally in biometric statistical models that address various assumptions, including measurement unreliability and rater biases.

Behavioral genetic studies have shown, unsurprisingly, that genetic influence on human variation is widespread. Most psychiatric disorders exhibit substantial heritability, as do most personality and temperament traits (Neale & Stevenson, 1989), including those discussed in Chapter 8. Bouchard (1994) provides a useful and readable overview of major findings over the past several decades in the field of behavioral genetics as a whole.

However, nonshared environment also plays a role in most temperament and personality traits. Though shared environment generally has a less clear role in psychopathology, shared environment effects are apparent in some psychopathological measures, such as oppositional, conduct, and antisocial behaviors (Eaves et al., 1997; see discussion by Nigg & Goldsmith, 1998). These effects probably reflect the causal contribution to aggressive behavior of family and peer socialization effects (Patterson, 1986; Snyder, Reed, & Patterson, 2003). There is also some evidence that the overlap of ADHD with oppositional and conduct problems is related to shared environment effects (Burt, Krueger, McGue, & Iacono, 2001), although other studies indicate that the specific overlap of ADHD and conduct problems is also related to shared genes (Silberg et al., 1996). ADHD may index a trait characteristic that in some situations gives rise to conduct problems, perhaps in instances of high parent–child conflict. Consistent with this picture, Burt, Krueger, McGue, and Iacono (2003) found that the overlap of ADHD with conduct and oppositional symptoms was related to parent–child conflict via both genetic and environmental effects.

In all, however, it is not clear that ADHD per se shows the same pattern of etiological effects in twin studies as do antisocial and oppositional behaviors. In the case of ADHD, over a dozen behavioral genetic studies of ADHD have established that when parent ratings of ADHD are studied, (1) heritability is substantial (many estimates range from .60 to as high as .90; Sherman, Iacono, & McGue, 1997a; Sherman, McGue, & Iacono, 1997b; Thapar, Harrington, Ross, & McGuffin, 2000; Faraone et al., 2000a), (2) nonshared environment effects are modest to small; and (3) shared environment effects are practically nil. These findings hold whether ADHD is viewed as a dimension or as a category, and heritability is similar throughout the distribution, suggesting a continuum structure (Levy, Hay, McStephen, Wood, & Waldman, 1997).

Heritability estimates for ADHD are somewhat lower when teacher ratings of ADHD are studied, however (Goodman & Stevenson, 1989; Sherman et al., 1997b; Thapar et al., 2000). This could be because teachers see a different universe of behaviors than parents see, or due to various types of rater biases in one or the other rater. Stevenson (1992) found that heritability was significant for parent-rated but not teacher-rated hyperactivity. However, Sherman et al. (1997b) looked at twin concordance by using a structured interview and parent and teacher ratings, which provided an appropriate analysis of ADHD as a clinical syndrome. They estimated heritability of liability at .79 and nonshared environment effects at .21 across all data sources. The estimates for teachers were similar (heritability = .73, nonshared environment = .27), although with the small sample, dropping of the heritability term entirely did not significantly worsen model fit. Relatively few studies have looked at twin concordance of ADHD diagnoses derived from full clinical evaluation and careful combination of parent and teacher input on symptoms and impairment.

It is also important to recognize that in addition to partitioning variance, behavioral genetic analyses are now asking advanced questions such as whether there are developmental changes in genetic effects and degree of covariation of genetic sources of influence on different disorders or traits (for excellent examples of these efforts, see chapters in Levy & Hay, 2001). However, for our purposes it is essential to grasp some basic points about the basic structure of influences as it has been established in ADHD as they have been described here, and to understand key cautions associated with those conclusions. These points set the stage for thinking about integrated gene–experience interplay in the development of ADHD.

CAUTIONS AND CAVEATS
ABOUT BEHAVIORAL GENETIC ESTIMATES IN ADHD

In addition to the relative shortage of twin or adoption studies of the full ADHD clinical syndrome (as opposed to trait ratings), at least two other key issues must be noted for the twin data. First, some question remains as to whether twin estimates of heritability are overestimates because of "rater contrast effects." That is, temperament studies find that parents rating twins' activity levels tend to emphasize *differences* between fraternal twins but *similarities* of identical twins, leading to an inflated heritability estimate (Saudino, 2003a, 2003b; Saudino, Cherny, & Plomin, 2000; Schmitz, Saudino, Plomin, Fulker, & DeFries, 1996). It is not entirely clear to what extent this problem pertains to ADHD ratings, but the somewhat lower heritability from teacher than from parent ratings in some studies is consistent with this likelihood (note that this discrepancy could be due to other effects, but appears to be due to parent contrast effects or rating bias; Simonoff et al., 1998). Two studies (Thapar et al., 2000; Simonoff et al., 1998) found significant contrast effects in maternal ratings of twins' ADHD symptoms, but the large Australian twin study (Levy et al., 1997) did not. Thapar et al. (2000) looked at parent and teacher ratings on two different scales (the ADHD Rating Scale and the Rutter A Scale). They fitted models that included maternal contrast effects (which were apparent on the Rutter A Scale but not the ADHD Rating Scale), and still found that heritability for teacher ratings of ADHD was about .60, with nonshared environment effects estimated at .23. Parent-rated estimates varied with the scale, but remained large even with contrast effects in the model. Both Sherman et al. (1997b) and Thapar et al. (2000) found a small but noteworthy contribution of *shared* environment in teacher ratings of ADHD symptoms. In all, rater bias effects may vary across

particular measures or scales; for example, shorter scales may introduce more bias, or asking parents to rate both children immediately
after one another may introduce additional bias (D. Hay, personal
communication, November 2005). Supporting this supposition, Hay,
Bennett, Levy, Sergeant, and Swanson (in press) found that contrast
effects were restricted to particular scale types

Simonoff et al. (1998), however, analyzed over 1,600 twins from
the Virginia Twin Study. They confirmed maternal contrast effects, but
also noted biases in teacher ratings due to twin confusion (known as
"correlated errors"), especially for MZ twins. In other words, many
twins have the same teacher, and teachers apparently have more difficulty keeping MZ twins straight in their minds. These investigators fitted a statistical model that included contrast bias effects (in effect, controlling for those effects). They still found that heritability was large.
Eaves et al. (1997), using the same Virginia Twin Study sample, estimated heritability at .60–.70, with the exact figure depending on
which rater bias effects were controlled. More comparative studies are
needed that examine rater differences in heritability estimates for
ADHD and evaluate contrast effects for ADHD symptoms in particular. Rietveld, Hudziak, Bartels, van Beijsterveldt, and Boomsma (2003,
2004) reported on a longitudinal study of a large sample of twins in
Europe, with maternal CBCL ratings at four age points (ages 3, 7, 10,
and 12 years). Rater contrast effects were only significant at age 3, and
even with controls for these, heritability was above .70 at each age.

Note, then, that although parent ratings appear to yield somewhat
inflated heritability estimates due to contrast effects, teacher ratings of
twins may also be biased, so that no one data source is a suitable "gold
standard" (Simonoff et al., 1998). Nonetheless, heritability estimates
for ADHD, often quoted in the range of .80, may be high estimates.
Better and more reasonable estimates are likely to be in the range of
.60–.70, depending on age and method of defining ADHD (Eaves et
al., 1997; Rietveld et al., 2004; Simonoff et al., 1998; Sherman et al.,
1997a, 1997b; Thapar et al., 2000). Concomitantly, shared or nonshared environment effects may be underestimated by those higher figures. That said, heritability remains substantial and clearly cannot be
ignored in models of ADHD causality.

A second issue, which has begun to be addressed, is that even
though very large population-based twin samples have been assem-
bled—notably in Australia (Levy et al., 1997; Levy & Hay, 2001) and in
the United States (Eaves et al., 1997; Simonoff et al., 1998)—many twin
samples do not include the entire population of twins in a region, and

thus may tend to represent only a subset of the population that is less exposed to environmental risk factors or without severe adversity. To the extent that this is the case, some estimates of heritability may again be somewhat high.

Consistent with that speculative possibility is a provocative initial finding by Turkheimer, Haley, Waldron, D'Onofrio, and Gottesman (2003) concerning IQ. They found that heritability of IQ was very high in samples with "normal" (middle to low) SES, but that heritability of IQ was low when SES was extremely low (adverse). This finding underscores the potential dependency of heritability estimates on the socioeconomic context of the twin samples being studied. As causal environmental variation goes up, heritability must, mathematically, go down (since all estimates are constrained to add up to 1.00). Note, however, that the Turkheimer et al. finding, while illustrative, has yet to be replicated for IQ. No such studies have been done for ADHD. But the possibility may warrant exploration, especially in light of the potential contributions to ADHD of severe adversity and of particular experiential injuries (which I consider later).

Despite these caveats and cautions, a large and well-replicated literature indicates that effects of heritability make the largest single contribution to liability to develop ADHD. Nonshared environment effects also appear to be important, but contribute only a modest portion of the total variance in liability. Thus causal models of ADHD must include substantial genetic influence, as well as notable nonshared environmental effects. Yet just as some seemingly environmental effects can reflect genetic influences, so these heritability effects do not preclude important environmental processes, which operate via genotype–environment interplay.

These behavioral genetic findings have had two powerful ramifications in the field of ADHD research. First, the very high heritability observed for ADHD in parent ratings of twins has spurred an intensive search for individual genes in ADHD. The results of this effort are summarized only briefly herein; new studies in this area are continually appearing, so early findings will certainly be qualified or amplified by rapidly emerging new data and methods.

Second, high heritability has tended to discourage the search for environmental contributors to ADHD. The moderate levels of neuropsychological impairment seen in ADHD are smaller than those seen in frank neurological injury, and thus are viewed as consistent with genetic effects. This line of thinking is probably mistaken, at least in its assumptions. I argue below and in Chapters 10 and 11 that experiential causes warrant more intensive investigation than they have received. However, the twin data can guide us as to which classes of environmental contributors are most likely to pay off.

In the next section, I comment further on these two issues. First, I briefly remark on the molecular genetic findings. Then I discuss in more detail the relatively neglected domain of experiential causes for ADHD, and note which kinds of experiential causes can be reconciled with the behavioral genetic discoveries.

MOLECULAR GENETIC FINDINGS: MANY GENES WITH SMALL EFFECTS

One single-gene mechanism related to ADHD has been identified. In the 1990s it was discovered that ADHD can be caused by a disorder called "resistance to thyroid hormone" (RTH), attributable to a single gene known as the thyroid hormone beta receptor gene (Hauser et al., 1993). It has an odds ratio of 3.2, far larger than that of any other gene for ADHD (see note 1 to Chapter 10 for an explanation of odds ratios and other statistics to capture risk). This finding is important because it shows that thyroid dysfunction can be a causal route to ADHD. As I note in the next chapter, insults to the thyroid system may warrant more consideration. However, RTH itself is not a major cause of ADHD. RTH has a population prevalence estimated at 1 in 2,500, or less than 0.04% (Elia, Gulotta, Rose, Marin, & Rapoport, 1994). Thus, even if 70% of children with RTH develop ADHD, RTH would still account for fewer than 1% of cases of ADHD. In the end, genetic liability for ADHD in most cases is probably due to many genes, each of which exerts a small effect.

Caution has been the watchword for interpreting molecular genetic findings in psychiatric disorders. The field has been plagued by a tendency for initial findings not to be supported or replicated over time (see Risch & Botstein, 1996, for an account of this frustrating early history in the study of the genetics of bipolar disorder). A bit more success appears to have ensued for ADHD, but caution may still be in order. Nonetheless, it is critical that readers recognize the advances underway in this domain, and what may emerge in coming years.

Two kinds of molecular genetic studies are noteworthy in the case of multifactorial disorders such as ADHD. A "whole-genome scan" searches the entire genome for "hot spots" that give a signal of association with a disorder. These regions of the genome can then be searched more intensively for individual genes. At this writing, only two projects have published whole-genome scans—one at UCLA (Fisher et al., 2002; Ogdie et al., 2003, 2004) and one in the Netherlands (Bakker et al., 2003). Fisher et al. (2002) examined 126 affected sibling pairs (in which both siblings had some form of ADHD), and suggested possible susceptibility regions on chromosome 5 (5p12),[4] chromosome 10 (10q26), chromosome 12 (12q23), and chromosome 16 (16p13). In a follow-up study, adding to the sample another 101 families, the same group (Ogdie et al., 2003) refined their conclusions to focus on 5p13, 6q14, 11q25, 16p13, 17p11, and 20q13. Finally, "fine mapping" of these regions (i.e., mapping with a higher density of markers) in the same sample again slightly expanded (by addition of another 39 sibling pairs, for a total sample of 308 affected sibling pairs) was conducted by Ogdie et al. (2004). They concluded that there were potential ADHD susceptibility regions on chromosome 5 (5p13—however, this effect was marginal, included only because of possible overlap with the Dutch sample), chromosome 6 (6q12, a region that includes two serotonin receptor genes), chromosome 16 (16p13), and chromosome 17 (17p11, a region that includes the serotonin transporter gene). In the Dutch study, Bakker et al. (2003) identified nonoverlapping regions of interest, including regions on chromosome 7 (7p13), chromosome 9 (9q33), chromosome 13 (13q33), and chromosome 15 (15q15). They obtained marginal effects at 5p13. A pooled analysis of these two samples showed, unsurprisingly, a significant effect at the 5p13 locus that had emerged (at least marginally) in each sample separately (Ogdie et al., 2006).

Thus these studies remain intriguing but preliminary. It was notable that no overlap was found with most of the regions identified in candidate gene studies (see below), and that almost no results were replicated across sites, but that some overlap *was* found with regions identified in autism (on chromosomes 16 and 17) and regions involving serotonin genes. All of these issues suggest that sample sizes probably remain too small for reliable whole-genome scan effects. Furthermore, the definition of ADHD can affect these findings; ascertainment differences across sites could also weaken the ability to replicate whole-genome scan results. Nonetheless, these intriguing initial findings should be followed up with additional studies.

In general, the whole-genome scan approach relies on identifying relatively large areas of the genome that may harbor susceptibility genes, or on using very large samples to locate smaller effects. However, these initial studies have generated new hypotheses that can be pursued in other research. Future whole-genome scans may prove decisive in identifying genes involved in ADHD, but breakthrough findings will probably await collaborative and consortium efforts pooling genetic data across many centers. Such efforts are already underway.

In the meantime, the second, more common, and more widely discussed approach is the "candidate gene" study. Candidate gene studies typically focus on polymorphisms in selected genes of *theoretical* interest. In the case of ADHD, the most common types of polymorphisms studied are either single-nucleotide polymorphisms (SNPs, pronounced "snips") or variable numbers of tandem repeats (VNTRs). The frequencies of different forms of the genes are then compared between affected individuals and controls. If the frequencies are higher or lower in the sample with ADHD than in the control sample, then the genes may be associated with the disorder.

In addition to perennial concerns about sample size, an initial problem with these studies was getting valid and defensible population matching of cases and controls. In other words, allele frequencies could be different in the ADHD and control groups due to population stratification (that is, the ADHD sample and the control sample derive from underlying populations that differ in allele frequencies, perhaps due to different ethnic group composition in the two samples), creating an artifact in which ADHD appears to be associated with a given allele or gene. That problem is addressed by newer within-family statistical techniques, such as the transmission disequilibrium tests. In the case of ADHD, most studies have looked at catecholamine-regulating genes, such as genes for dopamine or norepinephrine receptors. Figure 9.2 schematizes the catecholamine synthesis and activation pathways, illustrating the numerous genes that might be relevant to ADHD under a catecholamine theory. Such a theory, of course, is relevant to essentially all of the neuropsychological functions that have been discussed in Part II of this book.

Focusing on this pathway and candidate genes along it, several dozen candidate gene studies of ADHD have now been published (for additional review, see Faraone et al., 2005). However, the majority have addressed just two genes. The first of these is the dopamine transporter gene (SLC6A3 or DAT1), on chromosome 5 (Barr et al., 2001; Cook et al., 1995; Daly, Hawi, Fitzgerald, & Gill, 1999; Gill, Daly, Heron, Hawi, & Fitzgeralf, 1997), with a polymorphism (5p15.3) outside the region on 5p detected in the whole-genome scan. This "10-repeat" allele is associated with ADHD risk (Cook et al., 1995; Waldman et al., 1998). The second is the dopamine D4 receptor gene (DRD4), on chromosome 11 (Faraone, Doyle, Mick, & Biederman,

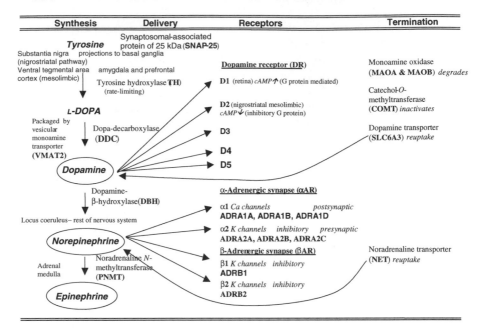

FIGURE 9.2. Catecholamine pathway. DAT1 (see text) is another name for the SLC6A3 gene or dopamine transporter gene. Courtesy of Karen Friderici, PhD, Michigan State University. Copyright 2005 by Karen Friderici. Reprinted by permission.

2001; Swanson et al., 2000a), with a polymorphism at 11p15.5. For DRD4, a receptor expressed primarily in prefrontal regions, the "7-repeat" allele is associated with risk for ADHD (LaHoste et al., 1996; Faraone et al., 2001). Well over a dozen studies for each of these two genes alone have yielded relatively striking replication in relation to ADHD. In fact, few psychiatric disorders have been the subject of such success in molecular genetic studies (Swanson et al., 2001a).

However, these do not appear to be genes with major effects. To quantify the size of these effects, meta-analyses indicate that the odds ratios associated with these genes are in the 1.2–1.4 range, meaning that the risk alleles increase the chances of having ADHD by 20–40% (Faraone et al., 2001). This is consistent with the idea that there are multiple genes influencing ADHD.

In aggregate, these molecular genetic data are consistent with the idea that multiple genes of modest effect may be involved in ADHD—or that other genes (such as those on the serotonin pathway; Ogdie et al., 2004) require more serious consideration in candidate gene studies. At the same time, the data are quite interesting, because researchers can develop plausible hypotheses about how malfunction or different functioning of these genes might connect to neuropsychological findings in ADHD. Thus DAT1 is important in reuptake of dopamine at the synapse, which in turn is important for regulating dopamine neural transmission. DRD4, important in prefrontal structures, could be subsensitive, leading to faulty cognitive efficiency in those networks (Swanson et al., 2000a).

In the meantime, a number of other catecholamine genes have been examined in fewer studies, including DRD2, DRD3, DRD5, the alpha-2-noradrenergic receptor gene (Park et al., 2005), and others (Hawi et al., 2003; Maher, Marazita, Ferrell, & Vanyukov, 2002), as described in Figure 9.2. These effects are still emerging, but it is likely that some of these genes will also be associated with ADHD (Lawson et al., 2003; Maher et al., 2002). In particular, it is clear that noradrenergic receptor function in the prefrontal cortices is involved in many aspects of cognitive control that are typically associated with executive functioning (Arnsten, 2001; Birnbaum, Podell, & Arnsten, 2000). Therefore, further scrutiny of noradrenergic genes is likely to prove useful. Moreover, the results of the initial whole-genome scans are likely to increase interest in serotonin-related genes, which have shown positive associations with ADHD in initial studies (Manor et al., 2001; Seeger, Schloss, & Schmidt, 2001).

It will be important to determine whether different genes are associated with different subtypes, and whether gene–gene interactions explain more variance in ADHD symptoms. It will also be of interest to discover whether different genes are associated with different neuropsychological functions, based on their differential regions of expression in the brain. For example, recent creative studies have begun to pair molecular genotypes with neural or pharmacological measures or both. In one intriguing report, Loo et al. (2003) found that children with two copies of the 10-repeat (risk) allele on DAT1 had more slow-wave brain activity on EEG recording. The 10-repeat carriers also showed a different pattern of EEG response to methylphenidate than did the other children. In another provocative study, Swanson et al. (2000b) divided children with ADHD-C from the MTA into those with and without the long-repeat allele of DRD4. They then compared these two groups to the healthy control children on a composite reaction time index averaged across multiple cognitive tasks. The group with the long-repeat (risk) allele had typical neuropsychological performance, whereas the group with ADHD but without that allele had impaired or slow reaction time performance. Swanson et al. argued that this might suggest two pathways to ADHD—one via neural insult (early brain injury, perhaps prenatally), and the other via inherited extreme temperament. Although that conclusion is speculative, the data do suggest multiple routes, one of which is characterized by particular neurocognitive deficits and marked by a particular genotype. However, Langley et al. (2004) reported that the high risk allele was associated with worse neuropsychological performance. Further such studies are needed to clarify the moderators or sampling variation that will link cognitive scores to genotype.

More studies pairing molecular genotype with neuropsychological, physiological, and other measures may clarify the pathways to ADHD and are a clear direction for next-generation research on ADHD. However, it will be even more crucial for such studies to include measurement of known experiential etiologies, as discussed later.

An interesting issue for these molecular studies is that many of the risk alleles examined so far in candidate gene studies occur in over 50% of the population. This state of affairs underscores the likelihood, already noted, that the genes are exerting their influence along with other genes or with experiential triggers. However, also important to recognize are the variations of genetic structure *within* the alleles being studied for each gene. These variations in structure are indicated by different sequences of DNA—making up, for example, a 7-repeat variant of a gene. These within-allele variations may be useful, or even crucial, in discovering the functional contribution of the genes to ADHD, and also may identify less common genotypes more specifically related to ADHD. To get at this and related issues, several new approaches are emerging.

One notable strategy entails "haplotype mapping" in an effort to better identify functional variants of the relevant genes, as well as more refined genotype definitions (Daly et al., 2001; Gabriel, 2002). A "haplotype" refers to a unique combination of alleles or markers (e.g., a pattern of SNPs) that tend to be inherited together (and therefore usually occur close to one another on the genome). Newly developed "haplotype maps" attempt to identify marker combinations that actually occur in the population; these are then used to narrow the range of the gene that may be involved in the disorder.

For example, Grady et al (2003) found that the particular haplotypes found in children with ADHD at the DRD4 7-repeat allele were in fact rare in the population—an observation that could not be made with the cruder single-marker approach. Likewise, our own group (Park et al., 2005) found that haplotypes of the alpha-2-receptor gene yielded a clearer association and linkage with ADHD than individual SNPs alone did.

For our purposes, the main message here is that we will see new advances in molecular genetic mapping of ADHD risk as these and other new techniques come into more regular usage. At the same time, they require complex analyses and, once again, larger samples than have often been used. Thus it may take some time for substantial breakthroughs to emerge.

Overall, it is striking that replicated findings have already begun to emerge for dopamine-related genes in ADHD. This makes it one of the few psychiatric disorders with replicated molecular genetic discoveries. Despite the large number of published studies, however, this field remains young. Very little is yet known about the effects of other potentially crucial genes, such as the alpha-2-noradrenergic receptor (influencing noradrenergic functioning in frontal cortex), genes that affect GABA-ergic transmission, and others. Newer, more refined approaches that examine haplotypes, as well as those that broaden the field of investigation beyond catecholamine genes, will be important in the next generation of molecular studies.

As well, whole-genome scans may become important as larger, pooled, multisite samples become available via collaborative networks of ADHD genetics researchers that are already in place. Notably, the National Institute of Mental Health Genetics of ADHD Network (Faraone, 2001) was recently renewed and brings together ADHD genetics researchers from around the world. It has already led to some initial data-pooling efforts. In Europe, a new initiative features collaborations from researchers in several countries to generate a very large sample of identical phenotypic and genotypic data for pooling purposes (Asherson & The IMAGE Consortium, 2004). Thus major collaborative analyses are inevitable and may shed new light on the molecular concomitants of ADHD, as well as their relations to neuropsychological functioning in the disorder.

GENOTYPE–ENVIRONMENT INTERPLAY: INTERACTIONS AND CORRELATIONS

When they hear about genetic influences, students or others may ask, "But what if the child has a very effective parent?" Parents often ask, "Why did my child with ADHD do so well with that great teacher in third grade?" or "Why doesn't my effective strategy for my other chil-

dren work on this child?" I now consider key conceptual issues necessary for a full etiological understanding of ADHD. In preparation, I
have already explained that genetic effects in ADHD are not the deterministic effects seen in classic metabolic diseases such as phenylketonuria or Huntington's disease. Rather, they are mediated and moderated by other biological and experiential mechanisms. Two very
general gene–environment interplay need to be understood at this
point—and are critical to evaluating the possible role of experiential
potentiators in ADHD.

Genotype–Environment Interactions

First, and perhaps easiest to grasp, are genotype–environment interactions. (In the remainder of the chapter, I abbreviated these as G × E
interactions.) The basic idea here is that two different children will
respond to the same environment in different ways, because they have
different temperamental predispositions (recall the pathways described
in Chapter 8) that are rooted in different genotypes. This can also be
thought of as genetic sensitivity to environmental effects or environmental activation of genetic effects (Purcell, 2002). For instance, a
loud, emotionally expressive home may be experienced as liberating
and energizing for a child with an extraverted, relatively fearless temperament, who therefore thrives; it may be experienced as stifling and
oppressive by a child with a temperamentally inhibited or anxious predisposition, who therefore develops psychopathology. Children born
into the same family may have very different temperaments, and may
respond very differently to that same home environment. As a result, a
child with an average temperament, paired with average parents, may
not be very likely to develop marked antisocial psychopathology (e.g.,
see Nigg & Hinshaw, 1998, for data indicating that parents of children
with ADHD generally had typical personality trait scores). However a
child with a very active temperament, or a predisposition to angry negative affect, may be at risk for developing antisocial behavior even in an
average home. We (Nigg & Hinshaw, 1998) found that for children with
ADHD, parent personality traits predicted their aggressive behavior,
but this was not the case for nondisabled children. These could be due
to or related to G × E interactions.

Thomas and Chess (1977) suggested long ago that the "fit"
between a child's temperament and his or her environment might
be important in understanding psychopathology (see also Lerner &
Lerner, 1994). With regard to temperament, Crockenberg and colleagues (e.g., Leerkes & Crockenberg, 2002; Crockenberg & Leerkes,

2003) have demonstrated that child behavior problems map onto particular configurations of early childhood temperament and parenting style or parent characteristics. Kochanska, Murray, and Coy (1997) have shown that children's internalization of conscience follows distinct pathways, with some temperament types responding better to a strict discipline style, and others responding better to a more reasoned discipline style. With regard to genotype, Cadoret, Yates, Troughton, Woodworth, and Stewart (1995) used an adoption study to show that negative parenting practices were associated with aggressive behavior only for children who had biological risk (defined as a biological parent with antisocial behavior).

Although we cannot equate individual genotypes with temperament, analogous to this conception is research that looks directly at the interplay of genotype and experience, bypassing temperament itself. Such studies have not yet been done for ADHD, but interesting findings have already emerged in molecular studies of depression and antisocial behavior. It is quite instructive to consider these direct genotype by experience findings to consider the potential for analogous research in ADHD (though, no doubt, with experiential factors distinct from those studied here). Caspi et al. (2002, 2003) showed that alleles of a monoamine oxidase-active gene moderated child aggressive behavior after abuse, and that alleles of the serotonin transporter gene moderated depressive response to trauma. Kendler et al. (2005) replicated this second result, finding that genotype was particularly important in modulating the effects of more common low-level stress events in the onset of episodes of major depression. Extreme stress level increased the risk of depression, regardless of genotype. Two studies replicated this result in adolescents and children, respectively (Eley et al., 2004; Kaufman et al., 2004). Kaufman et al. (2004) found a three-way interaction between genotype, trauma, and social support in children, such that the effects of trauma in the risk genotype (the short allele of the serotonin transporter gene) were dampened by social support. Chapter 12 discusses these findings in more detail.

Interactions between genotype and environmental activators or triggers may also exist in ADHD, but the appropriate environmental triggers have not yet been paired with the genotype. Indeed, little such research has even been conducted. If such interplay involves common experiential effects, but these are not explicitly searched for, then they do not automatically appear in behavioral genetic studies. Instead, they are "hidden" in the environmental or heritable effects, depending on the nature of the effect (Purcell, 2002). Let me explain.

Interactions between genotype and *shared* environment effects can masquerade as genetic (heritable) effects, because they tend to make MZ twins more alike than DZ twins. For example, if the entire population in a country is exposed to lead via auto exhaust, but its effects on learning disability interact with genetic ability to metabolize the lead, then learning disability will afflict genetically vulnerable individuals and will appear to be largely determined by genotype. MZ twins will tend to be affected together far more often than DZ twins. On the other hand, interactions between genotype and *nonshared* environment look like environmental effects in typical twin studies. Whether an experiential agent is "shared" or "unshared" is not always obvious. However, these principles indicate that we should carefully consider risk agents that might qualify as common and shared potentiators of ADHD. I take up this point again later.

Genotype–Environment Correlations

Second, and more difficult for students, clinicians, and even scientists to grasp, are genotype–environment correlations (Scarr & McCartney, 1983). (In the remainder of this chapter, I abbreviate these as (G)(E) correlations, to distinguish them more clearly from G × E *interactions*.) The basic idea here is that parents pass on both genes and environments to their children; thus genotype and environments usually cannot be separated when we conceptualize the effects on children in a family (even though they can be separated conceptually in the case of adopted children). These correlations are not all passive; they can be due to a child's eliciting or choosing different experiences. Misattribution of causal effects here is the opposite of what it is for G × E interactions. If genes are correlated with shared environment, the genetic effects masquerade in twin studies as shared environment effects. If genes are correlated with nonshared environment, the environmental effects are subsumed under the heritability term (Purcell, 2002). Allow me to explain further.

Scarr and McCartney (1983) suggested that three kinds of (G)(E) correlations exist. A "passive" (G)(E) correlation occurs when parents who raise their children pass on their genes to the children, as well as the environment in which they are raised. For example, intelligent parents pass on genes for high verbal ability to their children—and also surround them with books and learning opportunities. In the case of ADHD, we can imagine that some parents pass on genes leading to dopamine dysfunction and executive functioning problems in children, but that these same parents may also create an unpredictable home routine that dampens their children's ability to self-regulate.

An "evocative" (G)(E) correlation occurs when a child stimulates (evokes) a particular response from the environment. For example, a friendly child with a propensity for positive affect may evoke more positive responses from caregivers, than a more irritable sibling or cousin may. Powerful evidence for such effects comes from the Iowa Adoption Study. Ge et al. (1996) examined the parenting practices of adoptive parents with their adopted children. They divided the adopted children according to whether their *biological* parents had antisocial psychopathology. The children were adopted at birth, and the adoptive and biological parents had no knowledge of one another. Yet when the biological parents had antisocial behavior, the adoptive parents were more critical, hostile, and negative with the adopted children. Why would this be? Virtually the only possible explanation is an evocative (G)(E) correlation: The children of the antisocial parents had more difficult temperaments, and triggered more negative parental responses from the adoptive parents. Further support for these effects has emerged in subsequent studies (Riggins-Caspers, Cadoret, Knutson, & Langbehn, 2003). Such patterns no doubt occur even more powerfully in the homes of biological parents, who may have weakened parenting ability due to their own psychopathology (Bor & Sanders, 2004; Capaldi, Pears, Patterson, & Owen, 2003; O'Leary, Slep, & Reid, 1999; Patterson, 1986; Patterson, Forgatch, Yoerger, & Stoolmiller, 1998). Yet this effect, to the extent that interchanges are experienced uniquely by a child in a family, could appear as genetic effects in a twin design (Purcell, 2002). That is, these dynamics could magnify *differences* between genetically less similar children (i.e., DZ twins) and *similarities* between genetically identical children (i.e., MZ twins).

The third type of correlation is an "active" (G)(E) correlation, or what Scarr and McCartney (1983) called "niche picking." Children, and to a greater degree adults, select their own experiences and contexts—which in turn influence their development. For example, a very active or fearless child might be drawn to risk-taking peers, whose influence then contributes to further fearless, risk-taking, or impulsive behaviors. An active child might also expose him- or herself to more lead dust (e.g., by exploring more of the house). Such niche picking can be adaptive, as when persons with ADHD choose a profession that suits their abilities and limitations well (somewhat stereotypical examples might include actor, salesman, politician, or artist, but the possibilities are vast when one considers the broad heterogeneity of children—and adults—with ADHD). It can also be maladaptive, as in the example of choosing antisocial peers.

(G)(E) correlations can be captured in either the environmental term or the heritability term, depending on the type of correlation that occurs. When genotype is correlated with shared environment (e.g., an organized mother creates a structured environment for both of her twin children, who have also inherited a conscientious style), the effect inflates the role of environment by making both MZ and DZ twins more similar than would be expected by genetic effects alone. Thus what appears to be an environmental effect may include crucial genetic contribution. However, correlations between genotype and nonshared environment (e.g., genotype's influencing choice of peer group, or parents' expressing more negativity with the more difficult sibling) would contribute to heritability estimates by making MZ twins more similar than DZ twins. In that case it would be overly simplistic to conclude that environmental effects are unimportant simply because heritability is high. In fact, important environmental mechanisms would be mediating the genetic influences.

Implications of (G)(E) Correlations' "Hiding" in the Heritability Term

The fact that G × E interactions and correlations can be "hidden" in the heritability term in twin studies is extremely important. It means that if we draw overly simplistic conclusions about mechanistic genetic or environmental "main effects" on ADHD, without considering gene–environment interplay, we might easily "miss the boat" if these interaction, coaction, or correlation effects are present. Identifying these effects in biometric designs is complex, is difficult to do with certainty, and requires large samples (see Eaves & Erkanli, 2003; Turkheimer, D'Onofrio, Maes, & Eaves, 2005). However, they may be able to be teased out with molecular strategies combined with measures of environmental effect, so as to capture genotype-based variation in response to environmental risks (Rutter, 2001). Even those designs require consideration of the converse possibility that the environmental measure includes genetic influences. Overall, however, at least two broad implications follow.

With regard to (G)(E) correlations, at least one major implication is that socialization mechanisms require further scrutiny in ADHD (Nigg et al., 2006). Evocative and passive (G)(E) correlations can be expressed through children's interpersonal interactions and social experiences. Parent–child relations may influence a child's developing self-regulation, self-control, executive functioning, arousal state, and emotional reactivity throughout development, all without changing the high heritability of the condition—if those parenting effects are mediated via (G)(E) correlations. The example given earlier for aggressive behavior in children is a now-classic demonstration. Those mechanisms could be the means by which genetic influences on ADHD are, at least in part, expressed and actualized—and may therefore be a route by which causal sequences in development can be diverted or modulated. In short, the fundamental principles of behavioral genetic research call for a careful understanding of how genes and socialization work together specifically in giving rise to and maintaining the behavioral and self-control problems that constitute the hallmark of the syndrome.

Although (G)(E) correlations remain to be demonstrated in ADHD, child-elicited effects on parenting do appear to be important. Barkley and Cunningham (1979) looked at parenting behaviors when children with ADHD were on and off stimulant medication. When the children were on medication, parents showed more appropriate behavior with them; they provided more praise, more warmth, and less hostility and criticism. Subsequent work has borne out this observation (Danforth, Barkley, & Stokes, 1991). This finding is consistent with child-elicited effects in parent–child interchanges in ADHD. It is also consistent with the idea that evocative (G)(E) correlations may be an important element in the developmental processes involved in ADHD.

Johnston and Mash (2001) provided a cogent summary of the various family processes that require further study in ADHD. These include the ways in which parenting practices and parent–child conflict, marital/couple conflict, and parental psychopathology (among other potential mechanisms) may lead to ineffectiveness in structuring child development. The degree to which altering these processes could alter the trajectory of maladaptive development for a child with ADHD remains largely unknown.

If this conception is correct, then teaching parents to overcome such evocative influences in parenting guidance should alter the developmental course of ADHD. Follow-ups to study whether parenting interventions alter the course of ADHD have been quite limited. Clinical psychologists have known for over 20 years that short-term interventions teaching parents to manage oppositional and aggressive behaviors more effectively are effective for those behaviors (Bank, Marlowe, Reid, Patterson, & Weinrott, 1991; Forehand, Rogers, McMahon, Wells,

& Griest, 1981; Patterson & Reid, 1973; Wells & Egan, 1988). It has been more difficult to show such consistent effects on ADHD behaviors per se, although interventions that strengthen parenting practices nonetheless do have a positive influence on ADHD outcome and, in some studies, on symptoms of hyperactivity and inattention (Bor, Sanders, & Markie-Dadds, 2002; Dubey, O'Leary, & Kaufman, 1983; Hinshaw et al., 2002; Hechtman et al., 2004; Sonuga-Barke, Daley, Thompson, Laver-Bradbury, & Weeks, 2001). Furthermore, ADHD symptoms did improve with such psychosocial interventions—especially if these were combined with medication therapy—in both the MTA (Swanson et al., 2001b) and the Montreal multimodal treatment study (Hechtman et al., 2004).

The difficulty of altering ADHD's course via parenting interventions does not mean that (G)(E) mechanisms are unimportant. Rather, the canalizing effect of a child's temperament combined with a parent's vulnerability may be so powerful that any time-limited intervention has only a modest effect. These possibilities warrant continued investigation and more recognition than they have received in recent years.

Implications of G × E Interactions' Hiding in the Heritability Term

The major implication of hidden G × E interactions is a key focus in the remainder of this book. The present analysis tells us that interactions between genotype and common environmental potentiators may be hidden in the heritability term for ADHD. Because this effect is restricted to shared environment effects, it is most likely that they will be found in relation to risk agents that are very common, even ubiquitous, in children's development. As I show in the following two chapters (especially Chapter 11), many candidate risk agents exist, with varying plausibility as etiological contributors to ADHD.

In light of the preceding, then, it is useful to divide experiential effects into *common* effects (most likely to be shared) and *relatively uncommon* effects (most likely to be nonshared). The relatively *uncommon* agents, even if they interact with genotype, will still be more likely to show up as environmental effects in the twin data, and thus are already addressed by the search for those environmental triggers. Therefore, conceptual models of ADHD usually already consider these types of effects, albeit as part of nonshared environment rather than as interactive effects. However, the *common* agents will be easily missed, because their effects, when they interact with genotype, will be "hidden" in the heritability term. Thus these common G × E interactions have been generally overlooked in conceptual models of ADHD etiology.

Instead, the main research logic in the field has been to focus only on relatively *uncommon* environmental effects. Thus we know more about the influence on ADHD of these somewhat exceptional types of risks than we do about common risks. In general, clinical and medical professionals recognize that psychopathology and neuropsychological/cognitive disabilities can emanate from relatively rare (though still distressingly frequent) disastrous environmental risks, such as severe physical abuse, high levels of individual lead poisoning, serious perinatal complications, or significant head injury. They also recognize that children respond differently to these disasters. In most instances, these effects are probably nonshared and reflected in the modest (though not inconsequential) nonshared environment effects on ADHD, which are in the 20–30% range.

We cannot always be certain whether relatively uncommon effects are unshared and common effects are shared, however. For example, lead exposure might have similarly effects on children in the same family (e.g., if they are close together in age and play together often), even if it is uncommon in the population at large. Yet this "common" and "uncommon" dichotomy will provide us with a reasonable heuristic for considering the types of effects relevant to ADHD.

In all, nonshared environment *main* effects for ADHD are modest in size. As noted earlier, they account for 20% or perhaps 30% of variance in ADHD symptoms—an important percentage if the causal effects therein can be identified and prevented. Shared environment *main* effects are vanishingly small in ADHD, although they do emerge in some studies of teacher ratings. When it comes to common risk agents, however, our reliance on twin study estimates may lead us to overlook environmental mechanisms if G × E interactions are operative. Put another way, we do not know what proportion of ADHD's heritability is attributable to (1) extreme inherited temperament versus (2) common experiential mechanisms acting via G × E interactions.

I view option 2 in the prior paragraph as a "blind spot" in the nation's ADHD research portfolio, because in contrast to the recognition afforded relatively rare triggering events (such as severe abuse or injury), little attention has been paid to ubiquitous, common, and moderate-to-mild risk exposures. One reason for this blind spot is failure to recognize that heritability estimates encompass certain classes of G × E interactions and (G)(E) correlations. Interactions between genotype and shared environment factors (for which I will use the proxy term "very common" risk agents) will masquerade as genetic main effects in traditional twin designs, and thus be hidden from view in our research models.

The importance of this blind spot is substantial, because it leads to insufficient consideration of environmental mediators and moderators of genetic effects. One common-sense example of this is that if children in a population share exposure to environmental risks that interact with genotype, then their chances of developing a disorder will depend largely on their genetic differences in liability. This state of affairs will produce high-heritability estimates *even in the presence of important G × E interactions* that may have a major influence on the final expression of the disorder or disease. This is another way of saying that interactions between shared environment (and a ubiquitous risk exposure is a shared environment factor) and genes lead to "inflated" estimates of heritability (Purcell, 2002), compared to what one would expect from purely genetic main effects.[5]

It should be easy to recognize examples in which environmental effects can appear to be genetic at first glance. For example, political beliefs often run in families; however, twin studies show that they are largely a product of shared environment, not shared genes. More difficult to detect are those instances in which genes and environments combine to produce a disease, but the environmental effect at first looks like a genetic effect.

An example of the importance of this principle comes from the history of an infectious disease, tuberculosis (TB; this history was reviewed by Fine, 1981, whose presentation I follow here). In the 19th century, the intergenerational consistency of TB infection led some observers to speculate that the disease itself was inherited (Hirsch, 1986). By the mid-20th century, some twin studies were showing that TB had high heritability (Kallman & Reiser, 1943), though others yielded lower figures (Harvald & Hauge, 1956). Yet the unweighted average of five twin studies reported by Fine (1981) suggested an average MZ concordance of 51% and a DZ concordance of 16%, suggesting heritability between 60% and 70%—the same as what I've suggested for ADHD. (See Fine, 1981, for discussion of sampling biases, the meaning of susceptibility, and a range of unique issues pertaining to studying heritability of liability for infections disease, including differential social contact among MZ and DZ twins.) Of course, scientists knew by then that TB is caused by a bacterium, and that what the twin studies were revealing was heritability of liability—vulnerability—to the TB bacterium.

This instance has some limitations as an analogy to ADHD. In particular, for TB the bacterium is necessary for the disease to develop (this is sometimes called genotype–environment "coaction" to distinguish it from "interaction"). In the case of ADHD, we expect environmental triggers to act probabilistically, in concert with genetic influences, even if important G × E interactions are taking place.

Yet the example illustrates dramatically that in the presence of common exposure to the bacterium, genetic variability largely determined who became ill even when environmental triggers were essential to the disease. The same logic would hold with probabilistic effects and mental or behavioral disorders. Common environmental risk agents may be important, even in the presence of high heritability, via undetected G × E interactions.[6]

Are there plausible *common* risk agents that could affect children's development of psychopathology—in this case, ADHD? I scrutinize some possibilities in Chapter 11. In all, the plan for the next two chapters is to consider (1) relatively well-established yet mostly *uncommon* experiential causes of ADHD (which probably explain only a minority of cases and are likely to account for some of the nonshared environment influence on the disorder) in Chapter 10; and then (2) speculative, emerging, or as-yet-unstudied *common* experiential causes of ADHD, and their likelihood of leading to a payoff, in Chapter 11. The latter include common risk agents that could interact with genotype to cause ADHD. I argue that the most promising of these warrant consideration in terms of high-risk/high-payoff directions for future research.

CLINICAL IMPLICATIONS

"Is ADHD caused by genes?" "Did my child inherit the disorder from me?" "Is psychotherapy useless with hyperactive children, if ADHD is due to genetic effects?" These types of questions are often posed by parents, students, and others. First, despite some questions about the correct magnitude of heritability estimates in ADHD, variation in children's ADHD symptoms is due in substantial part (60–70%) to variation in their genetic makeup. Molecular studies are moving forward, with replicated findings for key dopamine-related genes—though these genes are not acting alone, but are moderated by other effects.

Yet it is important to recognize that genetic studies are not diagnostic of ADHD, unlike Huntington's disease or other single-gene disorders. Such studies cannot, in principle, become diagnostic until or unless the disorder is redefined to specify biological markers to which genes can be linked. Genetic testing for ADHD is therefore not possible at this time.

Second, the causal mechanisms involved in ADHD may differ from those involved in the closely related problems of oppositional and defiant behaviors, aggression, and conduct problems. These associated disruptive behaviors are under more direct shared environment influence, perhaps emanating from the types of coercive exchanges in families that Patterson and colleagues have documented (see, e.g., Snyder et al., 2003). Despite their frequent co-occurrence, differentiating ADHD from oppositional and aggressive behavior problems during evaluation and treatment is important for case conceptualization, intervention planning, and psychoeducation with parents.

With regard to parent psychoeducation, it may be of value to recognize the substantial heritable component of attention problems and hyperactivity. Recognizing that many of these problems may reflect an extreme temperament may help ease parental fears and insecurities, and thus may open the door to more productive parental counseling.

Third, however (and balancing this last point), these types of genetic influences on ADHD are probabilistic, not deterministic. They may be mediated through automatic, preconscious interchanges during children's early and ongoing socialization by parents and families as well as peers. These effects may be self-maintaining, and so may become canalized and difficult to change. Such effects could include (G)(E) correlations, some of which inflate heritability estimates. Thus these unfolding developmental effects would not be inconsistent with high heritability estimates.

Nevertheless, however, the emergence, continuation, and worsening of these behavior problems are not inevitable or predetermined even in the presence of substantial heritability. Parental guidance to manage the behaviors can have an effect. Still, as the intervention literature documents, these parental interventions are more clearly effective for oppositional and defiant behaviors (Wells & Egan, 1988) than for hyperactivity per se.

Moreover, a key finding is that shared environment effects are quite important in oppositional and aggressive behavior problems. In early childhood, these behaviors may be particularly susceptible to family socialization and parenting style. Children with ADHD are *at risk* of developing oppositional and conduct problems, even in the presence of normative parenting (Nigg & Hinshaw, 1998). Parental action can forestall these developments, so clinical intervention to prevent the potential complications of ODD or CD in cases of significant hyperactivity and inattention represents a key treatment target.

Fourth, aside from the misconception that genetic influences are deterministic and immutable, the most important misconception about genetic influence on ADHD is that it renders experiential influences of little importance. Although these assumptions may hold for some single-gene metabolic diseases, they are faulty for multifactorial disease generally (see Chapter 2).

In the case of ADHD, the genetic effects are probabilistic. They are likely to be mediated via downstream (G)(E) correlations in the following form: parent–child socialization and the child's eliciting of responses from others and the environment amplify the dysregulated developmental pathway on which the child's temperament may have launched him or her. Altering these canalized and automatized behavioral interchanges can be difficult, but at least in principle, it can be done. Thus findings that psychosocial interventions may help children with ADHD do not contradict the role of heritable mechanisms in the disorder. Indeed, the hunt for environmental interventions to prevent or ameliorate ADHD is as important as ever. See Paul Meehl's (1972) classic essay on the general point that cause and solution are not inextricably linked; genetic influence is no grounds for therapeutic or existential nihilism.

Most important to recognize is that heritability may reflect *liability* to disorder, rather than direct genetic *determination* of the disorder. This means that causal processes may well include certain kinds of G × E interactions—specifically, interactions with shared environmental effects. For the sake of simplicity, in this book I speak of "common" and "uncommon" environmental agents. The reason I do so is that whether a causal agent is acting as a shared or a nonshared agent is an empirical question. To avoid creating the illusion that we know which agents are shared and which are unshared, I speak of common agents (more likely to be shared) and uncommon agents (more likely to be unshared). In imagining the etiology of ADHD, it is essential that we not overlook these possible G × E interactions. The failure to consider this possibility is an important "blind spot" in the nation's ADHD research portfolio.

In all, clinicians can guide parents to the knowledge that (1) some of the behavior problems in ADHD reflect temperamental or genetic variation, and so are not the fault of poor parenting; (2) even these fewer effects may respond to effective parenting or other behavioral guidance; and (3) the potential for oppositional and antisocial behaviors to develop is an important target for psychosocial intervention.

TABLE 9.1. Frequently Asked Questions about ADHD and Genes

Question	Answer
Is ADHD inherited?	The propensity to develop ADHD is partially influenced by heredity.
Aren't there biases in twin studies?	Rater bias can and does occur, but this does not explain ADHD's substantial heritability.
Does this mean that my child cannot change?	No. Genes are expressed in context, and effects are supported by ongoing behavioral interchanges. These effects may be difficult to interrupt, but are not immutable in principle. Behavioral studies show effects on aspects of ADHD symptoms.
Does this mean that I have to medicate my child?	No. Causes and treatments have no necessary connection; some heritable conditions may respond best to psychosocial treatment, and vice versa.
Does a single gene cause ADHD?	Almost certainly not, except possibly in rare instances of a particular thyroid disorder.
Does high heritability mean that research should stop seeking experiential causes of ADHD?	No. Certain types of environmental effects remain in need of intensive investigation.

Table 9.1 summarizes key points made in this chapter as answers to frequently asked questions that often confront professionals working with ADHD.

CONCLUSION

It is impossible to ignore the role of genetic influences in any complete model of ADHD. Yet it is a major mistake to assume that experiential influences should not receive equal weighting in the scientific research agenda on ADHD. The most important environmental influences are those that (1) are mediating genetic effects via (G)(E) correlations, or (2) emanate from commonly occurring risk agents that interact with genetic liability. In sum, even as the behavioral and molecular genetic data point to potential breakthroughs in understanding the biological level of analysis in ADHD, they also show us that *certain kinds* of experiential influences require more investigation—and have probably been mistakenly ignored.

| C H A P T E R   1 0 |

Uncommon Experiential
Risk Factors

A mother may ask, "Did my child's early problems when I was pregnant cause ADHD?" A doctor may ask, "Did my patient's smoking when pregnant cause the child's ADHD?" A researcher may ask, "Is there any plausible explanation for the perceived increase in incidence of ADHD that would reflect a real increase?" or "What, besides genes, contributes to the etiology of ADHD?"

Several experiential risk factors for ADHD exist that are relatively uncommon. These are promising candidates to explain the *nonshared* environmental causes of the syndrome. Of course, some of the risks covered in this chapter may still cluster in families, and so may really function as shared environment effects even though they are relatively uncommon. However, this possibility does not prevent a general analysis of the likely direct effects of these potential causal agents. In addition, if relatively rare effects operate as shared effects via interaction between geneotype and shared environment, their influence on the heritability term is likely to be small because the events are relatively uncommon as noted. If, however, these effects operate as nonshared effects interacting with genotype, then they will still contribute to the nonshared term in twin studies. In all, even though classifying these risk factors is imprecise, the emphasis of this chapter is on risk agents that are plausible candidates to explain the nonshared environment etiology of ADHD.

Among these candidates are prenatal teratogens, such as prenatal alcohol exposure. Of particular recent interest has been prenatal nico-

221

tine exposure. Because so much controversy surrounds the topic, I devote some space to describing the state of knowledge about prenatal cigarette use on ADHD. A separate category of risk marker is represented by low birthweight (LBW)—itself multiply determined, with maternal smoking being one important contributor to it. LBW in turn is associated with increased risk of ADHD. Although LBW is not a single causal agent (but represents a clustering of risk agents), recognizing its role may shed light on the syndrome, and so I discuss that role herein. However, even for these rather heavily researched risk factors and/or risk markers, the *magnitude* of the contribution to ADHD is not always well described in the literature. I attempt to estimate it here.

Many questions are also asked about the role of prenatal stress and about traumatic disruptions in early development. Although these literatures are small, I will briefly note the preliminary conclusions from them. However, because the focus is on attempting to identify causes that could explain the *neuropsychological* weaknesses observed in ADHD, I emphasize early developmental insults. In this chapter, then, I describe the state of knowledge about these relatively well-studied risks. In describing magnitude of risk, the literature often presents data on "proportion of variance" in ADHD symptoms explained in a population sample. It is difficult to translate this figure into a "proportion of cases" that might be explained by a causal trigger. However, I attempt to summarize data about proportional and attributable risks when available; see Table 10.1 for an overview of key terms, and note 1 for further details.[1] These statistics, which derive from estimates of the degree to which a given risk factor or causal agent increases the chances of getting ADHD, will permit some rough estimate of what

TABLE 10.1. Key Statistics for Estimating Potency of Risk Factors

Term	Meaning
Relative risk	Proportion of cases in an exposed versus an unexposed population
Attributable risk	Rate of disease in the exposed group minus rate in the unexposed group
Population attributable risk	How much of the population is getting the disease because of this risk factor
Population attributable fraction	What percentage of cases can be attributed to this risk factor

Note. Data from Fletcher, Fletcher, and Wagner (1996). See note 1 for detailed explanation.

proportion of ADHD cases might be associated with a particular causal risk factor or risk marker.

Aside from prenatal teratogens such as alcohol, the neurotoxic effects of acute high-level exposures to environmental and industrial solvents, fuels, pesticides, and heavy metals are well documented in the neuropsychological literature (Lezak et al., 2004; Spencer & Schaumburg, 2000). The brain is especially vulnerable to such effects because of its rich fat content (e.g., myelinated fibers). Many of these substances are therefore potentially harmful even to adults. Children are more vulnerable still, and the developing fetus is most vulnerable of all—potentially harmed even at low exposure levels that have no discernible effect on adults (see Koger, Schettler, & Weiss, 2005, for more discussion). Yet for the most part their relations to ADHD are virtually unstudied and thus are still speculative, though worrisome. Importantly, however, many such exposures may be extremely *common*, placing them in a different class of risk factors from the point of view of causal models. For that reason, Chapter 11 addresses the toxicant effects that are (1) best studied; (2) most closely related to potential ADHD symptoms and the kinds of neuropsychological findings described in Chapters 4–7; and (3) extremely widespread, so that they could materially influence the heritability estimates for ADHD if genotype–environment interactions are occurring as explained in Chapter 9.

In this chapter, I consider major causal influences (whether established or disputed) that are relatively *uncommon* and might take up some percentage of the nonshared effect on ADHD etiology, but that probably have little influence on heritability estimates. My three goals here are to (1) acquaint readers with these probable etiologies and/or risk markers; (2) evaluate the status of knowledge about them and their potential magnitude of influence on the problem of ADHD; and (3) highlight potential high-risk/high-payoff directions for the public health research effort on ADHD's etiology.

LOW BIRTHWEIGHT

About 7% of children born alive in the United States are classified as having LBW (< 2,500 grams). LBW provides an entryway into a range of developmental problems, including ADHD. Before the findings related to ADHD are described, it is important to define the context: What is LBW, and why does it occur?

What Is LBW, and What Causes It?

LBW has multiple causes and often reflects an accumulation of psychosocial and physical risk factors that are difficult to tease apart. For example, it is more common in low-SES families. Furthermore, children born with LBW include two groups: (1) those born prematurely but with a typical rate of growth; and (2) those who experienced intrauterine growth delays (referred to as "intrauterine growth retardation" or IUGR), many of whom are also born prematurely. Premature birth in turn is due to a range of factors, such as maternal stress, physical activity, and infection; smoking has only a small effect on prematurity, and the majority of prematurity has unknown causes (Kramer, 1987).[2] However, of primary interest to us here is LBW due to IUGR (regardless of whether a child is carried to term or born preterm). This type of LBW is weight that is low for gestational age.

The causes in this latter instance remain multifaceted. Nonetheless, comprehensive reviews suggest that, at least in developed countries such as the United States, the largest single contributor to LBW is maternal smoking during pregnancy. Kramer (1987) conducted a comprehensive meta-analysis of studies to that time and concluded that the attributable risk (proportion of cases) due to smoking was about 22%. Other significant contributors to or causes of LBW were poor maternal nutrition/low calorie intake, low maternal prepregnancy weight, and a range of physical risk factors in the mother (e.g., small stature, prior LBW birth of the mother). Notably, maternal alcohol use during pregnancy accounted for only a little over 2% of the risk of LBW in Kramer's (1987) comprehensive review. However, psychosocial adversity and ill health obviously converge on a range of physical and emotional stressors that complicate the picture. This is relevant to ADHD because psychosocial adversity may increase risk of ADHD, over and above the effects of prenatal nicotine and alcohol (Biederman, Faraone, & Monuteaux, 2002).

In a more recent review, Chomitz, Chueng, and Lieberman (1995) reached conclusions similar to Kramer's (1987): Causes of LBW were viewed as including inadequate maternal health and nutrition, inadequate weight gain, nicotine or cigarette use, alcohol, or other substance use during pregnancy, maternal illness, domestic violence leading to fetal injury or to premature labor due to severe emotional stress, and possibly other significant maternal emotional stress. Yet Chomitz et al. concluded as well that the single largest and most preventable cause of LBW in developed countries is cigarette smoking during pregnancy. Their estimate of the attributable risk of LBW due to prenatal cigarette exposure was somewhat higher than Kramer's (1987); they concluded that cigarette smoking causes up to 30% of LBW cases, and that alcohol use accounts for a smaller percentage (and cocaine use a smaller percentage still).

When we take all of this together, it is apparent that although LBW is multiply determined, it is one pathway of risk for early developmental problems. Prenatal cigarette exposure is the single largest contributor in the developed world, although it accounts for only a minority of cases. Various other health and stress factors also contribute. In all, LBW is in part a pathway for several health-related risk factors; it is in part a marker of concentrated demographic risk.

What Are the Outcomes for Children with LBW?

Hack, Klein, and Taylor (1995) reviewed population outcomes associated with LBW, including the dramatic historical changes in medical care that have led to an increase in the number of such births. They noted that prior to the 1960s, newborns weighing below 1,500 grams (about 3 pounds, 5 ounces) rarely survived. Even then, children with "moderately low birthweight" (less than 2,500 grams but greater than 1,500 grams) had some adverse outcomes, such as mental retardation, developmental delays, and emotional and behavioral problems including "minimal brain dysfunction" and hyperactivity. That literature, however, was confounded by the often disastrous iatrogenic effects of early yet misguided treatment efforts with these children (Hack et al., 1995).

Advances in neonatal intensive care in the 1960s resulted in the survival of more children weighing less than 1,500 grams at birth, termed "very low birthweight," and at the same time a reduction in rates of cerebral palsy and developmental disabilities in these survivors. However, other adverse outcomes were noted for this group of children, who are now the focus of most of the medical literature on LBW. Beginning in the 1970s, further advances in neonatal intensive care led to the survival of children weighing less than 1,000 grams at birth (2 pounds, 3 ounces), termed "extremely low birthweight," as well as children weighing less than 750 grams (1 pound, 10 ounces). I use the generic term "LBW" when referring to all of these groups, unless specific subgroups are relevant.

After about 1980, rates of cerebral palsy and other disabilities stayed constant among children with LBW (about 1 in 12 of these live births), while survival rates increased. As a result, the total prevalence of disabilities in the general population steadily increased after 1980 in developed countries. Even after we eliminate cases with cerebral palsy and control for low IQ, other outcomes can include neurological soft signs; neuropsychological problems, including spatial, motor, and verbal deficits; and behavioral problems, including hyperactivity (especially among boys). This last group of problems is obviously the outcome of interest to us here (see Hack et al., 1995, for additional details).

If a percentage of children with LBW develop ADHD, then the greater survival of such children (and their protection from severe neurological injury) in the past few decades could have contributed not only to the prevalence of ADHD but to a secular trend of rising incidence over time (Mick, Biederman, Prince, Fischer, & Faraone, 2002b), even though some causes of LBW itself (such as smoking) have declined over that time. Recent studies establish that LBW is associated with increased risk of ADHD, perhaps more so than other psychopathologies (Pinto-Martin et al., 2004; Mick et al., 2002b; Whitaker et al., 1997; Szatmari, Saigal, Rosebaum, Cambell, & King, 1990; O'Callaghan & Harvey, 1997; Breslau, Klein, & Allen, 1988; Breslau & Chilcoat, 2000). How big is this effect—or, to put it another way, how prevalent are attention problems and hyperactivity in these children?

Magnitude of the LBW Effect on ADHD

In one of the first and most often cited studies, Szatmari et al. (1990) estimated that ADHD was present in 16% of children with extremely low birthweight (<1,000 grams), versus 7% of healthy control children at age 5. They did not find an increased risk of other psychiatric problems and so concluded that risk was relatively specific to ADHD; however, even this effect appeared to be largely explained by low IQ/developmental delay in this sample. Szatmari, Saigal, Rosebaum, and Cambell (1993) followed up this sample at age 7–8, finding that when parent and teacher reports were combined, ADHD was present in 18.5% (24.1% of boys, 13.8% of girls) of the sample with extremely low birthweight, versus 5.7% (consistent with population averages) in the control group. This represents a threefold increase in risk; again, ADHD was the only disorder that was significantly more likely in the risk group (CD, $p = .57$; emotional disorder, $p = .91$). Yet low IQ again statistically explained this effect. However, it is unclear whether covarying IQ is appropriate in this situation. Subsequent studies showed an effect of LBW on ADHD even when IQ was controlled for, both in retrospective case–control designs (Mick et al., 2002b) and in prospective population-based designs (Breslau et al., 1996).

Whitaker et al. (1997) and Pinto-Martin et al. (2004) reported on ADHD rates at age 6 and age 9, respectively, in their sample of children with LBW from New Jersey. When the children were 6 years of age, a structured parent interview yielded the conclusion that 15.6% (22% for boys, 9% for girls) of this sample had ADHD, which was the most common psychiatric outcome at this age. This increased risk was related to brain injuries identified at birth on cranial ultrasound (specifically, parenchymal lesions or ventricular enlargement). This type of injury would be expected to interfere with cortical organization during early postnatal development. At age 9, the overall rate of ADHD in this sample was estimated at almost twice the expected population rate (5.2% vs. 3%, according to these researchers' cutoffs on the Conners scales). Within the sample, rates of ADHD were directly related to severity of LBW, with higher rates among children with extremely low and very low than among those with moderately low birthweight. Several other studies with varying methodology yielded varying results with regard to magnitude of effect of LBW on ADHD (Botting, Powls, Cooke, & Marlow, 1997; O'Callaghan & Harvey, 1997; O'Keefe, O'Callaghan, Williams, Najman, & Bor, 2003), including some evidence that some of the association of ADHD with motor clumsiness (Chapter 7) may be related to LBW (Foulder-Hughes & Cooke, 2003).

In a well-controlled population-based sample in southeast Michigan, Breslau et al. (1996) examined psychiatric outcomes at age 6 years in urban and suburban children. Relying only on a structured parent interview, they identified a twofold increase in ADHD among inner-city (urban) children with LBW, but no increase in ADHD among suburban, middle-class children with LBW. To define ADHD better, they then classified children by both parent and teacher reports. That method showed no significant interaction with urban–suburban status, although in the urban group, the relative risk of ADHD was 3.4 (13.9% for LBW vs. 4.1% for average birthweight), whereas in the suburban group the relative risk was 2.3 (6.9% for LBW vs. 3.0% for average birthweight). Effects held independently of IQ. Although the potential moderation of LBW outcome on ADHD is important, as a gauge of overall risk we can pool these values to obtain a composite relative risk estimate of 2.85. Again, there was some specificity in the relation of LBW to attention problems: Teacher-rated attention problems on the Achenbach Teacher's Report Form (TRF) yielded a stronger association with LBW than any other behavioral scale on the TRF.

Breslau and Chilcoat (2000) reported on the same sample at age 11. Children with LBW in urban settings had more than a twofold risk of new cases of ADHD (over and above cases seen at age 6). This effect was independent of maternal smoking during pregnancy; indeed, consistent with some population-based studies (reviewed in a later section of this chapter), smoking during pregnancy was more clearly related to antisocial and conduct problems in children than to attention problems per se. Their finding on some measures of ADHD of an interaction effect with urban–suburban status is of interest, suggesting possible buffering or amplifying effects of other psychosocial adversity or protective factors.

Further evidence of moderating effects on the LBW - ADHD connection emerged from a study by Tully, Arsenault, Caspi, Moffitt, and Morgan (2004). They found that maternal warmth (rated in a parent–child observation) completely moderated the LBW effect. Thus children with LBW and high maternal warmth had rates of ADHD no higher than population base rates; those with LBW and low maternal warmth were at elevated risk of ADHD.

Despite wide variation in study methodologies, sampling, and point prevalence of ADHD, as well as occasional mixed findings, these studies together suggest the following: (1) LBW may convey a relatively specific risk of ADHD, but not so much other child behavioral or psychiatric disorders; (2) these children may also have motor delays or motor control problems; and (3) LBW may confer a doubling of risk of ADHD, or a tripling of risk in combination with other risk factors. Risk may be higher with very LBW. Several studies replicated findings that ADHD was the most common psychiatric outcome for children with low birthweights (excluding motor and coordination problems).

I now extrapolate from the best of these numbers to estimate what percentage of ADHD cases may be attributable to LBW in the population. I use the 1990 U.S. statistics for LBW (Hoyert, Mathews, Menacker, Strobino, & Guyer, 2006), which indicate that 6.97% of children in the population are affected by LBW (Hoyert et al., 2006); for present purposes, I assume an ADHD incidence of 6% (see Chapter 1); and I use a relative risk estimate of 2.85 (the composite of values reported by Breslau et al., 1996, as noted above; Foulder-Cook & Hughes, 2003, reported similar values). The attributable risk is therefore 11.1%; the population attributable risk is 7.7 per 1,000; and the population attributable fraction, or percentage of ADHD cases that could be attributable to (in this case) LBW, is 12.8% (Hoyert et al., 2006). (See note 1 to this chapter for fuller explanations of these last three statistics and how they are derived.) Note that low birth weight births continue to increase, and had risen to over 8% in 2004; this will lead to an increase in the attributable fraction of ADHD cases potentially related to low birth weight in the future.

These numbers can be placed next to those from the only case–control study to ask directly about frequency of LBW among children with ADHD (Mick et al., 2002b). Mick et al. examined the rate of LBW in their clinic series of 252 children with ADHD and 231 controls without ADHD. LBW was somewhat underrepresented (only 2% of controls and 7% of ADHD cases), perhaps due to the exclusion of children with IQ < 80. LBW contributed independently to ADHD risk (p = .04) even after the researchers controlled for prenatal exposure to cigarettes or alcohol (p = .016), parental ADHD (p <.001), child conduct problems, parent antisociality, and child IQ (p <.001).

They estimated that LBW could be a direct cause of ADHD (here undifferentiated by subtype, and defined by DSM-III-R criteria) in about 14% of cases. Despite some limitations in that study, their estimate of a 14% risk is similar to the 12.8% I have arrived at above.

To summarize, it appears that LBW explains a small but noteworthy proportion of ADHD cases. These would be expected to be cases with associated motor problems (Chapter 7). The increased survival of children with LBW has contributed to an increased incidence of cerebral palsy; speculatively, it may also contribute slightly to an increased incidence of ADHD (such an increase is not clear, however). Most importantly, LBW is a likely contributor to a portion of the nonshared environment effect on ADHD etiology.

A final question before we move on: Do these cases of LBW and ADHD account for the neurocognitive findings in ADHD samples? They may account for motor control problems, as already noted. However, they do not appear to account for deficits in other neuropsychological functions, such as alerting. Potgeiter, Vervisch, and Lagae (2003) used an elegant 2 × 2 design (ADHD yes–no, very low birthweight yes–no) and found that ERP responses on an "oddball paradigm" (a well-established procedure designed to probe alerting ability in children) were associated with a main effect of ADHD, but no interaction (performance was no worse in children with ADHD + LBW than in those with ADHD but not LBW). Thus, whereas children with ADHD with LBW may have the same neurocognitive deficits as other children with ADHD, they do not "explain" the neurocognitively impaired children in samples with ADHD.

PRENATAL ALCOHOL EXPOSURE

Alcohol is a teratogen when used in sufficient quantity during pregnancy. One outcome has been thought to be impulsivity, hyperactivity, or inattention (Mick, Biderman, Faraone, Sayer, & Kleinman, 2002a). These associations may be causal, due to the effects of alcohol on the early developing nervous system. Notably, prenatal alcohol exposure is not a major contributor to LBW (Kramer, 1987); instead, it appears to act directly on the developing nervous system even when birthweight may be average (Streissguth, Barr, Sampson, & Bookstein, 1994a).

Fetal alcohol syndrome (FAS), which was identified in Europe and the United States in the early 1970s, results from heavy alcohol use during pregnancy (e.g., 5 or more drinks per drinking day, drinking several days per week, or weekend binge drinking) in a minority of women who drink heavily. The reasons why some such pregnancies do not result in these devastating outcomes are unknown, but numerous moderators have been suggested, including maternal age, child and parent genetic makeup (e.g., alcohol metabolism), and a range of other health factors (Jacobson, Jacobson, Sokol, Chiodo, & Corobana, 2004). FAS, when it occurs, often results in mental retardation. It is defined by characteristic physical signs that are visible between late infancy and late childhood (Stratton, Howe, & Battaglia, 1996). These include three types of facial anomalies: (1) short palpebral fissures (i.e., narrow eyes or short distance from inner to outer edge of the eyes); (2) smooth or flattened philtrum (i.e., the typically curved skin between the nose and upper lip is flat); and (3) thin upper lip. For photographs illustrating these features, see Chudley et al. (2005).

FAS is often also accompanied by other neurological soft signs, by language and cognitive delays, and by some increase in hyperactivity or impulsivity. The prevalence and incidence of FAS have been disputed in the literature. Abel (1995), after pooling data from 29 studies, estimated its incidence at 0.97/1,000 live births in Western countries. However, his methodology was criticized by Sampson et al. (1997), who estimated the incidence at between 2 and 3/1,000. More recently, the Centers for Disease Control and Prevention (CDC) attempted to standardize methods of identifying FAS, so as to avoid the pitfalls of under- and overidentification present in many studies. A recent summary of those efforts concluded that FAS has an incidence in the United States of 0.3–1.4/1,000 live births (Meaney, Miller, & FASSNET Team, 2003). Although FAS may be associated with ADHD, and even though it is difficult for many clinicians (including many physicians) to confidently identify FAS, in principle FAS is identifiable as a condition distinct from idiopathic ADHD. Even if cases of FAS are widely missed in practice, however, its low incidence and prevalence mean that these "misdiagnosed" cases would account for less than 2% of cases of ADHD.

Therefore, in considering the role of prenatal alcohol exposure as a potential explanation for ADHD, of more interest are lower-level effects that fall short of frank FAS. In support of the idea of these more subtle alcohol effects even in the absence of characteristic physical anomalies, animal studies indicate that prenatal alcohol exposures too weak to cause any visible physical effects can alter neuronal cell migration and proliferation (Clarren et al., 1990; for a review, see Streissguth, Sampson, Barr, Bookstein, & Carmichael-Olson, 1994b).

To attempt to capture these more subtle effects that can be observed in animal studies, the term "fetal alcohol effect" was coined in the late 1970s. However, that term, though useful in animal studies and in some epidemiological samples, proved too vague to be of use clinically. In 1996, the Institute of Medicine issued a consensus report in which five levels were proposed for fetal alcohol spectrum disorders (Stratton et al., 1996; see Table 10.2). All but one of these levels requires the documentation of heavy maternal drinking during pregnancy (i.e., heavy daily drinking of 5 drinks or more, or heavy weekend binge drinking). The reason for this requirement is that even though some studies show behavioral differences between children of mothers who drank even a little alcohol and abstainers, consensus on those effects, and on the amount of

TABLE 10.2. Institute of Medicine Classification of Fetal Alcohol Spectrum Disorders

Category definition	Clinical description
Category 1: FAS[a]	Classic facial dysmorphologies; "full-blown FAS"
Category 2: FAS absent confirmed	Classic facial dysmorphologies; can be diagnosed maternal alcohol exposure even when fetal exposure is not documented
Category 3: Partial FAS[a]	Partial facial anomalies; associated cognitive and behavioral problems, including hyperactivity
Category 4: FAS and birth defects[a]	Some congenital anomalies due to alcohol exposure
Category 5: FAS with ARND[a, b]	Either CNS abnormalities (e.g., language, motor, cognition) or complex behavioral/cognitive problems, but no physical anomalies

Note. Data from Stratton, Howe, and Battaglia (1996).
[a]Requires documented or confirmed prenatal alcohol exposure in relatively heavy quantity (≥ 5 drinks per episode).
[b]Alcohol-related neurodevelopmental disorder.

drinking needed to cause behavioral problems in offspring, is lacking. The Stratton et al. (1996) report therefore requires documented heavy drinking for all of its classifications.

The fifth category in Table 10.2 is the one of most interest for our purposes, because it can include ADHD without obvious physical or congenital defects. However, these children must have at least three signs of "neurodevelopmental disorder" from a list that includes neurological soft signs, language delays, cognitive problems, and distractibility/attention problems. Moreover, even full-blown FAS is often missed in clinical practice and therefore could contribute to an inflated incidence of idiopathic ADHD due to misdiagnosis.

The frequency of these fetal alcohol problems is also difficult to establish. However, Sampson et al. (1997) estimated the total prevalence of all five of these conditions at 9.1/1,000, including 2.8/1,000 for FAS. If we use those numbers to subtract the cases of full FAS (categories 1 and 2) from the others, we can estimate prevalent non-FAS fetal alcohol spectrum disorders at about 6/1,000 at the time of their review. Of these, it is speculated that 40–50% may develop ADHD (Koren, Nulman, Chudley, & Locke, 2003). This prevalence of fetal alcohol spectrum disorders, though estimated from data now more than a decade old, may still be approximately the same today. The CDC (2004a) estimates that about 10% of pregnant women drink alcohol, and that 2% engage in binge or frequent alcohol use, with little decline in the past decade. If even 6% of the pregnant women who drink give birth to children with fetal alcohol spectrum disorders, then these estimates would hold. Furthermore, the same CDC (2004a) report estimates that 50% of women of childbearing age who are not using birth control drink, and that 12% binge-drink. Some of these women will become pregnant and drink heavily in the first month before they realize they are pregnant.

In all, lacking better data, I base my calculations here on an estimated prevalence of non-FAS fetal alcohol spectrum disorders of 6/1,000 births, with an ADHD risk among that group of 40% (I scrutinize the plausibility of that 40% estimate shortly below). Those figures, if correct, would yield an attributable risk of 40% – 6% = 34%, for a relative risk of nearly 6:1. Population attributable risk is then estimated at 6/1,000 × .34 = 2.04/1,000. This in turn would generate a population attributable fraction of 3.4% of cases of ADHD. If we assume a lower rate of 30% (see discussion later), then we arrive at a population attributable risk of 1.44/1,000, equivalent to 2.4% of ADHD cases. In short, if present, this effect is extremely important because it is preventable;

however, it is apparently modest in terms of explaining the overall incidence of ADHD. Despite widespread public education about the dangers of drinking during pregnancy, the incidence of FAS or fetal alcohol spectrum disorders is not decreasing. Rather, decreased drinking (e.g., in response to warning labels) tends to be limited to women who drank lightly; those who drank heavily have not decreased their use (Hankin et al., 1993).

Up to this point, I have emphasized heavy drinking during pregnancy and have not scrutinized the claim that a significant proportion of these children will have ADHD. Let us evaluate these two issues.

First, what about moderate or lighter drinking during pregnancy (e.g., fewer than 5 drinks per drinking day)? From a clinical viewpoint, risk drinking is often defined as 1–3 drinks per day (Sokol, Delaney-Black, & Nordstrom, 2003). However, this definition of risk drinking is problematic because women who drink during pregnancy typically drink in episodes, with many drinks on one day and none on other days (Jacobson, Jacobson, Sokol, & Ager, 1998). Moreover, retrospective reports of prenatal drinking are prone to error (Jacobson, Chiodo, Jacobson, & Sokol, 2002), but prospective studies often lack power to detect sufficient cases of ADHD if these effects are small. In all, demonstrating alcohol effects on ADHD in the lower range of alcohol use has been difficult. In a comprehensive review of prenatal alcohol use and ADHD, Linnet et al. (2003) identified nine studies looking at prenatal alcohol use and either ADHD or a proxy for ADHD (rated attention problems) in children. Five of these studies failed to find an association, leading Linnet et al. to question whether low levels of alcohol use contribute to ADHD when appropriate confounds are controlled for. Yet key studies did find an association of low-level alcohol use and behavioral or cognitive problems in childhood (Martinez-Frias, Bermejo, Rodriguez-Pinilla, & Frias, 2004) although whether those problems were classifiable as ADHD was unclear. Streissguth et al. (1994b) examined CPT performance at age 4 years in offspring of women who drank (some of whom drank more than 5 drinks per day while pregnant) but did not smoke, smoked but did not drink, both drank and smoked, and did neither. Children's CPT attention problems were independently related to both alcohol and smoking exposure during pregnancy, whereas fine motor problems and lower Performance IQ were related to alcohol exposure but not smoking exposure. At age 7, effects on measured attention were confined to alcohol exposure. The same result held for a latent variable summarizing teacher ratings of disruptive behavior.

Second, however, are these effects really severe enough or specific enough to equate to ADHD? Clearly, some children with FAS have severe behavioral impairments and impulsivity. However, (1) only a handful of these studies looked at formally defined ADHD as an outcome in relation to any level of prenatal alcohol use by the mothers, and (2) vanishingly few have directly compared children with ADHD and fetal alcohol spectrum disorders on neuropsychological measures. Mick et al. (2002a) reported that in their clinical sample, children with ADHD were likely to have prenatal alcohol exposure; the effect held even after the researchers controlled for maternal ADHD, smoking during pregnancy, and parental antisociality. However, this study was retrospective and "alcohol exposure" was defined as daily or binge drinking, which means that these children classified as "alcohol-exposed" were exposed to relatively heavy levels of alcohol use by their mothers. In a small population-based study, Hill, Lowers, Locke-Wellman, and Shen (2000) used a criterion of "any drinking" during pregnancy and failed to find an association with diagnosis of ADHD. Low power may have been an issue in that study (n = 150), however.

Relatedly, is the neuropsychological profile of children with fetal alcohol spectrum disorders similar to the profile for ADHD? Some researchers have conducted behavioral and cognitive comparisons of children with fetal alcohol exposure and children with frank ADHD. Nanson and Hiscock (1990) found that children with FAS or fetal alcohol spectrum disorders had similar behavioral problems similar to those of a group of children with ADHD, and lower IQ and attention scores on cognitive testing. However, Coles et al. (1997) found that 25 children with FAS or fetal alcohol spectrum disorders had ADHD symptoms (defined by the Achenbach TRF Attention Problems Scale) that, at T = 61.5, were worse than those of the control group, but significantly less elevated than those of the group with ADHD (T = 72.1). On a neuropsychological battery, they found more evidence of verbal learning problems in the group with ADHD, and of spatial and math problems in the FAS/spectrum group. They also reported a qualitative difference in the pattern of scores on their extended battery, but significance values for those comparisons were not reported. Coles, Platzman, Lynch, and Freides (2002) reported on a larger sample of adolescents with fetal alcohol spectrum disorders. They had more difficulty on visual sustained attention (vigilance) than a special education comparison group, who had more difficulty on auditory vigilance.

Yet other studies have found executive dysfunctions—in particular, working memory and planning problems—in children with fetal alcohol spectrum disorders (Kodituwakku, Handmaker, Cutler, Weathersby, & Handmaker, 1995; Olson, Feldman, Streissguth, Sampson, & Bookstein, 1998). These dysfunctions are consistent with the pattern noted for ADHD in Chapter 5. More recently, Burden, Jacobson, Sokol, and Jacobson (2005) factor-analyzed their test battery and created factors for working memory (a blend of spatial and verbal short-term and working memory tasks), sustained attention (reliant on CPT variables), set shifting (on the WCST), and CPT commission errors. Only the working memory factor was uniquely related to prenatal alcohol exposure, but in children of older mothers (older than age 30), the sustained attention factor was also related. However, ADHD diagnosis was not reported, and comparison groups with ADHD were not examined, in those studies.

Thus these studies collectively suggest that there may be some parallels in the cognitive deficits associated with fetal alcohol spectrum disorders and ADHD. However, they call into question (1) whether most children with fetal alcohol spectrum disorders have behavior problems severe enough to qualify for a diagnosis of ADHD, and (2) whether the neuropsychological deficits are sufficiently similar to those of children with ADHD to create a mimicking condition. In particular, the fetal alcohol effects may tend to affect spatial and math abilities, at least in some samples. It will be necessary to separate ADHD from verbal learning disabilities (e.g., reading disorder) to clarify these differences. Learning disabilities were not controlled for in these studies.

In all, despite relatively clear findings that moderate to heavy alcohol use during pregnancy results in FAS (which includes significant behavioral and cognitive delays), and despite clear evidence that other fetal alcohol spectrum disorders also cause cognitive delays, still unclear are (1) the likelihood that fetal alcohol spectrum disorders may contribute to cases of ADHD per se, and (2) the magnitude and specificity of this effect if present. Population-based studies of prenatal alcohol exposure and ADHD with adequate controls do not allow firm conclusions as yet about the effects of fetal alcohol spectrum disorders on ADHD. Furthermore, effects of poorly defined low-level alcohol use during pregnancy are unconvincing in relation to ADHD. Crucially, parents with ADHD may be more likely to drink during pregnancy than other parents. Aside from the case–control study by Mick et al. (2002a), no population-based studies that found an association between prenatal alcohol exposure and later symptoms of inattention in children controlled for maternal ADHD. Whether these are mediated genetic effects thus remains unclear. When ADHD and fetal alcohol spectrum disorders have been directly compared in neuropsychological testing, it has appeared that the neuropsychological profiles may differ, but inadequate controls for learning disabilities leave that state of affairs in question.

Because moderate drinking during pregnancy remains relatively common (at about 12% of women who know they are pregnant, and perhaps double that rate in women who are not yet aware they are pregnant), clarifying the matter of low-level alcohol effects on development is important generally, regardless of the effect on ADHD. If this relatively light or moderate drinking has even a slight association with increased risk of ADHD, it could contribute to ADHD's incidence and could be preventable. Yet at present, even the specificity and magnitude of association of heavy drinking and fetal alcohol spectrum disorders with ADHD (rather than nonverbal learning disabilities, mathematics disorder, and other developmental delays) remains in dispute. The potential for specific effects of fetal alcohol exposure on visual processing is supported by experimental animal research showing specific disruption of visual cortical organization (Medina, Krahe, & Ramoa, 2005). Clearly, it continues to be advisable for pregnant women to avoid alcohol. Yet whereas the link between drinking during pregnancy and a range of developmental and cognitive delays is well established, the link to ADHD per se is not as clear as for other developmental and cognitive delays.

In summary, although FAS leads to severe behavioral and cognitive impairments, the specific association of fetal alcohol spectrum disorders and ADHD remains in question. Whereas additional controlled studies may overturn this conclusion, it may be that heavy alcohol use during pregnancy contributes in some instances to ADHD when it does not result in full-blown FAS. These cases of ADHD may be characterized by a neuropsychological profile similar to that for nonverbal learning disabilities, with problems in vigilance, math, and spatial ability. Specific problems in visual processing may contribute to this profile. Thus these children are likely to differ in cognitive and learning characteristics from the main group of children with ADHD. Whether their profile matches the neuropsychological profile described in Chapters 4–7 is unclear, because few studies have looked at such skills as response inhibition, spatial working memory, or temporal information processing in offspring of mothers who drank while pregnant; no studies have done so in comparison to a sample of children with frank ADHD. These effects on ADHD, if present, would account for about 2% of cases of ADHD, probably separately from the effects of LBW. However, numerous cautions remain as to whether fetal alcohol effects lead to ADHD rather than to other types of learning and developmental delays.

PRENATAL NICOTINE EXPOSURE

Overview

Because the role of prenatal smoking in ADHD is so widely discussed, considerable space is allocated here to updating readers on the status of knowledge about it, as well as on several ancillary issues that complicate our ability to draw definitive conclusions in this area. First, nicotine use during pregnancy has been identified for over 50 years as a risk factor for child developmental problems. Since 1979, the U.S. Surgeon General has warned that smoking during pregnancy can harm the fetus and retard growth (Chomitz et al., 1995; Ernst, Moolchan, & Robinson, 2001; Streissguth et al., 1994b). In the 1970s, cigarette use during pregnancy was associated with a wide range of child developmental anomalies, including LBW, reductions in growth, learning or cognitive problems, and increased locomotor activity. These effects, proven causal in animal studies, were identified as clear correlates in humans despite difficulties in controlling for a range of confounds (for reviews, see Ernst et al., 2001; Streissguth et al., 1994b).

Second, as noted earlier, one route for these effects is via LBW. We would expect to find an association between maternal cigarette use while pregnant and ADHD in the offspring, because cigarette use can cause LBW, and LBW increases the risk of ADHD. However, many studies have controlled for birthweight in an attempt to evaluate whether nicotine exposure causes ADHD independently. Such studies may have underestimated the full impact of nicotine use on ADHD, if a portion of that effect is via LBW.

Third, prenatal nicotine exposure has been associated with child externalizing behavior problems in several well-controlled, prospective population studies that included multiple methods of assessing child behavior problems, and that controlled for SES, other demographic factors, maternal use of alcohol and other drugs, and maternal depression (Brook, Brook, & Whiteman, 2000; Fergusson, Horwood, & Lynskey, 1993; O'Connor, Heron, Golding, Beveridge, & Glover, 2002;

Williams et al., 1998). However, even that well-controlled association has been called into question by recent genetically informative twin studies (Silberg et al., 2003).

Fourth, the specific linkage between ADHD and prenatal nicotine exposure has been less well studied, because many of the largest population-based studies did not include an assessment of ADHD criteria (many focused instead on conduct problems). However, prenatal nicotine use was among the strongest of a range of retrospectively assessed pre- and perinatal correlates of ADHD in the Massachusetts General Hospital series of children with ADHD and pediatric controls (Milberger, Biederman, Faraone, Guite, & Tsuang, 1997b). Linnet et al. (2003) reviewed 24 studies of smoking and child externalizing problems; they concluded that despite numerous cautions in this literature, a link between maternal smoking in pregnancy and child ADHD was likely, in view of several well-controlled replications using both prospective population-based designs and retrospective case–control designs. These studies in aggregate controlled for a number of confounds (e.g., low SES, maternal IQ, and in some instances maternal psychiatric symptoms, but not maternal ADHD). In any event, the effect of maternal smoking was far clearer in their review than the inconclusive effects for low to moderate maternal alcohol use on ADHD.

A series of issues, however, complicate the interpretation of this association. These issues include (1) evaluating the magnitude of the association apart from confounds such as prenatal alcohol exposure; (2) isolating an effect of cigarette use on ADHD from the effects of antisocial or conduct problems in parents and children; (3) the overlap of maternal smoking and maternal ADHD; and (4) the issue of whether smoking relates to ADHD after controls for genetic effects on ADHD.

Magnitude of Smoking's Effects
Apart from Common Confounds

Is smoking associated with hyperactivity after the effects of heavy prenatal drinking have been controlled for? In the section on prenatal alcohol exposure, I have noted that at least one study (Streissguth et al., 1994b) concluded that alcohol use but not cigarette use carried the prenatal risk effect on attention problems. Similarly, Hill et al. (2000) followed children from families with a high family history of alcoholism. ADHD in the children was related to family history of alcoholism, but not to prenatal cigarette exposure when family alcoholism history was controlled for. Parental antisocial behavior, but not ADHD, was also controlled for.

However, both of those studies selected their samples on the basis of heavy drinking. A larger number of population-based studies counter these findings and suggest that when cases of FAS or very heavy alcohol use are excluded, prenatal cigarette use is an independent predictor of child ADHD or ADHD symptoms when mild or moderate prenatal alcohol use is controlled for. Linnet et al. (2003) identified 11 studies that looked at these two risk factors together. They concluded that smoking was related to later ADHD after drinking was controlled for.

In a subsequent large population-based prospective study, Kotimaa et al. (2003) followed a population cohort of over 9,000 children in Ireland. They found that maternal smoking during pregnancy was associated with offspring hyperactivity even after adjustments for SES, other covariates, and maternal alcohol use. Thus the main population-based evidence suggests that the correlation of maternal smoking during pregnancy with later child hyperactivity is not an artifact of co-occurring prenatal exposure to alcohol.

Other issues, however, complicate conclusions from this literature: Definitions of smoking varied widely; relative risk or odds ratio values were often not reported; and parental ADHD status was almost never controlled for. With regard to relative risk, I have pooled the handful of relative risk and odds ratio values available in the tables provided by Linnet et al. (2003) to arrive at a composite relative risk of 1.53 for ADHD when mothers smoked (any amount) during pregnancy and common confounds were controlled for. However, there was some suggestion in this literature that the effect on boys may be larger, whereas the effect on girls may be smaller or nonexistent. These figures are summarized in Table 10.3.

However, several studies with negative findings did not report odds ratios; most of the studies in Table 10.3 are those with positive findings. Therefore, the odds ratio estimate there may be considered a high estimate. If we assume an average odds ratio of 1.0 in three additional (null) studies with 2,000 per sample, then the effect size would drop to an odds ratio of 1.4. Yet if a smoking main effect of even 1.4 exists in the population, it would be significant to understanding nonshared environment effects in the etiology of ADHD.

Some 18% of women in the United States reported smoking during pregnancy in 1990 (CDC, 2004c); it was thought that about 15% of

TABLE 10.3. Studies of Prenatal Smoking and ADHD That Used DSM or Equivalent Definitions of ADHD, and That Reported Relative Risk or Odds Ratios

Study	Definition of smoking	RR/OR	n	Comment and controls
Mick et al. (2002a)	≥ 20 cigs/day/3 mos	2.1^a	522	OR = 4.4 for boys
Landgren et al. (1998)	More than occasional	2.5^b	103	Not DSM-based
Hill et al. (2000)	Smoking or not	1.38^b	109	n.s.
Weisman et al. (1997)	≥ 10 cigs/day	$0.44^{a,\,b}$	147	OR = 2.26 for boys
O'Connor et al. (2002)	Smoking or not	$1.42^{a,\,b}$	7,447	For boys only
Williams et al. (1998)	1–9, 10–19, or ≥ 20 cigs/day	1.52	4,879	n.s.
		2.03		$p < .05$
	Average	2.16		$p < .05$
		1.91^b		
O'Callaghan and Harvey (1997)	4 levels	1.3^b	5,005	Composite value, dose effect
Weighted composite				
Any smoking		1.53^b		
Any smoking, boys		1.62^a		

Note. The first two studies listed are case–control studies; the rest are population studies. Only the first study controlled for maternal ADHD. RR, relative risk; OR, odds ratio. Data from Linnet et al. (2003).
[a]Pooled for the "boys" total.
[b]Pooled for the "any smoking" total.

women in the United States smoked but did not drink during pregnancy, in surveys up to the early 1990s (Chomitz et al., 1995). These rates have been dropping. They were estimated at 12% in 2000 (Cnattingius, 2004), and overall smoking in pregnancy had dropped to 11.4% in 2002 (CDC, 2004c). These estimates, however, rely on self-report. Underreporting is estimated at about 20% when checked in studies that use physiological measures to confirm nicotine use (Russell, Crawford, & Woodby, 2004). Thus for the sake of our estimates, sticking with an estimate of about 14% of women smoking during pregnancy at present in the United States appears reasonable. Those figures generate an attributable risk of 3.2%, which translates to a population attributable risk of 4.2/1,000 (Table 10.4).

This effect in turn would mean that 7.0% of ADHD cases are attributable to maternal smoking during pregnancy, if we assume straightforward main effects. Therefore, this possibility warrants fur-

TABLE 10.4. Percentage of ADHD Cases Attributable to Prenatal Nicotine Use

	Children exposed	Relative risk[a]	AR	PAR	PAF
Prevalence of ADHD				60.0/1,000	100.0%
Cigarettes (1991, self-report)	18.4%	1.53	3.2%	5.9/1,000	9.8%
Cigarettes (2002, self-report)	11.5%[b]	1.53	3.2%	3.7/1,000	5.8%
Cigarettes (2002, if underreport)	14%	1.53	3.2%	4.2/1,000	7.0%
Other drugs (without cigs or alc)	5/1,000	1.5	3.0%	1.5/10,000	<1.0%

Note. An incidence of ADHD of 6% is utilized here; see text in Chapter 1 and note 1 to this chapter for more detailed discussion of ADHD prevalence rates. Substance use data from Johnson, McCarter, and Ferencz (1987). AR, attributable risk (increased odds of ADHD from smoking in pregnancy); PAR, population attributable risk (incidence of ADHD in population due to smoking); PAF, population attributable fraction, or how many cases of ADHD may be due to smoking. If a lower incidence of ADHD is assumed (say, 2%), PAF increases.
[a]Cigarette relative risk effects are based on pooled odds and risk ratios taken from tables in Linnet et al. (2003), with confounds adjusted in logistic regression models (see Table 10.4). Dose–response effects are ignored.
[b]Rates of self-reported smoking during pregnancy are provided by CDC (2004c). Corrections for underreporting are as discussed in the text.

ther scrutiny for its potential to contribute to prevention. But how clear is it that this effect exists apart from genetic transmission of ADHD or antisocial behavior?

Parental ADHD and Smoking

ADHD and Antisocial Behavior in Parents

If we set aside issues such as definitions of smoking, the overarching issue in this literature is the almost universal failure to control for parental (especially maternal) ADHD in population-based designs. This prevents detection of possible genotype–environment correlations in the data. Smoking and alcohol use could lead to ADHD via mediation of genetic effects (women with ADHD tend to smoke or drink; this in turn contributes to ADHD in offspring and to the observed familial nature of the syndrome). If so, this would be an effect well worth knowing about and trying to prevent. However, alternatively, smoking could be a noncausative correlate of the ADHD genetic transmission. This seems to be the case, for example, with prenatal cigarette exposure and antisocial behavior; the association apparently can be accounted for by a child's genetic inheritance of a mother's antisocial traits. Silberg et al. (2003) demonstrated this effect in a genetically informative twin design in which they assessed antisocial traits in mothers and offspring; once the genetic transmission of antisocial traits was statistically controlled for, there was no independent association of maternal smoking with offspring conduct problems at age 6 years. This weighs against viewing smoking as causal in relation to conduct problems, if it holds up at older ages.

However, maternal ADHD (and, by extension, genetic effects) may operate separately from conduct problems. Ideally, both would be included in statistical models. Yet parental ADHD and antisocial behavior generally were not both controlled in the studies just noted or in those reviewed by Linnet et al. (2003).

Are Parents with ADHD More Likely to Smoke?

The confound between parental ADHD and parental smoking is important, because numerous studies in recent years have suggested that ADHD is associated with a greater chance of beginning to smoke in adolescence and/or adulthood (Burke, Loeber, & Lahey, 2001; Pomerleau et al., 2003; Tercyak, Lerman, & Audrain, 2002; Whalen, Jammer, Henker, Delfino, & Lozano, 2002). It is important to pause a moment to scrutinize this "side issue" of whether ADHD leads to increased risk of smoking in the parent, before returning to prenatal cigarette exposure and ADHD. If parents with ADHD are far more likely to smoke, then control of parental ADHD is critical in studies of prenatal smoking and offspring outcome. If, on the other hand, parents with ADHD are not more likely to smoke, failure to control parental ADHD status is less of a "fatal flaw" in those studies.

With regard to whether ADHD leads to smoking, many studies again failed to control for comorbid CD in the smokers, making it difficult to disentangle ADHD from antisocial behavior as a risk factor for smoking—and thus for smoking while pregnant. Milberger, Biederman, Faraone, Chen, and Jones (1997a), in their clinical series, found that children's smoking was predicted by CD, but that ADHD predicted smoking onset even after the CD effect was controlled for.

Yet that sample was selected for ADHD. Prospective longitudinal population studies indicate that comorbid CD accounts for the risk of smoking in children with ADHD (see Klein, 2002). For example, Lynskey and Fergusson (1995), in their study of the New Zealand birth cohort, concluded that ADHD did not predict smoking independently of CD or other indices of antisociality. Kodl and Wakschlag (2004) found that maternal history of conduct problems, but not ADHD, independently predicted persistence of smoking during pregnancy. They also found, however, that those with comorbid ADHD + CD were at most risk and most likely to persist in smoking. This pathway from ADHD to smoking is thus mediated or amplified by comorbid antisociality in population studies.[3] Although these findings provide some assurance that ADHD is not a primary driver of smoking in parents, still needed are studies that (1) control for parent ADHD and antisocial traits, and/or (2) are genetically informative. Such studies can verify that effects are not due to (G)(E) correlations (Chapter 9) in which ADHD or ADHD + antisocial traits in parents are passed on to children, with both parents and children then more likely to smoke. The few such studies available are considered next.

Results of Studies That Controlled for Genetic Effects

Only a handful of studies controlling for genetic effects have been reported. Milberger, Biederman, Faraone, Chen, and Jones (1996), again looking at the clinical series at Massachusetts General Hospital, found that 22% of boys with ADHD had a history of maternal smoking during pregnancy, versus only 8% of control boys; this association held after controls for SES, parental IQ, and (crucially) parental ADHD, with an odds ratio of 2.7—suggesting that the estimates of smoking's effects on ADHD in Table 10.3 may hold. A subsequent study looked at siblings of the boys with ADHD (i.e., siblings at "genetic risk" for ADHD). That study revealed that when siblings developed ADHD, they were twice as likely to have been exposed to prenatal smoking by their mothers (Milberger, Biederman, Faraone, & Jones, 1998), again even after control for maternal ADHD. Yet these studies did not control for parent antisocial traits or prenatal alcohol exposure, were not genetically informative, and relied on retrospective assessment of prenatal exposure.

Thapar et al. (2003) examined 1,452 twin pairs in the United Kingdom. Genetic factors explained most of the variance in parent and teacher ratings of children's ADHD symptoms, but maternal smoking during pregnancy still had a significant, environmentally mediated effect on ADHD symptoms after genetic factors and other confounds (including parent rater bias, social adversity, birthweight, and child CD), were controlled for. Smoking accounted for about 1% of the variance in ADHD symptoms, independently of genetic and other effects. Note that the full effect of smoking could be larger; for example, some effects might have operated through birthweight. However, even that careful study did not include a measure of parental ADHD or assess whether transmission of ADHD from parent to child (via nongenetic means) would account for the observed effect.

However, the most parsimonious conclusion from the Milberger et al. (1996, 1998) studies, together with the Thapar et al. (2003) study, is that maternal smoking during pregnancy exerts a small but reliable effect on development of ADHD in offspring. The upper-bound estimate on this effect is probably an odds or risk ratio of 1.4. Note that this same conclusion may not hold for CD.

Prenatal Nicotine Exposure and ADHD: Summary

Despite the complexity of this problem, the connection between prenatal exposure to nicotine and ADHD continues to survive the available statistical controls, albeit with a very small effect. For present purposes, then, it can be tentatively concluded (1) that prenatal nicotine exposure is related to later ADHD independently of the transmission of CD in families, as well as of most other confounds; (2) that the relationship is not due merely to more smoking by mothers with ADHD than by other mothers; and (3) that it is independent of genetic influences on ADHD. Nevertheless, the remaining effect may be quite small.

In short, the potential link of prenatal nicotine use to ADHD has been difficult to dismiss. The effect has survived in the most well-controlled studies. However, these well-controlled studies are few, and no one study was able to institute all of the controls that ideally would have to be considered. The negative results obtained by Silberg et al. (2003) for CD stand as a caution in this regard. Furthermore, the literature has scarcely begun to consider whether prenatal cigarette exposure affects cognitive development in a manner consistent with that described for ADHD in Chapters 4–7. Overall, key questions for the field concern (1) the size of these effects (in terms of relative risk), (2) the possibility of genotype–environment interactions in their expression, and (3) the possibility to explaining any ADHD-related cognitive effects by prenatal nicotine exposure.

HIGH LEVELS OF PRE- AND POSTNATAL EXPOSURES TO LEAD

High levels of exposure to lead, mercury, or other heavy metals cause multiple motor, sensory, and cognitive impairments that differentiate these conditions from ADHD per se. Of interest to us, then, is the potential contribution to ADHD of exposures that are insufficient to cause a full neurological syndrome, but could be sufficient to cause an ADHD syndrome. I begin with lead, the best-recognized of these risks in relation to hyperactivity and ADHD in children.

The neurotoxic effects of prenatal and postnatal lead exposure, known for millennia, have been documented in detail in the past century (Needleman, 1990; Bellinger & Needleman, 1994). Blood lead levels of 80 micrograms per deciliter (mcg/dl) are fatal; 60 mcg/dl cause encephalopathy; 25 mcg/dl was the WHO "safe" level until 1991, when it was lowered to its current level of 10 mcg/dl. The neurotoxic effects of even nonlethal lead exposures on the developing brain are extensive (Bellinger & Needleman, 1994). For example, lead can interfere with synapse formation—a critical element in the development of appropriate self-regulatory control in the first months and years of life. Recent work extends the risk range even below 10 mcg/dl, with recent calls to lower the "safe" threshold to 5 mcg/dl. In recent years, emphasis has been placed on the toxic effects of these so-called "minimal" or "background-level" exposures.

Between 1970 and 1991, the level of lead exposure considered "safe" continued to drop as studies of milder exposure levels went forward. Many studies were done in the 1980s, when lead poisoning was more common than it is today. In part because of aggressive U.S. Environmental Protection Agency (EPA) abatement efforts in response to the early rounds of research (notably elimination of leaded gasoline from much of the U.S. auto fleet), lead poisoning or exposures above "acceptable" levels (i.e., 10 mcg/dl) has dropped in incidence in the United States in the past 20 years. Yet renewed discoveries about aging lead water pipes in the United States have revived this issue as a major national concern (CDC, 2004b), and high-level lead exposure remains very common in children in many other nations (Fewtrell, Pruss-Ustun, Landrigan, & Ayuso-Mateos, 2004).

In support of the *causal* role of these lead exposures, lead exposure in animals creates cognitive deficits relevant to our interest in the cognitive profile of ADHD—in particular, deficits in handling reward delay (Brockel & Cory-Slechta, 1998) and on some attention tasks (Bellinger, Hu, Titlebaum, & Needleman, 1994). However, in a detailed review of experimental studies, Cory-Slechta (2003) argued that memory and vigilance are largely spared in lead exposure. The most reliable experimental finding noted in her review was excess responding during fixed-ratio reinforcement schedules, which was associated with poor impulse control and poor management of temporal intervals.

Thus an intriguing suggestion from that review was that the most important effect of high-level lead exposure on neuropsychological functioning pertinent to ADHD may be on reinforcement learning and impulsive behavior (as described in Chapter 7), rather than on executive functioning (as described in Chapter 5).

Also supporting a causal role is the finding that hyperactivity after lead exposure was reversed after lead chelation in animals (Gong & Evans, 1997). Is this a potential treatment option for children? Initial promising trials in children led Arnold (2002) to note that chelation is considered a viable treatment for lead poisoning, and may therefore be a possible treatment for children with ADHD who have levels of lead exposure over 10 mcg/dl. However, a more recent trial in children with quite high blood lead levels (20–44 mcg/dl) was unsuccessful in reversing hyperactivity and cognitive problems, even though it did succeed in lowering blood lead levels (Dietrich et al., 2004). It appears that those levels of lead poisoning caused irreversible effects on neural development, so that merely removing the lead was not sufficient to ameliorate all symptoms.[4]

As a result of all of these developments, it is established that lead ingestion above 10 mcg/dl (1) increases the risk that a child will develop behavior problems (perhaps including but not necessarily specific to hyperactivity, impulsivity, and aggression); (2) leads to a lowering of IQ (by over 7 points on average, vs. children with no lead exposure); and (3) leads to weakened response control, perhaps because of problems with reward delay and reinforcement response (Needleman, 1990; Bellinger & Needleman, 1994). In relation to disruptive behaviors, far more work has looked at antisocial behavior than at ADHD until recently. The earlier work is relevant, due to the high overlap of ADHD and conduct problems. For example, elevated lead levels have been found in samples of delinquent youth, with a fourfold risk of lead levels above a toxic threshold (Needleman, McFarland, Ness, Fienberg, & Tobin, 2002). Correlations with attention problems, delinquency, and aggression have also been reported in longitudinal studies (Needleman, Riess, Tobin, Biesecker, & Greenhouse, 1996). Nonetheless, specific relations to ADHD symptoms in this established literature have formerly been lacking, because most studies did not specifically assess ADHD. That situation has since been remedied by more recent work on low-level lead exposures (see the next section).

If there are effects of high-level lead poisoning on ADHD what would be the magnitude of these effect? To answer this question, it would be helpful to know what percentage of children with exposure above a given lead level develop ADHD, as well as the extent to which elevated lead levels are found in samples of children with ADHD. Data on these crucial questions are scarce. As noted above, Needleman et al. (2002) reported a fourfold risk of lead toxicity in samples of behaviorally disordered youth, which may serve as an upper-bound estimate for our purposes in relation to ADHD. My estimates here assume linear dose–response effects and no subgroups with especially adverse reactions to lead. Exposure above 10 mcg/dl is now estimated at 400,000 children (Meyer et al., 2003), or about 4.4% of children in the United States.[5] Although this figure is disturbing in light of the vast lost potential in the affected children, it indicates that unless a high percentage of these children develop ADHD, lead exposures above 10 mcg/dl account for only a small minority of cases of ADHD in the United States.

With a relative risk of 2.0 (doubling of risk for ADHD in children with lead exposure above 10 mcg/dl vs. those with no exposure), we would have a population attributable risk of 2.6/1,000, accounting for 4.3% of cases of ADHD (see Table 10.5, below). A relative risk of 3.0 (Needleman et al., 2002) would double this impact to 8% of cases of ADHD, whereas a conservative estimate of relative risk of 1.5 would drop this to 2% of cases. The few studies to check lead levels in samples of children with ADHD have found that levels above 10 mcg/dl were rare among these children (Eppright, Vogel, Horwitz, & Tevendale, 1997), and not far above population base rates, suggesting that these lower estimates may prove correct.

Furthermore, lead poisoning is usually accompanied by other clinical signs. Thus clinical guidelines currently suggest that routine screening of lead levels in the absence of environmental or other indicators of lead exposure is not warranted (Barkley, 2006). This guideline may be headed toward revision, however (Bernard, 2003).

LOW-LEVEL LEAD EXPOSURES

The most pressing question now with regard to lead exposure and ADHD is whether so-called "low-level" lead exposures (below 10 mcg/dl) could be contributing to ADHD in the population. Because the history of research in this area has been one in which each level of lead investigated (even levels once thought safe) has been found to result in neural damage, scientists and toxicologists have remained concerned, and authorities are discussing whether to further lower the CDC and/or WHO acceptable lead exposure limit (Bernard, 2003).

The reason this question has some urgency is that large swaths of the population still experience these lower exposure levels, even in the United States. Children continue to be exposed to lead in contaminated house dust, soil, and water. The average blood lead level among children in the United States is 2–3 mcg/dl. At a blood level of 5 mcg/dl, 25% of 1- to 5-year-old children in the United States would meet the exposure cutoff (Bernard & McGeehin, 2003).[6] Those rates climb to 47% among African American children and 28% among Mexican American children, and exceed 42% among children living in older housing (built before 1944).

Is there any evidence of cognitive decline, executive function problems, impulsivity, or other ADHD symptoms within this lower range of 1–10 mcg/dl? Unfortunately, recent data suggest quite a clear effect even at these lower levels. In a national survey data set, Lanphear, Dietrich, Auinger, and Cox (2000) found associations with cognitive delays in children with exposures even below 5 mcg/dl. Those findings were challenged on reanalysis of the data (Stone & Reynolds, 2003); however, supporting Lanphear et al.'s findings, Tuthill (1996) found that in 277 first graders with hair lead levels from 1 to 11.3 ppm, these levels showed a dose–response relationship with (1) teacher ratings of attention problems and (2) physician diagnosis of ADHD. The authors concluded that even low levels of lead exposure were unsafe with regard to ADHD symptoms. Canfield, Kreher, Cornwell, and Henderson (2003b) also found that lead levels in the range of 1–10 mcg/dl were associated with attention problems, in the form of difficulty with focused attention and ability to inhibit automatic responses; however, lead levels were not associated with poor task switching. Thus these findings seem consistent with the idea that low-level lead exposure may affect impulse control and reinforcement learning, while having relatively less effect on executive functioning.

In ADHD, we tend to see clearer deficits in response suppression than in task switching (see Chapter 5), consistent with this latter result. Even so, Canfield, Gendle, and Cory-Slechta (2004) found clear associations between lead exposure and executive functioning in spatial working memory, attention shifts, and planning in 5-year-old children with blood lead levels ranging from 0 to 20 mcg/dl, even after controlling for IQ and other covariates. Minder, Das-Smaal, Brand, and Orlebeke (1994) found that lead levels were related to children's poor performance on laboratory measures of reaction time and set shifting. Thomson et al. (1989) found a dose–response relationship between blood lead levels and teacher ratings of hyperactivity in a general population sample of 501 children (Edinburgh, Scotland), with no threshold observed.

In one of the most ADHD-relevant studies of low-level exposure, Chiodo, Jacobson, and Jacobson (2004) examined neuropsychological and behavioral scores in a population of children with lower average lead levels than most other studies (average of 5 mcg/dl). Teacher ratings on the Achenbach (1991) TRF indicated specific associations with ADHD symptoms (only the Attention Problems scale and the Withdrawn scale were uniquely related to blood lead level). On a DSM-IV ADHD symptom checklist, lead level was uniquely related to symptoms of inattention–disorganization, rather than hyperactivity–impulsivity. Thus, in this low-level range, the impression was that exposure was associated with low energy level and not hyperactivity. Chiodo et al. found cognitive deficits in visual–motor ability (recall the discussion of motor problems in Chapter 7) and on short-term memory (digit span), but not on set shifting (as measured by the WCST) or on CPT commission errors. The authors examined these correlations, using a threshold of 3 mcg/dl; even at that cutoff, significant associations were observed. Thus they were unable to locate a "safe" exposure level for these cognitive and behavioral effects. Although that sample was also exposed to prenatal alcohol, those effects were controlled by removing children with high exposure levels and covarying when necessary. This study provides one of the clearest findings that inattentive symptoms of ADHD are related to these low levels of lead exposure.

Amplifying this concern about very low exposure levels, Canfield et al. (2003a) found that the correlation of blood lead level with lowered IQ was *greater* between 1 and 10 mcg/dl of lead than above 10 mcg/dl. They concluded that as blood lead increased from 1 to 10 mcg/dl, IQ dropped 7.4 points. Needleman and Landrigan (2004) interpreted this finding as evidence that the majority of the harm done by lead exposure occurs in the initial exposure levels (1–10 mcg/dl). Supporting this scenario, Lanphear et al. (2000) found correlations between lead levels of even 1–5 mcg/dl and lower cognitive scores. As a result of all these findings, a recent expert review by Koller, Brown, Spurgeon, and Levey (2004) concluded that no safe level of exposure to lead can be established for children. However, they also argued that lead accounts for only a small percentage of the variance in IQ. The latter point may be true, but this would not prevent such exposures from accounting for a large percentage of the extreme cases and, in more vulnerable individuals, for cases of ADHD (see Stein, Schettler, Wallinga, & Valente, 2002, for an illustration).

The implications of these findings are potentially dramatic. As shown in Table 10.5, if we suppose a twofold risk increase of ADHD at lead levels above 5 mcg/dl, low-level lead exposures would account for 25% of the cases of ADHD in the United States! Even at a more cautious projection of a 25–50% increased risk of ADHD with these levels of exposure, 6–12% of cases of ADHD would be preventable by eliminating the exposure. In the absence of genotype–environment interactions, these effects would be shared or nonshared environment effects, arguing for the lower estimates.

However, if there is no safe level of lead, but if ADHD can be influenced by levels ranging from 1 to 10 mcg/dl, then low-level lead exposure is a common risk agent. If it functions as a shared environment effect (i.e., affecting all children near the same age in a family) and interacts with genotype, then its effects can be hidden in the heritability term (see Chapter 9). In that event, the magnitude of influence of lead exposure on ADHD could be significantly greater and could approach or exceed those higher estimates shown in Table 10.5. In vulnerable populations (inner-city children, minority children), the effects could well be larger.

Thus low-level routine exposures to lead (from 1 to 10 mcg/dl) do lower IQ and appear to be correlated with symptoms of ADHD and attention problems. Many of these initial studies controlled for obvious confounds such as low SES (which is correlated with maternal smoking,

TABLE 10.5. How Many Cases of ADHD Are Attributable to Lead Exposure?

Type of exposure	% exposed	Putative RR	AR	PAR	PAF
I. High-level lead exposure (>10 mcg/dl)					
If relative risk = 3.0	4.4%	3.0	12%	5.2/1,000	8.6%
If relative risk = 2.0		2.0	6%	2.6/1,000	4.3%
If relative risk = 1.5		1.5	3%	1.3/1,000	2.6%
II. Low-level lead exposure (>5 mcg/dl)					
If relative risk = 2.0	25.0%	2.0	6%	15.0/1,000	25%
If relative risk = 1.5		1.5	3%	7.5/1,000	12.5%
If relative risk = 1.25		1.25	1.5%	3.75/1,000	6.25%

Note. RR, relative risk (which is speculative and used for illustrative purposes here—see text); PAR, population attributable risk; PAF, population attributable fraction, or percentage of ADHD cases potentially explained by lead exposure. See note 1 of this chapter for explanation of how these are calculated. An ADHD incidence of 6% in unexposed children is assumed (Chapter 1 and note 1 to this chapter).

for example), although continued carefully controlled studies will be needed to verify this effect. Because lower-level exposures are so widespread, if the increased risk of ADHD due to lead exposure in this range is even at a risk ratio of 1.25 or 1.5, then these lead exposures could account for a substantial percentage of cases of ADHD. Again, this has been illustrated in Table 10.5. This possibility has not been seriously examined, however, and data with which to evaluate it are lacking. It remains a speculative but important possibility that should be examined.

Adding to the importance of this hypothesis is the possibility of interactions between risk factors in a subset of the population (Schettler, 2001; Stein et al., 2002), or significant adverse reactions in a subset of children. Interactions with genotype may be particularly important, as I detail later in this chapter. Overall, determining the extent of ADHD (as well as other adverse reactions) among children with lower-level lead exposures warrants public health attention, from the viewpoint of a high-risk/high-payoff research strategy to understand causes of ADHD. It is a plausible, common, and preventable (albeit at substantial cost) potential contributor.

EXPOSURES TO OTHER TOXICANTS

Mercury

Mercury is another toxic metal for which the so-called "acceptable" exposure levels have dramatically dropped as research has accumulated. Mercury might, in theory, be considered another potential culprit in ADHD, because it is also among the most widely recognized, chemical poisons to which children in industrial nations are exposed. No longer widely dispersed via auto exhaust, it is still relatively widely dispersed via air pollution from waste incinerators and coal-fired power plants. It then settles in soil and water supplies, and so can reach developing children via air, water, and food, particularly fish.[7] Exposures among fish eaters result in either shared or nonshared environment effects (the latter if some children are more vulnerable than others). Mercury has relevant neurodevelopmental toxic effects, in that exposure *in utero* can disrupt cellular migration (essentially disrupting typical brain formation), and postnatal exposure can disrupt synaptic transmission (Myers & Davidson, 2000).

As has happened with lead levels, the definition of an acceptable level of methylmercury exposure has dropped dramatically with accumulating research. As summarized by Stein et al. (2002), the scientific literature on mercury exposure was really begun in 1972, with studies of victims of a population exposure in Iraq. The conclusion then was that infants had a toxic threshold of 34 mcg/kg/day. Subsequent studies resulted in lowering of this threshold by orders of magnitude. EPA and WHO "acceptable"levels are now between 0.1 and 1 mcg/kg/day. Prenatal exposures of 0.8 mcg/day appear to cause later deficits in language, memory, and attention (Grandjean et al., 1997). The causal effects of these exposures are confirmed in animal studies, which show subtle cognitive deficits (including deficits in reinforcement learning and avoidance learning) in instances of even modest or low-level exposure (reviewed by Weiss, 1994). Developmental effects of mercury exposure are able to be detected in infants born to mothers with less than 10 parts per million (ppm) in hair (corresponding to about 300 parts per billion [ppb] in the fetal brain). Recent EPA guidelines suggest even lower levels, at about 1 ppm in hair (corresponding to 0.1 mcg/kg/day), and these levels have been endorsed by the National Academy of Sciences (2000; see also Schettler, 2001). Stein et al. (2002) note that a woman of childbearing age would exceed this limit by consuming 7 ounces of tuna or 1.5 ounces of swordfish per week; a child would exceed it by consuming 2.5 ounces of tuna per week.

If mercury is an important influence on ADHD, we might expect regional variability. For example, exposure might be higher in the U.S. Northeast (the Great Lakes area and New England) because of the prevailing winds and the heavy use of coal-fired power plants, the greater rate of eating freshwater fish, or both in those regions. Therefore, if mercury exposure is a major cause of child attention and learning problems, we might expect varying incidence or prevalence by region of the country. Data to test that hypothesis are lacking. Indeed, good survey data on the extent of mercury exposure in the population are scarce (see Stein et al., 2002). However, EPA estimates based on dietary surveys suggest that 7% of U.S. women of childbearing age and as many as 20% of children ages 3–6 may exceed this recommended limit (EPA Mercury Study Report to Congress, 1997, cited by Schettler, 2001). The National Academy of Sciences (2000) estimates that 60,000 children are born per year at risk due to mercury exposure *in utero*, which is a lower estimate. These data need further clarification as to the actual degree of risk in the population. Nonetheless, they suggest that *in utero* mercury exposure has the potential to be an important contributor to learning disabilities and ADHD.

The neurodevelopmental effects of mercury in early development are most notable on motor and visual–spatial processing. A specific influence on attention and activity level is less clear, even though ADHD often co-occurs with motor delays. ADHD is more common in males, and (as in the case of LBW and possibly that of prenatal nicotine exposure), males may be more vulnerable to neurodevelopmental delays after routine dietary mercury exposure (Weiss, 1994). At this time, however, data that would clearly link mercury exposures to ADHD per se are not in hand. It remains important to examine this question further, in light of the prevalence of mercury exposure in the general population and its established neurodevelopmental harmful effects.

Manganese

At high exposure levels, manganese is a neurotoxin that targets the striatum, resulting in initial hyperactivity followed by a parkinsonian syndrome (Centonze, Gubellini, Bernardi, & Calabresi, 2001; Nachtman, Tubben, & Commissaris, 1986). More subtle effects are observed during neurodevelopment, wherein excess levels reduce striatal dopamine levels and affect working memory and avoidance learning in rodents (Tran, Chowanadisai, Crinella, Chicz-Demet, & Lonnerdal, 2002; Tran et al., 2002b). Manganese is an essential dietary trace element, and is found in human breast milk at naturally occurring levels of about 6 mcg/liter. Children receive excess exposures to manganese postnatally from two major sources: auto exhaust (because manganese is used as an octane enhancer in gasoline) and soy-based infant formula. The latter may contain 200–300 mcg/liter (50 times the levels in breast milk). Controversy over soy-based infant formula has been enhanced by these and other concerns. Older studies have historically identified elevated manganese in children with learning disabilities (e.g., Pihl & Parkes, 1977) or with learning disabilities and hyperactivity (Collipp, Chen, & Maitinsky, 1983). These studies, however, tended to have small and non-representative samples; recent replications using more contemporary measurement tools have not been forthcoming. Therefore, it is unclear whether these effects are specific to ADHD or what the level of risk is. The population prevalence of exposures is unclear, and it is unclear to what extent manganese exposure may overlap with other risk factors. Overall, more work is needed to determine the level of risk of ADHD or other neurodevelopmental problems at higher exposures to manganese, and to rule out confounding explanations. However, excess manganese exposure's action on developing striatal dopamine neurons suggests a plausible hypothesis of potential influence on symptoms of ADHD, especially when ADHD is comorbid with motor control problems or learning disabilities.

PSYCHOLOGICAL TRAUMA, EARLY PARENTAL DEPRIVATION, AND ATTACHMENT PROBLEMS

Can ineffective parenting cause ADHD? Is it true that if only some parents would be more strict, children's attention and activity problems would vanish? Because of the small role found for shared environment and the large one for heritability in ADHD, most commentators consider it unlikely that parenting problems are a major factor in causing ADHD. Indeed, now-classic studies showed that child behaviors tended to drive parenting effects, rather than the other way around. Barkley and Cunningham (1979) found that when hyperactive children were switched from placebo to medicated status, negative parenting behaviors improved. Those types of findings have supported the view that parenting problems are more likely to be reactions to ADHD than causes of it. This information may be a relief to parents who have "tried everything" with their children or who feel inadequate as parents; such a negative self-image among parents of children with ADHD is an underappreciated clinical problem in its own right (Podolski & Nigg, 2001). This picture is also quite distinct from the picture for oppositional and aggressive behaviors, where breakdown in parenting skills appears to play a causal role as already noted (Snyder et al., 2003).

Yet nearly any theory of how children develop self regulation includes a role for adequate parental or caregiver attunement to the child. The child's internal regulatory systems—including executive functioning, motivation, arousal, and language (see Chapter 8)—develop in an "expectable context" in which caregivers are present to mirror, to support, to scaffold, and to provide external regulation until the child gains the ability to self-regulate (for more theoretical discussion, see Calkins & Fox, 2002; Rothbart & Bates, 1998; Nigg & Huang-Pollock, 2003). Based on these general developmental theories, then, we might expect that one route to a self-regulation disorder such as ADHD would be through insufficiencies in parental caregiving—specifically, failure to provide support for self-regulation to develop.

Indeed, we know that children exposed to sexual abuse can exhibit heightened activity and impulsivity (Glod & Teicher, 1996), and that in addition to being diagnosed with PTSD, children who have been sexually abused are often diagnosed with ADHD (Famularo, Kinscherff, & Fenton, 1992; McLeer, Callaghan, Henry, & Wallen, 1994). Glod and Teicher (1996) concluded that abused children who develop PTSD exhibit activity profiles similar to ADHD, whereas abused children who do not develop PTSD exhibit a more depressive profile. Thus, at least for clinicians, there is a danger of misdiagnosis if an overactive child is assessed for ADHD and an adequate history of potential trauma or abuse is not collected (Weinstein, Staffelbach, & Biaggio, 2000).

Significant early trauma can also disrupt neural development, affecting the systems that are involved in self-regulation; thus this effect does not conflict with the neuropsychological findings in ADHD. For instance, it is notable that early trauma may alter development of the hippocampus, amygdala, and frontal cortex (Teicher et al., 2003), and potentially also of the cerebellar vermis (Teicher, Andersen, Polcari, Anderson, & Navalta, 2002). These regions are important in various conceptions of inhibitory control of behavior and affect (Nigg & Casey, 2005). In all, the plasticity of the early-developing neural networks in the brain allows many avenues for alterations in brain structure and function secondary to early trauma (Cicchetti, 2002; Cicchetti & Rogosch, 2001; Pollak, Cicchetti, Klorman, & Brumaghim, 1997; Rinne, Westenberg, den Boer, & van den Brink, 2000). As outlined elsewhere (Nigg, Silk, Stavro, & Miller, 2005c), these effects may suggest some overlap between instances of ADHD and later personality disorder, perhaps mediated by traumatogenic disruptions in self-regulation.

Such disruption of the expectable environment (Cicchetti & Lynch, 1995) for learning self regulation during early development, if the cause is a parent's disability (e.g., a mother's depression) should emerge in either the shared environment (affecting both children in a family and causing them to be more similar to one another) or the nonshared environment (affecting children differentially, causing them to be less similar)—depending on whether they interact with children's constitutional vulnerability to ADHD. Yet, despite this logical theoretical framework, demonstration that breakdowns in family socialization may actually lead to ADHD have been few. As with parenting breakdowns generally, early attachment disruption appears to be associated with oppositional, conduct, and aggressive behavior problems rather than with attention and impulse control problems per se (Greenberg, Speltz, DeKlyen, & Jones, 2001). However, other characteristics of the caregiver–child relationship have received initial investigation in relation to ADHD.

More generally, child characteristics may interfere with socialization and thus consolidation of regulatory abilities (Johnston & Mash,

2001; Kochanska et al., 1997) particularly if the caregiver environment is limited and unable to scaffold the child's particular needs (Greenberg, Kusche, & Speltz, 1991). Conceivable, but not well supported by data as yet, is the possibility that breakdown of parenting ability due to psychopathology, impulsivity, marital/couple conflict, or other problems may impede the child's ability to develop adequate self-regulatory ability (Johnston & Mash, 2001).

Carlson, Jacobvitz, and Sroufe (1995) found that mothers who were intrusive and insensitive were more likely to have children who were insecurely attached and who went on to have problems with inattention and overactivity. However, parental ADHD was not assessed, so it is unclear whether this effect was an epiphenomenon of an inherited trait of overactivity in mothers and children, whether the attachment problems mediated the genetic effect (genotype–environment correlation), or whether the attachment effect independently predicted ADHD symptoms. A related study suggested that hostility between family members in the toddler years predicted ADHD symptoms in grade school in a small sample of nondiagnosed children, although toddler levels of behavior problems were not controlled for (Jacobvitz, Hazen, Curran, & Hitchens, 2004) and so conclusions about direction of effects cannot be drawn. Further research on these possibilities will be of interest. Of particular interest will be work that can examine individual differences in children's vulnerability, control for parental ADHD status or use genetically informative designs, and evaluate whether unique contributions of socialization breakdown to children's insufficient self-regulatory control can be identified. Such effects would have to be independent of the established family effects on aggression and antisocial behavior.

Our research group at Michigan State carried out one such longitudinal study with interesting results (Jester et al., 2005). We followed children of alcoholic parents and matched control parents from preschool to age 18, assessing (1) early home stimulation, via maternal report; (2) family conflict, via maternal report; and (3) parent and teacher ratings of inattention, overactivity, and aggression on the Achenbach (1991) CBCL and TRF. We found that the developmental trajectory of aggression was moderated by within-home conflict. In contrast, the developmental trajectory of inattention and overactivity was moderated by within-home stimulation, even with levels of aggression held constant. This is perhaps the first longitudinal evidence that home environment may moderate the trajectory of the development of attention problems. Effects held even after covarying for parental

ADHD status. Nonetheless, this still was not a genetically informative design.

Other work suggests that even though parenting problems may not cause ADHD, the secondary breakdown in parenting may contribute to maintenance of ADHD over time. Campbell (2002) reviews evidence that those children who persist in ADHD symptoms from preschool into early childhood are more likely than children whose symptoms desist to have parents with ineffective parenting skills. And Hinshaw et al. (2000), in the MTA, found that an intervention to improve parenting skills, though targeted at oppositional and noncompliant behaviors, also helped to maintain a reduction in disruptive behavior and improvement in children's social skills over time.

Thus it is noteworthy that (1) parenting interventions are helpful for children with ADHD, albeit these are primarily aimed at associated disruptive and social problems rather than inattention or hyperactivity per se; and (2) specific family correlates may yet emerge related to the consolidation of self-regulation apart from aggression. Further work along these various lines may help in the eventual development of more targeted prevention interventions with caregivers—in particular, interventions that may specifically address inattention and overactivity apart from oppositional, conduct, and aggression problems.

More extreme disruption of parenting has been examined in a handful of studies of institutionally reared children. The best and most recent of these come from studies in England comparing children adopted after institutional care in England to children adopted after institutional care in Romanian orphanages during a period of extreme social dislocation in that country (O'Connor et al., 2000; O'Connor & Rutter, 2000; Kreppner, et al., 2001). The children in England received sound care during their preadoptive lives, whereas the children from Romania experienced severe caregiving deprivation prior to their adoption (e.g., they were confined to their cots for most of the day). After adoption in England, the children were assessed at ages 4 and 6 years.

Children with severe early deprivation had higher levels of inattention and overactivity, and more often displayed these symptoms pervasively, than did other adoptees. Moreover, this pattern of differences was *not* seen for conduct problems or emotional disturbance, although elevated rates of attachment disorders and autistic-like symptoms were seen (Rutter et al., 2001). Thus there seemed to be a preferential effect of this early caregiver disruption on inattention and overactivity. These effects held after controls for LBW (rather common in these samples), poor nutrition, and IQ. Notably, these children also displayed attachment difficulties, and therefore their clinical phenotype was somewhat different from that of most children with ADHD.

Kreppner et al. (2001) stressed that they did not believe these findings were informative about most cases of ADHD. However, the results do show that one possible route to ADHD, even if an uncommon one, is severe deprivation. Such extreme effects may not be common enough to account for a large percentage of cases, but when such a history is encountered (as it occasionally is in clinical practice), consideration of the fact that this route can lead to ADHD or an ADHD-like syndrome, along with attachment problems, can be important for clinicians.

Less clear, but of considerable theoretical interest, is whether prenatal stress on the mother can lead to ADHD in the child. The mechanism here would be via stress hormone exposures *in utero,* which might alter neurotransmitter firing thresholds and influence neural development. Of the few studies that have investigated this question in ADHD (reviewed by Linnet et al., 2003), nearly all failed to control for prenatal smoking or alcohol use or for parental ADHD. However, O'Connor et al. (2002) did control for prenatal smoking and alcohol use, and still found an association between mother-reported prenatal stress and mother-reported child ADHD symptoms at age 4 years. In children, evidence about this possibility is limited in relation to ADHD per se. van den Bergh and Marcoen (2004) followed 71 children from pregnancy to ages 8–9 years. Maternal prenatal anxiety predicted ADHD symptoms at ages 8–9, even after controls for postnatal maternal anxiety, maternal cigarette use during pregnancy, and birthweight. However, these findings were nonspecific, in that several other areas of psychopathology were also elevated at ages 8–9. Failure to control adequately for maternal psychopathology (and attendant genetic influences on child symptoms) limits conclusions from this interesting study. In all, the possible role of prenatal maternal stress levels may warrant more research exploration, even though data are insufficient to permit any conclusions at this stage.

CLINICAL IMPLICATIONS

The material in this chapter on prenatal teratogens carries obvious implications in counseling pregnant or sexually active women about prenatal care. Good prenatal care, avoidance of substance use during pregnancy (including tobacco as well as alcohol), good diet and maternal health, and healthy delivery could both (1) reduce LBW and thus chances of ADHD; and (2) reduce additional risks associated with these factors, over and above their influence on birthweight. Health care professionals and mental health workers thus do well to assess for alcohol use, diet, and availability of prenatal care when working with young families, expectant parents, and parents of children with ADHD who expect to have more children. In some respects, this prevention concern is relevant to counselors and therapists working with women who become pregnant. In other respects, these are health care policy needs for society's policy makers to consider. However, these types of counseling considerations may be especially important in women with ADHD and antisocial histories (e.g., histories of CD), who are at greatest risk of continuing to smoke and drink while pregnant.

For the clinician working with parents of a child who is already born and now appears to have ADHD, the uncertainty of effects in individual cases would suggest a focus on the future rather than the past. Many parents, aware of the literature on teratogens, anguish over the possibility that their past behavior has contributed to their child's current problems. Clearly, this is a possibility, but it is virtually never certain in a particular case at present (cases of frank FAS aside). Even when exposure may be causal, it may cause disturbance in only a minority of cases. Thus, it is important for parents to refocus on what they can do for their child, rather than on what cannot be changed. It may be relevant to point out, for example, that even after heavy alcohol use in pregnancy, fewer than half of children develop significant behavioral problems.

Of course, counseling on this sensitive topic requires particular clinical skill when parents who may have had substance use during pregnancy are considering having another child. Clearly, taking fewer chances about substance use during a second pregnancy is advisable, especially if the first child has ADHD. (Because there is evidence that children born to older mothers are at greater risk, caution is even more essential if the mother is over 30.) Encouraging care for their health for the sake of the child will be understandable to all parents, but they may have difficulty implementing this suggestion if they themselves are impulsive or overwhelmed and disorganized. Intervention programs to help pregnant women stop smoking are growing in sophistication and effectiveness (Ershoff, Ashford, & Goldenberg, 2004; Melvin & Gaffney, 2004), but are underutilized by primary care providers. Clinical and therapeutic support may be useful to support abstinence in relation to such programs by helping to maintain impulse control, focus, and organization during the risk period of pregnancy and the early postnatal period.

During the postnatal and early childhood periods, social work and nursing interventions to assess risk of head injury, lead poisoning, mercury exposure, and major dietary deficiency (hunger and/or malnutrition) may be useful prevention steps for at-risk families. If symptoms of lead exposure, or known significant lead exposure, has occurred historically in a case of ADHD, Arnold (2002) suggests that a chelation trial (removing lead from the blood) be considered, under careful medical supervision (see his discussion for an overview of medical risks to these procedures); however, not all professionals are in agreement about this. Thus a review of potential lead exposure in history taking is something that clinicians may wish to consider. Such a review is particularly justified for ethnic minority children and children living in older housing, for whom base rates of lead exposure above 10 mcg/dl can be significant.

Parents can reduce lead exposure by keeping homes free of dust, filtering tap water, repairing any chipped or peeling paint (especially in older homes), and monitoring young children's placement of nonfood items (including dirt) into their mouths. More extensive prevention efforts include testing dirt in children's play areas for lead. It remains important to recognize that the CDC and WHO have yet to endorse calls for clinical action at lead exposure levels below 10 mcg/dl (although this could change in the near future, as noted earlier). At this writing, clinical guidelines continue to call for lead screening in children with ADHD only when other signs of lead toxicity are present. These other signs include upset stomach, tiredness, loss of appetite, constipation, hearing problems, weight loss, sleep problems, and irritability (in addition to hyperactivity). However, not all children with toxic lead levels will display these symptoms. Clinicians will be well advised to track developments in this literature. Again, the lead screening standards could be revised in coming years if the initial evidence for potential harmful effects of even lower levels of lead exposure continues to be replicated. If so, more aggressive screening of children will be called for.

In terms of other evaluation considerations, Aylward (2002) recommended that children known to have had LBW or preterm birth should be assessed for cognitive difficulties, including executive dysfunctions, nonverbal learning disabilities, attention problems, and motor delays. Thus, if a child presents with symptoms of ADHD and a history of LBW, a complete neuropsychological evaluation can provide valuable assistance in designing appropriate comprehensive treatment planning.

Similarly, children who have ADHD and may have been exposed to heavy prenatal alcohol use may warrant neuropsychological evaluation.

As reviewed by O'Malley and Nanson (2002), these children are likely to have learning disabilities (potentially including math learning problems or nonverbal learning disabilities), working memory problems, and communication and language disorders. Streissguth et al. (1994b), in summarizing their groundbreaking longitudinal study in Washington State, documented nonverbal learning problems (arithmetic) among the core cognitive findings. Full evaluation of these associated problems is essential to adequate management and intervention with these children. As should be apparent, identification of mathematics disorder or nonverbal learning disabilities (a less frequent syndrome than mathematics disorder; see Drummond, Ahmad, & Rourke, 2005; Rourke et al., 2002) would have important ramifications for educational and treatment planning.

Many clinicians (including many pediatricians) feel ill equipped to evaluate FAS or fetal alcohol spectrum disorders as part of the differential diagnosis with ADHD. As a result, it is believed that these disorders are often overlooked in clinical practice. Detailed clinical guidelines are provided by Hoyme et al. (2005); see also Sokol et al. (2003) and O'Leary (2004) for more clinically relevant background information. Consultation with a clinician experienced in identifying these conditions is another option to be considered if a clinician does not feel able to make this diagnosis. Many commentators suspect that the associated neuropsychological problems, potential medical problems (e.g., skeletal, renal, eye, cardiac problems), and potential differential response to medication of ADHD or ADHD-like symptoms when FAS or fetal alcohol spectrum disorders are present warrant careful scrutiny of this possibility in the differential diagnosis (O'Malley & Nanson, 2002). One key question is whether stimulant medication has a lower rate of effectiveness in children with fetal alcohol spectrum disorders, due to the neuropsychological effects of these disorders on learning, encoding, and memory rather than on vigilance and executive functioning.

As children with ADHD enter adolescence, a secondary point that emerges from this literature concerns their elevated risk of alcohol and cigarette use as well as illicit drug use, particularly if those youth also have conduct problems. Counselors working with teenagers with ADHD should routinely consider this possibility and assess accordingly.

It is noteworthy that the DSM-IV-TR (APA, 2000) does not list PTSD as a differential diagnosis when possible ADHD is being evaluated. Yet, as argued by Weinstein et al. (2000), it is important to rule out abuse or trauma history. Children with PTSD have elevated activity levels, and some of their symptoms can overlap with those of ADHD.

TABLE 10.6. Frequently Asked Questions about ADHD and Uncommon Experiential Risk Factors

Question	Answer
Does faulty parenting cause ADHD?	No, but is related to aggression.
How common is ADHD with fetal alcohol problems?	Probably 2–4% of cases.
Could prenatal smoking be a cause of ADHD?	Possibly yes; evidence is still accumulating.
Is lead poisoning a cause of ADHD?	Yes; findings on the magnitude of low-level effects are still emerging.
How many cases are caused by lead?	Perhaps 2–4% by today's standards, but potentially as many as 12–15% if lower-level lead exposures prove to be important in ADHD.
Can we relax now about lead and mercury?	No. Children remain at substantial risk.
Why would ADHD be increasing?[a]	One reason might be the increased survival of children with LBW.
Is LBW associated with ADHD?	Yes; a two- to fourfold risk increase occurs with LBW.

[a]It is actually unclear whether ADHD incidence is increasing.

The key suggestion is to take a careful history to rule out significant traumatic events; this should include asking the child about thoughts that distract him of her, and interviewing multiple informants.

Finally, several questions that clinicians are often asked to address have been answered in this chapter. The most significant or frequently asked of these are summarized in Table 10.6.

CONCLUSIONS AND FUTURE DIRECTIONS

What we can conclude, cautiously, at this point is that several known prenatal exposures (most importantly heavy alcohol use and possibly cigarette use), perinatal problems (most notably LBW), and postnatal exposures (most notably high- and low-level lead exposures) may each increase to a small extent a child's chances of developing ADHD, and probably do so via causal action on the developing brain. A conservative to generous range of estimates would be that elimination of all of these causes would reduce ADHD incidence by 10–15% (see Table 10.7). The estimates would go much higher if it is determined that low-level lead exposure leads to increased risk of ADHD by even a small margin, either via direct effects or via genotype–environment interactions. Whether the target range is 10–15% or whether it ultimately goes higher, this is a target well worth pursuing in view of the preventable nature of these experiential agents. Encouragingly, with the exception of nonspecific LBW, alcohol, cigarette, and lead exposures are in decline (at least in the United States) because of public health efforts to address these issues. These efforts are to be encouraged, and it is to be hoped that other toxicants will be targeted for more aggressive scrutiny and for elimination from children's environments.

Note that some of these cases would represent genotype–environment correlations, in which the early brain injury is mediating a genetic effect (e.g., maternal ADHD → smoking → fetal neural injury → child ADHD → smoking). All the same, some of these effects are doubtless being picked up by the nonshared environment term in twin studies, the value of which ranges around 25–30%. Although some effects in this table may prove high estimates (e.g., the smoking effect apart from LBW and genetic effects may be smaller), others may well prove low estimates (e.g., low-level lead effects appear increasingly likely in ADHD, yet are excluded entirely from the table). In all, these effects appear well positioned to help us begin to understand the nonshared environment effects in the etiology of ADHD.

We also know that extreme psychological trauma early in life can cause an ADHD syndrome. However, it seems likely that this sort of trauma is accounting for only a very small minority of cases, and that these cases are atypical (i.e., accompanied by attachment problems). Because these cases are rare and atypical, they are excluded from Table 10.7. More subtle traumatic effects (including extreme maternal emotional stress during pregnancy) may also contribute, but data to support this supposition are scarce. Other parenting effects in ADHD are generally nil; parenting breakdown is related instead to oppositional and aggressive behavior in children.

It will be important in etiological studies to identify these likely contributors and to include them routinely in research designs, so that they can be integrated with other causal mechanisms. For example, studies to look at how pre- and perinatal effects relate to both neuropsychological dysfunction and ADHD in the same samples have yet to be reported to any extent. Kristjansson, Fried, and Watkinson (1989) reported some time ago that maternal smoking during pregnancy lowered child vigilance. By the same token, lead exposure may not affect vigilance, but may affect impulse control while waiting for reward (timing of reward response). Several of these routes may affect motor or

TABLE 10.7. Low (Conservative) Estimates of Contribution to ADHD of Key Causal Agents Discussed in This Chapter

Agent	Estimated PAF	Comment
Heavy prenatal alcohol exposure	2.4%	Visual–spatial, math disabilities
Prenatal nicotine exposure (not resulting in LBW)	3.4%	Estimate may be high
LBW (due to cigarette use)	3.6%	Motor and coordination delays
LBW (due to other causes)	8.6%	Motor and coordination delays
High-level lead exposure (>10 mcg/dl)	2.6%	Reduced IQ, physical symptoms
Total	20.6%	
Total preventable causes (excluding nonspecific LBW)	12.0%	

Note. PAF, population attributable fraction, or percentage of cases of ADHD attributable to this risk factor; these figures may overlap among different agents.

visual–motor control. These distinct etiological agents thus may be differentially related to elements of the ADHD neuropsychological profile. Accordingly, studies that integrate these neurocognitive mechanisms with ADHD or ADHD-like outcomes will represent a key "next generation" of studies in the area.

A key theme in this book is the importance of identifying "high-risk/high-payoff" research directions, or research that has a chance of yielding a major breakthrough in understanding even if that chance is deemed less than 50% likely to succeed. A crucial direction for high-risk/high-payoff studies of environmental toxicants, which I emphasize in both this chapter and the next, concerns interactions of genotype with exposures. Susceptibility genes have already been identified in some instances. For example, two genes—the vitamin D receptor gene and the delta aminolevulinic acid dehydratase gene—affect lead absorption and metabolism, and may confer vulnerability or protection in response to low-level lead exposure (for a reviewed, see Stein et al., 2002). Kahn, Khoury, Nichols, and Lanphear (2003) reported that ADHD was found in children who had the dopamine transporter long (risk) allele and exposure to prenatal maternal smoking, but not in those with the risk allele and no exposure to maternal smoking. These sorts of interactions with specific genotypes are of paramount importance and urgently require further study. Their importance is particularly great in light of the potential effects of "subthreshold" exposures. Their systematic identification would potentially enable the identification of children at greatest risk from these exposures. Those data could then be utilized in a complementary prevention–intervention approach that reduces exposure levels overall in the environment, while also providing additional screening and intervention to children with vulnerable genotypes.

Although this chapter has referred to all of these mechanisms as "experiential" causes, they may reflect genetic effects (genotype-environment correlations, or experiential mediation of genetic influence) to varying degrees. For example, perinatal complications may be partially heritable (Magnus, Gjessing, Skronda, & Skjaerven, 2001), indicating that variation in those complications depends in part on variation in genotype. Thus we must use caution and avoid artificially separating these proximal triggers or causes from potential "upstream" or intergenerational mediation of genotype effects. From an intervention point of view, of course, this distinction is academic. Preventing perinatal complications should still interrupt the causal stream, at least for some children.

In summary, prenatal exposure to alcohol and cigarettes, perinatal problems (especially LBW), and postnatal exposures to lead appear to contribute to behavioral and neuropsychological problems that include ADHD symptoms. Indeed, they may cause some cases of ADHD by causing some of the neurocognitive problems that I have reviewed in earlier chapters. These mechanisms doubtless overlap with genetic transmission of risk traits. At the same time, they appear to have an effect that is at least partially independent of genetic effects, and so may contribute to a significant portion of nonshared environment effects on ADHD. Yet, even if they are viewed as mediators of heritable effects and as nonshared environment effects together, these environmental causes probably account for fewer than a quarter of the cases of ADHD; some authorities would argue that the percentage is substantially lower than that. These factors are well worth addressing in public health and prevention efforts (indeed, it is distressing that hundreds of thousands of children are still exposed to known toxic levels of lead and mercury, not to mention the widespread lower levels officially labeled as "safe" but likely to be proven harmful with time and more research). But they do not fully explain ADHD. We must consider other possible etiological mechanisms as well. Unfortunately for children, we have not yet exhausted the range of potentially harmful experiential causes. We now move to common risk agents, with the potential for interactions between shared environment and genotype, which can inflate heritability estimates.

|C H A P T E R   1 1|

Common Experiential
Risk Factors

In Chapter 10, I have discussed experiential risk factors that are likely contributors to the nonshared environment aspect of ADHD etiology. With the possible exception of low-level lead exposures, they fall into that group because the majority of children do not experience these risk agents. Of course, some of these agents might actually work as shared environment effects, but this possibility does not change the basic argument that (again with the exception of low-level lead exposures) they are not candidates to explain much of the heritability effect in ADHD.

In contrast, other experiential risk factors are very common in children's lives. If these common agents were to influence ADHD via genotype–environment interactions, they would inflate the heritability term in twin studies (see Chapter 9 for explanation). As a result, they may operate powerfully in the population, yet may be undetected in behavioral genetic designs. This possibility means that these common risk agents may prove to be even more important than the uncommon agents in explaining ADHD. However, each of these candidate risks requires evaluation. Those that are promising may fall into the category of "high-risk/high-payoff" etiological possibilities. They are high-risk to the society that invests in these studies, because investment in studies of any one particular such risk factor remains somewhat speculative; chances of a discovery or payoff may be deemed well under 50–50. Thus the investment, which could have gone elsewhere, may not pay off. On the other hand, they are potentially high-payoff because if a discovery is made, the breakthrough in understanding and prevention of child ADHD may be enormous, paying enormous dividends on the research investment for society.

Thus studies of the putative causal agents discussed in this chapter may be well worth undertaking, despite their potential to include many blind alleys and failed hypotheses. The purpose of this chapter is to update readers and provide comment and evaluation on three classes of such possible etiologies. I have chosen the topics for this chapter with an eye on both what is most discussed in popular parlance, and where I believe cutting-edge research may be headed. Not all of these candidate triggers are equally promising.

The three potential etiological candidates that I discuss in this chapter are (1) diet, (2) the electronic media, and (3) selected environmental toxins. I have selected these three domains for review in this chapter because all meet the following criteria: (1) They are ubiquitous in children's lives in the countries that have reported twin studies to date (i.e., they could be affecting most or all twins in a study); (2) theoretical hypotheses anchored in neuroscience and/or developmental theory can be advanced to support their potential links to ADHD; (3) animal studies are favorable; (4) at least a few pilot or initial correlational studies in humans have been conducted; and (5) many questions about their role persist in Western society. Yet not all of these hypotheses are equally promising, either theoretically or empirically. All are common, and most have a plausible (if in some instances essentially speculative) neural mechanism of action. But they vary extensively in actual empirical support in relation to ADHD, its neuropsychological mechanisms, or both. I now consider each in turn.

COULD DIET CAUSE ADHD?

"Could food allergies cause ADHD?" "Is my son deficient in a dietary mineral or vitamin that is causing his attention problems?" "Are pesticides in our food harming my daughter's learning?" These questions are difficult for clinicians (or scientists) to answer. Yet they persist, and so some attempts at answers are incumbent on the field. Indeed, the appeal in thinking of dietary contributors to the condition is obvious: If they can be substantiated, then treating the problem can be very economical and low-risk. Those who are uneasy with medication for children are often more comfortable with the idea of dietary intervention. Moreover, the Western diet is, sadly, infamous for its many nutritional deficiencies. These appear to be contributing to an epidemic of child-hood and adult obesity and diabetes, as well as rising rates of cardiovas-cular disease. All of this lends a certain degree of "face validity" to the idea that diet may also play a role in behavioral and mental disorders. Could ADHD be among the consequences of a nutritionally inade-quate diet?

Several distinct dietary-related hypotheses have been proposed. Yet the story of possible dietary influences on ADHD is in some ways a treacherous one that many scientists who study ADHD are reluctant to reenter. The reason is that many dietary hypotheses initially greeted with popular enthusiasm have proven, upon careful study, to be of little use in explaining ADHD. For example, in the 1980s it was popular to speculate that dietary sugar and candy contributed to ADHD. Con-trolled studies disproved this claim (Wolraich, Wilson, & White, 1985). Sugar ingestion led to increases in parental attributions of ADHD symptoms (similar to a placebo effect), but did not show an effect in observer ratings. Indeed, it is difficult to see how sugar intake could lead to the extensive neuropsychological profile that has been de-scribed in this book. Thus many scientists are reluctant to "cry wolf" again on the topic of diet and ADHD. Moreover, the high heritability of ADHD and the lack of shared environment effects have led many to conclude that diet is not a promising explanatory route for this disor-der. Barkley (2006) has provided a terse summary of this early history of dietary theories; Arnold (2001) has provided a somewhat different view of this history.

For our purposes, however, what is of interest is the possibility that interactions are occurring between genotype and extremely common or widespread environmental triggering agents. In light of the criteria described above for such high-risk/high-payoff ideas, this chapter con-siders these hypotheses afresh—beginning with historical suggestions that many in the field feel have not been supported, and then moving on to newer, still speculative, yet interesting hypotheses for the 21st century.

Food Additives and Allergies

In the 1970s, strong claims were made that food additives (salicylates, dyes, preservatives) were to blame for many cases of ADHD (Feingold, 1975). The logic was that allergies to food-borne chemicals would lead to toxic reactions affecting behavior. These types of additives have become ubiquitous in Western society, and therefore they constitute a viable candidate risk category from the behavioral genetic perspective I have outlined in prior chapters. Early controlled studies and, especially, authoritative meta-analyses failed to substantiate this idea (Conners, 1980; Kavale & Forness, 1983; National Advisory Committee on Hyperkinesis and Food Additives, 1980). However, a National Institutes of Health (1982) consensus panel concluded that more research was needed, due to what were seen as limitations in the studies conducted up to that time. More recently, Arnold (2001, 2002) has reviewed this literature in further detail and concluded that it merits more attention, based on positive findings from several more recent and putatively better-designed studies (Boris & Mandel, 1994; see Breakey, 1997).

An even more recent meta-analysis was completed by Schab and Trinh (2004). They identified 15 studies that met their criteria of being double-blind, placebo-controlled, and focused only on artificial food colors and not other dietary elements. Each of these studies looked at whether ADHD symptoms worsened in children with ADHD on the challenge diet with food coloring. The aggregate effect size on behavioral ratings was $d = 0.28$ (claimed to be about one-third the size of effects observed with stimulant medication). Although this modest effect was statistically significant, it masked a discrepancy between parents' ratings ($d = 0.44$), which were significant, and teachers' ratings ($d = 0.08$) and health professionals' ratings ($d = 0.11$), which were nonsignificant. The fact that the effect was carried by parental ratings suggests either that parent expectancy effects could have been operating, or that parents and teachers/professionals were assessing different aspects of children's behavior. Effects were also carried by the subset of studies in which children were preselected, based on parent report or challenge, as responsive to food coloring ($d = 0.53$); when that was not done, the effect was trivial ($d = 0.09$). Schab and Trinh concluded that further work to identify this responding subgroup was warranted. Arnold (2002) also concluded in his review that a subset of children may have allergic reactions to food additives; he suggested that these children are likely to exhibit atopy, irritability, sleep disturbance, and prominent hyperactive–impulsive symptoms.

Taken as a whole, then, this literature has historically described mixed results. Further work to determine whether a subset of children with ADHD may be reacting allergically to ubiquitous food additives, and to identify that subgroup, may warrant continued investigation.

The focus on allergic reactions, however, is a key complication for this theory. Despite reports of elevated ADHD + allergy comorbidity, data linking ADHD to asthma and other allergies remain mixed in both clinical samples (Biederman, Milberger, Faraone, Guite, & Warburton, 1994) and population samples (McGee, Stanton, & Sears, 1993). Past findings linking ADHD with allergies may have been artifacts of clinical ascertainment. Nonetheless, the potential link between ADHD and allergic reactions remains of theoretical and clinical interest.

Marshall (1989) theorized that some types of allergic reactions disrupt cholinergic (and adrenergic) neural transmission. Cholinergic activity, along with noradrenergic activity, is important in arousal and is also marked in the striatum (related to the frontal–striatal circuits described in Chapter 3). Moreover, cholinergic activity in ADHD, though underemphasized, is of considerable interest. For example, the potential link between ADHD and smoking (recall the discussion of this in Chapter 10), sometimes thought to be a "self-medicating" effect (but note questions about this in the prior chapter), would be mediated by nicotine's effect on cholinergic systems. Levin et al. (1996) found that adults with ADHD experienced improved cognitive functioning on nicotine, presumably due to enhanced cholinergic functioning. Therefore, a neural link via allergic reactions and cholinergic systems is plausible. Marshall (1989) therefore suggested that children who have ADHD in relation to allergic reactions should exhibit cortical hypoarousal (see the discussion of arousal in Chapter 4). That in turn suggests a neuropsychologically defined subgroup to scrutinize.

Subsequent EEG studies, though very preliminary due to small samples, provide initial support for this idea: Slow-wave activity (i.e., low cortical arousal) was related to food allergic reactions in children with ADHD (Uhlig, Merkenschlager, Brandmaier, & Egger, 1997). Such studies on relevant subgroups warrant replication attempts before a final verdict on food allergies and ADHD can be offered. In the meantime, caution remains the predominant approach toward this hypothesis in the field.

Fatty Acid Metabolism and Omega-3 Fatty Acid Deficiency

The story of food allergies and ADHD has been checkered by controversy, yet remains a topic of refined studies that may yet prove relevant to defining a subgroup of children with ADHD. In the meantime, newer dietary hypotheses have subsequently emerged.[1] Perhaps the most striking of these new hypotheses concerns the role of highly unsaturated omega-3 fatty acids—an idea that has been popularized in the United States by Andrew Stoll's (2001) book *The Omega-3 Connection*. These particular fatty acids play a variety of health roles, but may also affect mood and behavior via their involvement in neuronal membrane health. They therefore have drawn interest in relation to schizophrenia, learning disabilities, and ADHD, in addition to their somewhat better-established relevance to preventing cardiovascular disease. What is the hypothesized source of risk here? How well does this hypothesis meet our criteria as a potentially promising clue to ADHD?

Omega-3 fatty acids are highly unsaturated fatty acids from what is known as the omega-3 and omega-6 series. They are most commonly found in fish oil, certain plant oils (such as olive oil and canola oil), and some types of nuts (such as flax seeds and walnuts). Two of these highly unsaturated fatty acids are thought to be particularly important to neuronal membrane health (these cell membranes are composed of phospholipids, including the omega-3 and omega-6 molecules), signal transduction, and neural development: arachidonic acid (AA) and docosahexaenoic acid (DHA). Also important are dihomo-gamma-linolenic acid (DGLA) and eicosapentaenoic acid. These fatty acids are distinct from the types of fatty acids that *contribute* to heart disease; instead, these are thought to counteract and *reduce* heart disease and to improve immune function. They are hypothesized to have been common in the evolutionary diet of early humans, and to be essential for organ health (including neural transmission). A key reason for this supposition is their role in the health of neuronal cell membranes. Because humans cannot manufacture the precursor essential fatty acids, they must be ingested.

With regard to the ubiquity of this dietary deficiency, support is relatively good for the claim that dietary shortage of omega-3 fatty acids is widespread in Western industrialized societies, including Europe, North America, and Australia (Holman, 1998). Investigation of this shortage continues in relation to cardiovascular disease. Thus, if low intake of these elements is to be a candidate for ADHD in terms of undetected genotype–environment interactions, it meets the test of being a very common experience that could affect most or all twins in behavioral genetic studies. In short, it meets our first criterion. What about the second criterion: Is there a plausible neurodevelopmental method of action that could lead to ADHD?

Richardson and Puri (2000) summarize the neurodevelopmental hypothesis at issue here, and I largely follow and paraphrase their argument. As noted already, fatty acids and their long-chain derivatives make up neuronal cell membranes. Alterations in their composition therefore should be able to affect membrane receptors and neurotransmitter functioning, as well as cell second-messenger systems. Thus their absence from a child's diet during early development is hypothesized to compromise the efficiency of neural transmission, neural development, and therefore learning and behavioral control. AA and DGLA are viewed as particularly important in the brain, because they make up a substantial percentage of neuronal mass, and their derivative molecules are thought to be involved in brain regulatory functioning.

Key in terms of ongoing neural health are both (1) the availability of the basic precursor molecules in the diet, and (2) the ability of the body to convert these precursors into the derivative molecules (AA and DHA) that are most actively used in the brain. These conversion processes apparently can be disrupted by still other dietary deficiencies (excess saturated fats, zinc deficiency, alcohol), and notably by stress hormone activity. In theory, genetically influenced variation in efficiency of conversion processes exists in the population. Therefore, some children—those with the least efficient conversion abilities—would be vulnerable to any dietary shortage of the precursors or to disruption in the conversion mechanisms (Horrobin, Glen, & Hudson, 1995). This effect, in turn, would provide the genotype–environment interaction needed to influence the heritability term in ADHD studies. In other words, with nearly all children receiving a shortage of dietary precursors, a subset of children will have behavioral difficulty due to genetically influenced problems in efficiently converting this diet to maintain neuronal health. Because nearly all children receive the inadequate diet, which ones develop problems will be determined largely by genetic factors and will appear as heritability in twin designs.

With regard to how such disruption might specifically lead to ADHD, it is notable that dietary fatty acid deficiency may disrupt the functioning of the neurotransmitters in the indolamine class (which includes serotonin, as well as the catecholamines serotonin and dopamine). In particular, disruption of dopamine functioning in frontal regions has been observed in at least initial animal studies (Delion et al., 1995). The effects appears to result in reduced dopamine availability in the synapse (perhaps via disrupted storage)—an effect consistent with what might occur in ADHD.

Richardson and Puri (2000) go on to hypothesize that these effects may be most pronounced in the inattentive features of ADHD, but one could also argue the opposite. They also postulate that males are more vulnerable to effects of dietary fatty acid deficiency than females, making this theory consistent with the observed gender differences in

ADHD. Finally, they review evidence indicating that disruption of these essential fatty acids may disrupt sleep regulation and may lead to atopic conditions (allergic reactions).

Once again, then, we have a dietary theory predicting that the subgroup of children with ADHD to which this hypothesis applies will include both those with sleep difficulties (see the discussion of this issue in ADHD in Chapter 4) and/or those with allergic reactions. In addition, this particular theory predicts weakened immune functioning if fatty acid deficiency is contributory. In other words, if this theory is right, we should see a subgroup of children with ADHD who also experience (1) excessive rates of infections and digestive disorders; (2) atopic reactions (e.g., eczema, asthma); and (3) dry skin and dry hair, excessive thirst, and frequent urination. They may also experience motor coordination problems—an important clue in light of the discussion in Chapter 7.

What are the results of initial animal or other pilot experiments? Although this literature is in its infancy, initial animal studies indicate that neural development and neural function are permanently disrupted by dietary deficiency of omega-6 and omega-3 fatty acids during the neonatal period. It is thought that neuronal migration, as well as synaptic pruning, can be influenced by metabolism of these fatty acids (Crawford, 1992). The omega-3 acids (e.g., DHA) are thought to be particularly relevant to cognitive impairments (Neuringer, Reisbeck, & Janowsky, 1994). Thus considerable importance may accrue to maternal dietary status and even the role of breast feeding during early life. However, ongoing dietary availability of these molecules is apparently also important to maintain healthy neural functioning.

In humans, preliminary studies of ADHD and fatty acid metabolism are mixed but intriguing. At least two studies have now found that when compared to age- and sex-matched controls, samples of children with ADHD had lower serum free fatty acid levels (Bekaroglu, Aslan, Gedik, & Deger, 1996; Stevens, Zentall, Abate, Kuczeck, & Burgess, 1996), as well as some of the physical symptoms noted above (i.e., dry skin, thirst, frequent urination). Their findings led those investigators to speculate that the observed effects might be due to faulty conversion of precursor chemicals to AA and DHA, consistent with the idea that a subgroup of children are genetically vulnerable to disruption in the supply of these building blocks.

However, initial efforts to alter ADHD symptoms by dietary supplementation have had mixed success, including frankly negative findings (Voigt et al., 2001). Yet these initial findings were criticized because trials were too brief and/or failed to include the full array of the omega-3 acids thought to be relevant to attention problems (Richardson & Puri, 2000). More recently, Richardson and Puri (2002) conducted a randomized, double-blind, placebo-controlled trial of dietary supplementation for 12 weeks with a full array of fatty acids. They noted significant improvements in Conners ADHD and Global Index scores over that time in the treatment group, but not the placebo group (the latter showed slight worsening of ADHD symptoms). Limitations were noteworthy: The sample consisted of children with learning disabilities; blood levels were not obtained; and persistence of benefits over time was not assessed. The last of these is an important issue, because early attempts to use amino acid supplementation in ADHD appeared to show effects, but it then became apparent that the effects did not persist (reviewed by Arnold, 2001).

A further limitation of this general argument is its nonspecificity. In addition to ADHD, fatty acid deficiency is thought to be related to mood and learning disorders. Thus an additional hypothesis is that this mechanism may be most relevant to children with ADHD who have comorbid difficulties in mood or learning problems. Once again, this may implicate the subgroup with ADHD-PI somewhat more heavily than the subgroup with ADHD-C.

In all, dietary fatty acid deficiency is an intriguing idea that meets many of our criteria for a promising candidate in a high-risk/high-payoff paradigm. Additional and confirmatory pilot studies are now needed to evaluate whether a more ambitious investment is justified. Those studies ideally should focus on identifying whether a reliably identifiable subgroup of children with ADHD meet criteria for a problem with converting these fatty acids, and then whether it can be replicated that they may benefit from dietary supplementation.

Sugar and Caffeine

I include a brief comment here on dietary sugar and caffeine, because inquiries about their roles are among the most common questions asked about ADHD and diet. Despite this high level of interest among the lay public, convincing evidence for a significant role of these two dietary agents is lacking. With regard to caffeine, concerns have been raised about the rising popularity of caffeinated soft drinks and potential heavy use by some children. Indeed, caffeine use among children and adolescents can affect the amount of sleep they obtain (Pollack & Bright, 2003) and may contribute to symptoms of anxiety (Broderick & Benjamin, 2004). Overall rates of caffeine consumption among children in the United States, however, remain within ranges usually considered to have little effect on behavioral adjustment (Knight, Knight, Mitchell, & Zepp, 2004). Furthermore, relatively recent reviews of the rather scant literature on children's caffeine use and ADHD symptoms have tended to conclude that there is no clear relation between caffeine use and ADHD-related problems (Castellanos & Rapoport, 2002; Leviton, 1992). Instead, questions remain as to whether caffeine may in some instances benefit children with ADHD (Castellanos & Rapoport, 2002). Thus, with very limited data available, it is difficult to make a case that rising caffeine use among children is an important contributor to ADHD.

Findings for glucose (sugar) intolerance have been decidedly mixed. Acute sugar intake does not explain ADHD symptoms (Milich, Wolraich, & Lindgren, 1986; Wolraich et al., 1985). However, still in question is whether chronic sugar intake interacts with excessive antibiotic use in early development (e.g., for treatment of otitis media) to influence ADHD symptoms. The argument here is that a combination of chronic sugar overload with repeated antibiotic use alters intestinal bacterial flora, interfering with absorption of nutrients (Arnold, 2002). It is unclear, however, that we would expect neuropsychological effects from this pathway. In short, caffeine and acute sugar intake both show little promise in explaining ADHD. Chronic sugar use remains a "longshot" explanation for a subset of cases—one that will only pay off when better integrated with newer designs to identify vulnerable subgroups.

Dietary Exposure to Organophosphate Pesticides

Exposures to pesticides and other household chemicals are a growing concern in the industrialized world. Thousands of pesticides, measured in the billions of pounds, are dispersed in the United States alone annually, and they include several classes of chemicals that might be expected to have adverse effects on the developing nervous system (Koger et al., 2005). Whereas particular exposure risks have been well identified for agricultural/farm workers, for others who face occupational hazards (e.g., those in the pest extermination business), and for their families and children, other, lower-level environmental exposures may be far more widespread among children. The main route of exposure is via food, because of the extensive use of these pesticides in mainstream industrial agriculture in the United States and worldwide. Organophosphate pesticides are the most commonly used, since the banning of dichlorodiphenyltrichloroethane (DDT) in many countries.

With regard to neural pathways, these chemicals' mechanism of action is cholinergic. As discussed in the prior section, potential cholinergic influences on ADHD are underexplored but potentially promising. Links to arousal and cognitive control are beginning to emerge. Therefore, dietary exposure to pesticides involves a plausible mechanism of neural action.

It is now well recognized that developing children are particularly vulnerable to these environmental exposures because of their rapid metabolism; the vast amount of food they consume per unit of body weight, compared to adults; their proximity to the ground (Weiss, 2000); and the relative volume of fruit and vegetable products in their diet (Goldman, 1995a, 1995b). Related sources of risk to children include household cleaning agents and insecticides, and other routine but potentially poisonous products that may not have a discernible effect on adults but may have an effect on the rapidly developing nervous system of young infants or toddlers (see discussion by Koger et al., 2005).

The EPA lists over 30 fungicides, herbicides, and pesticides as teratogens; concentrated exposures *in utero* (which may happen, for example, to a pregnant farm worker) can cause damage to the fetus. Risks to children outside the United States remain great in some cases, because products now banned in the United States are still in use in some other nations (Yanez et al., 2002). Thousands of other products are in widespread use, with no prior evaluation of their potential effects on neural development, cognition, or behavior in developing children (Koger et al., 2005). Exposures therefore may well be very common and work as shared environment effects (a key feature for potential genotype–environment interactions). One survey (cited in Schettler, 2001) concluded that 90% of U.S. children had detectable urinary levels of organophosphate pesticides (a known neurotoxicant class). A study in Germany produced similar findings, although average exposure levels appeared to be far lower than currently accepted toxic levels (Heudorf, Angerer, & Drexler, 2004). However, recall that even these "safe" levels have often not been evaluated in young children, and that the history of research on lead and mercury (Chapter 10) is one in which each decade has brought new discoveries of harm at levels previously thought to be safe. Thus caution remains necessary with regard to safe exposure levels for young children.

In light of all this, the potential field of risk to children with regard to organophosphate pesticides in food is both vast and unstudied. The health effects of these exposures are diverse, and specificity of any effects to ADHD is unclear at best. Even so, these agents appear to meet our criteria of (1) being extremely common in the experiential context of young children, and (2) having a plausible mechanism of action that could lead to ADHD (in this case, via cholinergic action on the developing nervous system; Eriksson, Ankarberg, Viberg, & Fredriksson, 2001). What do initial pilot studies indicate?

In human children, the causal effects on neural development of routine background pesticide exposures (e.g., eating food from the grocery store with pesticide residues on it, contact with lawn care products, and general household use) as well as excess exposures (e.g., spraying of a crop near a child) have been essentially unstudied because of the tremendous technical problems entailed in identifying actual exposure levels, complicated by the rapid dispersal of these chemicals from the body after ingestion (Wessels, Barr, & Mendola, 2003). Yet, although the EPA lists these chemicals as teratogens for the developing fetus when exposure occurs directly in the environment (e.g., to farm workers), the U.S. Food and Drug Administration has judged that routine exposure via food is not classifiable as a teratogen.

Nonetheless, a small number of initial studies again provide potentially disturbing evidence that this route may warrant more study. As a result of the difficulties in studying exposure reliably in children, researchers have turned to controlled animal experiments. The majority of these studies document that marked growth problems and mental retardation result from relatively high exposures. A few studies, however, have investigated effects of lower-level exposures on behavior, cognition, or subtle neurodevelopmental changes in animals—in other words, the sorts of effects that would interest us in relation to their potential contribution to ADHD. These have been suggestive. At least four animal studies have linked organophosphate pesticide exposure in early development to later behavior interpreted as a model of human hyperactivity (Ahlbom, Fredriksson, & Eriksson, 1995; Eriksson & Fredriksson, 1991; Icenogle et al., 2004; Winrow et al., 2003). Problems in an experimental task designed to probe working memory were identified in one animal study (Icenogle et al., 2004). These studies used low doses, so that major effects on health and development were not seen in the animals; they thus roughly mimicked the likely situation in children ingesting the substances postnatally on a routine basis via their food, or experienced prenatally via their mothers' diet.

As noted, measuring these effects in children is fraught with technical difficulties. Studies of human children must consider the critical period of exposure and the appropriate duration of measurement. In spite of these issues, one reasonably well-controlled study found that children with typical diets had "unsafe" urinary levels of these toxins according to the EPA standard, whereas children eating organic diets had urine levels well within the EPA's current guidelines (Curl, Fenske, & Elgethun, 2003). Thus, based on this initial study, it appears that organic diets may provide an effective remedy for parents who are concerned about the potential effects of these pesticide products on food in their children.

Overall, there is no question that these exposures in children are an important public health concern generally, due to their ubiquity and a disturbing lack of information about the effects of many of these chemicals (especially their interactions) on developing children. Yet data that could clarify whether these exposures may be specifically related to ADHD symptoms are limited. Future studies to explore this state of affairs therefore are extremely important.

Diet and ADHD: Conclusions and Cautions

Many dietary theories of ADHD involve factors or mechanisms that lack promising pilot data (e.g., amino acid deficiency), that have failed in controlled trials (e.g., acute sugar intake), or that are probably insufficiently ubiquitous in children's lives to show effects in the face of behavioral genetic findings. Their continued study and occasional positive findings testify to the potential myriad routes to ADHD that may be relevant in a given case. However, with regard to major, ubiquitous effects that may be interacting with genotype in virtually the entire population, two candidates stand out in the dietary universe.

One is the potential role of a dietary shortage of omega-3 fatty acids. This possibility now has the support of a small number of animal studies and positive findings in one well-controlled human intervention trial. It therefore warrants more extensive high-risk/high-payoff investigation. A caution is appropriate here: It remains possible that the nascent study of fatty acid metabolism may eventually fall to the same fate as other dietary hypotheses of ADHD and be mired in inconclusive controversy. However, this hypothesis has unique strengths, including (1) the pervasiveness of children's exposure to the problem, (2) the neuronal effects of shortages of these dietary molecules in animal studies, and (3) recent positive findings in a double-blind intervention trial in children. Another obvious caution is that there is now a "bandwagon effect," in which shortages of omega-3 fatty acids are cited as culprits in heart disease, cancer, asthma, mood disorders, and schizophrenia, as well as learning disabilities and ADHD—in short, a majority of the maladies of modern society. Such a broad-spectrum risk seems too nonspecific to account for the majority of cases of ADHD (in which there is no heart disease, mood disorder, schizophrenia, or even learning disability). Thus more refined arguments that target a subset of the population with ADHD, or that specify key developmental periods, developmental markers, or particular genotype–environment interactions related to ADHD and fatty acids, will be needed. On the other hand, the proof would be "in the pudding" in high-risk/high-payoff studies: If a link is identified and initial studies are replicated, we can work backward to understand how it operates.

The second potentially viable route to ADHD via diet involves the role of organophosphate pesticide residues in food. This possibility has achieved rather consistent support in small numbers of animal studies linking early exposure to animal models of hyperactivity. Appropriate exploratory trials in humans are as yet largely lacking, in part due to the daunting technical difficulties in such studies, and will need to be carried out before a major high-risk/high-payoff investment can be justified. Support for such studies in children should be provided, and those initial studies should be carried out.

Lacking overall are epidemiological studies to determine what percentage of children with clinical-level problems can be explained by any of these candidate dietary contributors. In other words, the relative risk or attributable risk of these factors (if any) is impossible to quantify at present. In most cases of dietary problems and ADHD, treatment is expected to be appropriate only for those with deficient or excessive levels of the relevant substance (although some clinical trials have applied the relevant treatment to all diagnosed children in a study without regard to deficiency or excess, these results generally appear less suggestive than those of studies that selected children with problematic levels for treatment). However, controlled, double-blind replication trials are generally lacking.

That said, these theories have the advantage of making testable predictions about the characteristics of the subgroup of children who might be affected, notably including a role for allergic markers in most instances. Therefore, the most optimistic picture for proponents of these hypotheses of ADHD is that children with ADHD may include one small subgroup with a history of otitis media and glucose intolerance (which seems unlikely at this point), and another subgroup with atopy and somatic problems who have deficient brain fatty acid levels (because of either dietary deficiency, poor metabolism, or their interaction). A third subgroup with atopy and other food allergies is also possible. It will be useful to see future studies that consider these mechanisms together in the same samples of children, to clarify whether they are distinct or overlapping. Finally, integration of these potentially interrelated dietary factors with neuropsychological measures—in particular, with measures of cortical arousal—may help to map the relevant subgroups. By these means, future studies may be able to make clearer advances than have yet been achieved, to justify further high-risk/high-payoff studies with larger population samples.

COULD ELECTRONIC MEDIA CAUSE ADHD?

Specific suggestions have been made that television, via its rapid alternating stimulation of the developing nervous system, could alter neural development in very young children and thus contribute to children's attention problems and ADHD (Healy, 1990). The fact that electronic media can influence children's behavioral development is in fact quite well established in a realm closely related to ADHD: the development of aggression (Anderson et al., 2003). However, in that domain, the emphasis is entirely on the programming *content* (i.e., violent television programs and video games lead to more aggressive behavior). In the case of ADHD, hypotheses center as much on the physiological and psychological responses to the *media* (regardless of content) as they do on questions of content (Healy, 1990).

Still further specificity of analysis is necessary, because some aspects or types of electronic media may be beneficial for children, and other aspects may be harmful. Some interactive video games, for example, may have positive effects on motor coordination and even on attention and problem solving, whereas some television programs may have a deleterious effect. Or perhaps computer and Internet usage are associated with enhanced learning, whereas television usage may have the opposite effect. Therefore, the types of electronic media, the types of programming, and the content versus form of the media are important considerations in evaluating this question.

I focus here primarily on television viewing, simply because it is the most pervasively used electronic medium for children and is the most often questioned in relation to ADHD. Similar arguments to those outlined here may apply to some types of video games (and may or may not be relevant to computer activity). Before proceeding further, let me consider the criteria I have suggested for a promising experiential risk agent in ADHD.

Television as a Ubiquitous Experiential Influence for Western Children

First, with regard to ubiquity, the widespread exposure to electronic media among children growing up in Western societies is so extensive as to meet this criterion easily. In particular, television has now become a ubiquitous part of children's experience not only in the United States, but in all of the countries where twin studies of ADHD have been conducted (Larson & Varma, 1998). Not counting "secondary viewing" (being in a room while a TV is on, but not watching it as the main activity), one large household survey in 1997 in the United States found that children ages 0–2 watched an average of 644 minutes (10.7 hours) of television per week, whereas older children averaged 828 minutes (13.8 hours) per week, or approximately 2 hours per day (Wright et al., 2001). Other surveys, which included secondary viewing in their totals, put these numbers slightly higher, concluding that children spend about 3 hours per day with a television (Huston & Wright, 1998). Developmental trends show variation in viewing, but the crucial point for us is that viewing begins very early (including the 0–2 age range) and persists throughout preschool, dropping somewhat at school entry (Wright et al., 2001). Wright et al. (2001) observed that, on the basis of sampling on 2 days, 88% of children watched some television. A major Kaiser Family Foundation (1999) report concluded that across all ages, only 5% of children spent less than an hour per day with some form of electronic media. Again, the majority of this time is likely to be spent in television viewing, with children averaging 2 hours and 46 minutes of television time per day in the Kaiser survey.

Crucial to theories of ADHD is children's exposure to television in the preschool years. The Kaiser Family Foundation (2003) conducted a randomized telephone survey of some 1,000 households in the United States, addressing electronic media use patterns in the all-important of 0–6 years. This survey found that in 2003, on a typical day, 89% of children in this age range used screen media (the same percentage as played outside); 79% watched television on a typical day (the same percentage as read or were read to). And children in this age range spent an average of nearly 2 hours per day in front of electronic screen media—equivalent to the time spent playing outside, and three times more than reading or being read to. Although an increasing percentage of this media time is spent with interactive media (video games, computers), the vast majority continues to be passive viewing—either watching television programs or watching movies/videos played on the television (I refer to both of these passive forms as "television viewing" herein). The Kaiser Family Foundation (2003) found that 66% of children in this age range lived in homes in which the television was on more than half the time; 36% lived in homes in which the television was on "always" or "most of the time." Secondary viewing is not incidental to developmental theories, as noted subsequently, so these numbers with regard to total "television on" time are quite relevant. Indeed, when secondary viewing is included, some surveys have placed television exposure levels very high. Nonsystematic convenience sample surveys have suggested that the average home has a television on 6 hours per day, and that preschool children, including toddlers and infants, are exposed to up to 2 hours per day (Anderson & Evans, 2001). These exposures include children under the age of 2 years, 43% of whom watch television "nearly every day," even though the American Academy of Pediatrics recommends no television in that age range (Kaiser Family Foundation, 2003).

Altogether, although methodologies have varied and surveys have relied heavily on self-report, the data suggest that television exposure qualifies as an essentially ubiquitous experiential effect on children in the United States and in other Western societies. This common exposure is widespread even in the very early developmental periods, when one could most readily argue that it might disrupt the consolidation of self-regulation (Jensen et al., 1997b). Admittedly, we do not know how much viewing (if any) is needed to influence attentional development, or at what ages, or how many children would exceed such a hypothetical viewing "threshold."[2] Nonetheless, at an average of 2 hours per day for electronic media and most of this for television, these *potential* effects are probably widespread. The developmental concern of theorists at these levels of electronic media engagement is that they rival the time spent with peers and in the play and socialization activities widely agreed to be integral to cognitive, emotional, and regulatory development (Kaiser Family Foundation, 2003). Thus, in theory, these media may have a substantial influence on socialization and cognitive development (Anderson & Evans, 2001; Jensen et al., 1997b). Not all of these influences are negative (as we will see), and the role of television viewing in social development is unclear and probably varies from home to home. For example, in some homes television viewing may serve as a social organizer that brings parents and children together socially, whereas in other homes it may displace such interaction (Larson & Varma, 2003).

Nonetheless, the logical possibility of influence on ADHD development in the early years is clearly sufficiently real to warrant scrutiny, in view of the high volume of television viewing that young children experience. Could children with high liability to ADHD be affected? Are there plausible developmental theories by which television viewing could lead to ADHD?

Developmental Theories of Television's Influence on Cognitive Control

What is the developmental hypothesis as to how television might influence children's arousal regulation, executive functioning, reinforcement response, temporal information processing, or other neuropsychological mechanisms in ADHD? Because development of regulatory abilities in relation to arousal, affect, attention, and executive functioning depend both on language and on the scaffolding of parent–child interactions in early life, it has proven relatively easy to generate hypotheses about how disruptions in language or social development could be caused by television, leading in turn to weakened consolidation of self-regulatory capacities. Anderson and Evans (2001) outline some of these possibilities; Jensen et al. (1997b) outline others. Many of these hypotheses relate to the *form* of the medium, regardless of the *content*. However, observers have noted that form and content are correlated. For example, public television programs tend to involve longer attention periods and less frequent shifts of focus than commercial television (Hooper & Chang, 1998). Also in question is whether very young children are vulnerable to television content because of their immature cognitive development. Here is a list of these various hypotheses:

1. Television's frequent auditory and visual changes prompt frequent, automatic reorienting of attention even during secondary viewing; these changes disrupt play and other interactions, and as a result potentially disrupt consolidation of cognitive development.

2. Television's demand for visual processing weakens language development, with a cascade of negative effects on social, language, and self-regulatory development. Most relevant to ADHD would be television's disruption of self-talk and then internalized speech, which the child would ordinarily be using during play and which are essential elements of the emergent role of language in self-regulation.

3. The constant stimulation of the television disrupts temporal information processing, making attention, motor control, and other abilities weaker in turn.

4. Parental attention is frequently distracted by the television, leading to failures of needed regulatory interactions with young children.

5. The hypnotic state induced by the television's flickering high-frequency refresh rate leads to greater slow-wave brain activity, with negative effects on consolidation of effortful attention.

6. Relatedly, the rapid pace of attention shifting demanded by the medium up-regulates some forms of attention (e.g., scanning) and down-regulates others (e.g., focusing; Jensen et al., 1997b).

7. A final hypothesis pertains to content: Arousing (e.g., violent or gripping) content maintains higher levels of emotional arousal than the child would otherwise have, making it difficult for the child's self-regulatory systems to adapt properly to ordinary social interaction and ordinary learning.

In short, developmental theory can accommodate (albeit with the aid of considerable speculation) a prediction that excessive television viewing interferes with social, language, and cognitive development and the consolidation of self-regulation, leading vulnerable children to develop ADHD. Yet demonstrating that such causal effects occur is difficult, and to this point evidence for them is lacking.

For one thing, genotype–environment correlations are likely to be ubiquitous in this domain. For example, higher parental intelligence and education may lead to less television viewing, and vice versa. Alternatively, difficult-to-manage toddlers may be placed in front of the television more often by parents, perhaps in some cases because parents themselves have limited coping skills. In those scenarios, television viewing would be correlated with ADHD symptoms, but might have no causal influence on it.[3] Experimental studies that can address such possibilities are in hand for some related effects—notably the effect of violent television content on child aggression—but are in short supply in relation to ADHD. Nonetheless, let us examine such data as are in hand.

Effects of Television on Related Behaviors: Aggression and Social Development

Data are far clearer for the effects of television (and other electronic media) on behavioral and social development than they are for effects on the kinds of neuropsychological mechanisms involved in ADHD as discussed in this book. These data suggest that behavioral and social effects are influenced by electronic media *content*, rather than by the nature of the media themselves. Because media use is not homogeneous but is quite varied, children are influenced in various ways, depending on what content they watch or engage with (Anderson, Huston, Schmitt, Linebarger, & Wright, 2001). For example, viewing of educational television in preschool is associated with better educational attainment (Anderson et al., 2001). Likewise, some evidence suggests that certain games can enhance cognitive skills; for example, the computer game Tetris appeared to enhance visual–spatial and visual reasoning ability, perhaps even influencing Performance IQ scores (Okagaki & French, 1996).

Effects of television viewing (regardless of content) on reduced language development, shortened attention spans, or intellectual passivity have not been as clearly demonstrated. No negative effects were seen, for example, in the Anderson et al. (2001) monograph. Although language development and attention spans were not directly measured, Anderson et al. found that total amount of television viewing in preschool (or in adolescence) did not strongly predict harm to academic achievement (in fact, for boys, more viewing was associated with better achievement; the negative association for girls was generally nonsignificant). These findings render it doubtful that there were major negative effects on language or attention span.

However, negative *content* is clearly harmful. Viewing of violent television programming is associated with development of behavior problems and aggression in children (Anderson, 2004; Anderson et al., 2001, 2003). This literature is so massive and so often reviewed that Bushman and Anderson (2001) provided a review of meta-analyses. Their "review of reviews" covered correlational and experimental evidence. They concluded that violent television viewing causes more aggressive behavior in children, with a main effect comparable in magnitude to that of cigarette smoking on lung cancer. Experimental studies indicate that these effects are carried by children who are vulnerable to aggression; some children are not at risk for aggression and are apparently fairly immune to these effects, though they may still experience heightened arousal and other negative effects of such programming. In fact, this causal effect between media violence and child aggression has now been accepted by public health authorities: it was accepted by the Congressional Public Health Summit (2000), which included the American Academy of Pediatrics, the American Academy of Child and Adolescent Psychiatry, the American Psychological Association, the American Medical Association, and other groups;

and the U.S. Surgeon General (U.S. Department of Health and Human Services, 2001).

The ability of violent television programming to cause increases in aggressive behavior in children (and adults) is a genotype–environment interaction, in that many children (and adults) watch violent television without becoming aggressive—just as many people smoke cigarettes without developing lung cancer, and many people are exposed to the TB bacterium without developing TB. Anderson and Bushman (2001) reviewed the more limited evidence on violent video game use (now increasingly common among preschoolers). The evidence pointed in the same direction as the data for television viewing, but evidence about this newer medium is still accumulating (Anderson, 2004).

Specific Studies on ADHD

Thus we know that television viewing (1) is extensive in young children, (2) can cause changes in behavior, and (3) can lead to the development of behaviors we associate with psychopathology. Is there any evidence linking it with ADHD specifically? The evidence here is quite limited. I have noted throughout this book that key to theories of ADHD are effects during early development (i.e., the infancy, toddler, and pre-school years). In general, evidence that concurrent television viewing shortens attention spans has not been forthcoming, in part because few studies have specifically examined ADHD-related symptoms. However, most research has not considered the television viewing of preschool children, and essentially none has examined the effects of viewing prior to age 2. Moreover, few if any studies have considered the effect of television on temporal information processing or advanced measures of cognitive control. For that matter, few studies have even checked for correlations with symptoms of ADHD per se.

Geist and Gibson (2000) looked at 4- to 5-year-old children (not diagnosed with ADHD), whom they randomly assigned to 30 minutes of (1) no television; (2) "slow" television (*Mister Rogers' Neighborhood*), which was believed to require less frequent attentional shifts; or (3) commercial "fast" television (*Power Rangers*), which was believed to require many and rapid attentional shifts. Children were then observed in a free-play period for the degree of time they spent on the same task and the number of times they changed activities in the immediately ensuing period. Children in the fast-viewing condition changed activity more often and stayed on each activity for less time than the children in the control condition. These findings could be consistent with a theory that the rapid pace of commercial television programs (as opposed to educational programming) disrupts attention and/or heightens arousal, causing children to be less likely to remain on the same task for an extended period of time. This study had some important limitations, however. Most notably, it was not clear that behavioral observers were unaware of the study condition of the children they were observing.

In the most recent and best correlational study to ask whether television viewing is associated developmentally with symptoms of ADHD per se, Christakis, Zimmerman, DiGiuseppe, and McCarty (2004) analyzed data from the National Longitudinal Survey of Youth, a nationally representative sample from which data on over 2,500 children were available. They found that number of hours of television viewing at ages 1 and 3 years (as reported by mothers) was associated with mother-rated attention problems on a behavioral rating scale at age 7. Numerous covariates were controlled for, including maternal depression, maternal education level, degree of stimulation in the home, gestational age, and alcohol or tobacco use during pregnancy. The effect size was expressed in terms of an odds ratio of 1.09, indicating that each hour of television viewed conferred a 9% increased risk of crossing the threshold Christakis et al. used for "attention problems" (not formal criteria for ADHD). For the typical child who watches 3 hours of television, this would amount to approximately a 30% increase in risk over the risk for a child watching no television. This is on the same order of magnitude as the effect of the DRD4 gene (a 40–50% increased risk; Chapter 9), or the figures I have provided, speculatively, for lead toxicity at the low end of the range (Chapter 10). In short, the magnitude of the effect was modest, but similar to that for other causal risk factors in ADHD. These findings thus were provocative.

However, again, significant limitations have to be noted. The main limitation in that study was that genotype–environment correlations were not considered, so that toddler attention problems (highly correlated from age 3 to age 7) were not controlled; nor were parental attention problems assessed. As noted earlier, children who have higher activity levels or who are difficult to manage (and who will go on to develop ADHD) may be placed in front of the television more often by parents. Those same parents may also have weaker coping skills. Nonetheless, this correlational finding may spark further experimental studies that may yield more definitive evidence one way or the other. A key gap so far in these initial studies is that they do not look at interactions (i.e., whether some children are vulnerable to more negative responses to television, whereas others are relatively unaffected by extensive viewing).

Electronic Media and ADHD: Summary

The effects of electronic media *content* on behavioral development appear to be robust and extremely important in several domains. Some of these effects can be positive, which seems to be the case with some aspects of educational media. Others can be quite deleterious—in particular, aggressive behavior in the case of violent television programming, and probably also in the case of violent video game content. Children with ADHD may be vulnerable to developing aggression, so this latter finding about aggression is hardly an aside. Yet, although aggression and learning are both relevant to ADHD, neither domain reflects the core dysfunction in ADHD per se. Initial exploratory studies provide intriguing potential links between early television viewing and symptoms of inattention/overactivity. However, these initial links are quite tenuous because of methodological limitations; certainly no causal conclusion can be drawn at this point. These preliminary findings require evaluation in better-controlled studies, including studies that control for parental ADHD, before they can be considered strong enough to justify an all-out investment in a high-risk/high-payoff research strategy focused on early childhood television viewing and ADHD. It is hoped that those follow-up studies will be conducted, so that the wisdom of such an investment can be fully evaluated.

COULD ENVIRONMENTAL TOXINS/CONTAMINANTS CAUSE ADHD?

I have already noted that a vast array of environmental contaminants may affect child development (Koger et al., 2005). Some effects are long studied and well known, including the dangerous effects on neural development of lead and mercury. The vast majority of toxicants being released into the environment and taken up into children's developing nervous systems are totally unstudied, and so cannot be suggested yet as targets of potential high-risk/high-payoff research strategies. In this section I emphasize the most advanced toxicant hypothesis about ADHD—that pertaining to a family of persistent organic pollutants (POPs). These compounds include polychlorinated biphenyls (PCBs) and related contaminants, such as polybromated biphenyls

(PBBs), dichlorodiphenyldichloroethylene (DDE), DDT, and hundreds of other chemicals. Because PCBs are the most well studied, I sometimes refer to all of these effects for simplicity as effects of "PCBs" (rather than the more inclusive term "POPs"). PCBs include 209 different cogeners (i.e., specific chemicals within this class), whereas inclusion of PBBs, DDT, DDE, and the others adds many more. How does this class of compounds meet our criteria for a causal agent that could be influencing ADHD via widespread, undetected genotype–environment interactions? First of all, are they common?

Ubiquitous Dispersal of POPs and PCBs in the Human Population

PCBs are industrial compounds, once widely used in a variety of applications. In the United States, they were widely used from the 1930s to the 1970s, when their manufacture was banned. However, they are extremely persistent and remain pervasive in the environment—including in soil, water, sediment, and air, in addition to their still-common presence in plastic products, buildings, and electrical equipment. PCBs and the other POPs are lipophilic (i.e., stored in human fat tissue) and have long half-lives (Kamrin, 1997; Matthews & Dedrick, 1984). These contaminants from water and sediments tend to accumulate in aquatic life. Because they are lipophilic, their concentration increases as they go through the food web (Kamrin, 1997). We humans are at the upper end of the food web; thus we often have significant exposure to these chemicals (Longnecker, Rogan, & Lucier, 1997). PCBs are found in many human tissues, including adipose (fat) tissue, blood, and (perhaps most significantly for their impact on human development) in umbilical cord plasma and breast milk (Longnecker et al., 1997). Extremely high exposures of adults, such as those after an industrial accident, lead to clear dermatological signs (dysmorphologies) as well as to cognitive delays in the offspring of women exposed (Chen, Guo, Hsu, & Rogan, 1992; Longnecker et al., 1997; Rice, 1997a, 1997b; Yu, Hsu, Gladen, & Rogan, 1991).

The focus here, however, is not on relatively rare extreme exposures after industrial accidents, but on ubiquitous, low-level, background exposures. Such low-grade exposures have been identified in all populations sampled and so are thought to be nearly universal, due to the wide dispersal of PCBs in industrialized countries (Longnecker et al., 2003; Schecter & Piskac, 2001). These exposures occur due to the previously mentioned passing of PCBs through the food chain, beginning with water and soil. The average levels of accumulation in the human population have begun to be quantified in some epidemiological studies. A number of issues make it difficult to compare these estimates—including different numbers of cogeners assessed, methods of assay, prenatal versus postnatal exposure levels, type of tissue sampled, and changes in population exposure levels over time, among others. Nonetheless, Rice (1997b) concluded in her review that the average level of PCBs in the population ranged from 2 to 10 ppb (see also Longnecker et al., 2003, for comparison of levels in different samples). In all, it seems that low-level, background exposures at these levels meet our test of being very common, even ubiquitous potential risk agents in children's development. Animal and human studies have now looked at the effects of these exposure levels on the developing nervous system. What would be the basic mechanism (or, more likely, mechanisms) of action for effects on neural development?

PCBs' Probable Mechanisms of Action: Hormonal and Dopaminergic

PCBs are known to be neurotoxic, and so several hypotheses for their mechanisms of toxic action in the developing brain have been investigated. One suspected mechanism entails occupation of estrogen receptors. This action in the fetal brain is theorized to disrupt endocrine activity and thus to influence neural development, which is hormonally modulated (Bonefeld-Jorgensen, Andersen, Rasmussen, & Vinggaard, 2001; McKinney & Waller, 1994). Another possibility is that some of these compounds are suspected of disrupting thyroid systems during fetal development (Osius, Karmaus, Kruse, & Witten, 1999; Zoeller, 2001). This potential mechanism of action is significant, because of emerging evidence that prenatal disruption of thyroid action may be one route to ADHD (Hauser et al., 1993; Vermiglio et al., 2004). A third hypothesis is that PCB-type compounds affect dopamine systems in development, either via early hormonal effects or via a separate route. A dopaminergic effect, of course, is relevant to several of our neuropsychological findings in ADHD (Sagvolden et al., 1998). Therefore, the possibility that these compounds have important effects on dopaminergic systems (Seegal, Brosch, & Okoniewski, 1997) provides a plausible neural and developmental argument that might link these contaminants to ADHD. If the route of influence is fetal estrogen effects' influencing later attention problems, these compounds would potentially be relevant (at least at a conceptual, global level) to understanding the role of sex hormones and sex differences in the development of ADHD.

The specifics of these effects are complex for several reasons. Effects may differ from one cogener to another and even from one type of tissue to another. For example, PCB-77, one well-studied cogener, can have both estrogenic and antiestrogenic effects under different conditions (Nesaretman, Corcoran, Dils, & Darbre, 1996). Moreover, the effects of different chemicals may interact. Combinations of chemicals may have synergistic negative effects on development, or, alternatively, may have protective effects (in which one compound counteracts another). Nonetheless, a number of important animal and human findings suggest that these compounds can disrupt neuropsychological development. The hypothesis explored here is that they may be pertinent to the inattentive and disorganized (executive function) symptoms of ADHD. In children, relatively low-level exposures (at the high end of the typical background range) appear to be related to inattention and impulsivity, but not to hyperactivity (Jacobson & Jacobson, 2003).

Evidence from Animal Studies

To evaluate whether low-level PCB exposures may *cause* behavioral or cognitive deficits, animal studies use experimental designs in which PCB exposures are randomly assigned. Rice (1997a) provided a detailed review of nearly two dozen such studies, most of them in either rodents or monkeys. Despite some inconsistent findings, she concluded that the PCB exposures caused later differences in the animals' behavior, as well as difficulties on cognitive paradigms designed to probe animal analogues of working memory (e.g., the delayed response alternation task).

Researchers in Norway have used a rodent model of ADHD called the "spontaneously hypertensive rat" (mentioned in Chapter 6). They compared such rats to animals exposed to PCB *in utero*, and concluded that the behavioral response style (excess responding to an operant reinforcement schedule) was similar in both sets of animals. They interpreted this as an influence on an animal analogue of impulsive behavior (Holena et al., 1995; Holena, Nafstad, Skaare, & Sagvolden, 1998).

Rice (1997b) also reviewed a series of studies by her group examining cognitive and behavioral effects in monkeys of maternal exposure to background levels of PCBs (i.e., similar to the levels observed in

the general human population in Canada and other Western countries). They reported two sets of findings. First, basic orienting of attention appeared to be intact in exposed rodents (Bushnell & Rice, 1999),
and perceptual and attentional functions were apparently typical in
exposed primates as well (Rice, 1997a). Second, functions that depend on prefrontal structures in humans—notably working memory as
assessed by delayed response alternation, and reinforcement response
as assessed by conditioning procedures—were affected in the offspring
of the mothers with routine exposure levels (Rice & Haward, 1997;
Rice, 1999). Effects were also observed with postnatal exposure (Rice,
1997a, 1998). Generalizing from animal to human effects is not
straightforward, but these findings are nonetheless consistent with predictions that PCBs have a preferential impact on dopamine-dependent,
prefrontal cognitive abilities.

As noted, several complications remain in pinning down the mechanisms of action of these effects. One issue is the question of single-
versus multiple-chemical studies. Studies of single chemicals allow
better isolation of cellular mechanisms. On the other hand, studies of
multiple compounds are likely to reflect real-world effects more accurately (whether these be synergistic, protective, or both). Many animal
studies have looked at only one or two compounds. Human studies
often assay a large number of cogeners and look at total exposure to
the most common elements. Another complication is that it is unclear
from animal data whether the mechanisms of effect are all directly neural or are also mediated behaviorally. Although PCB cogeners concentrate in fetal brain tissue when administered to mothers during
pregnancy, they also appear to alter maternal behavior (Simmons,
Cummings, Clemens, & Nunez, 2005). Maternal postnatal behavior
(e.g., extra grooming or licking), in turn, has effects on offspring neural development in animals. Therefore, this effect is significant in looking at moderators of outcome. Cross-fostering studies in animals may
be useful. Finally, the effects of prenatal versus postnatal exposures are
disputed by different investigators.

Nonetheless, the animal literature as a whole provides evidence
that early, low-level PCB exposures (both prenatal and postnatal) cause
impairment in animals' performance on tasks that are analogues for
human prefrontal functioning, including working memory and reinforcement learning. Evidence of impairment in other functions, such
as attentional orienting in space, does not seem as clear. This picture is
congruent with what would be expected if these animal PCB exposures
were to serve as a model of the development of ADHD-related cogni-

tive problems in humans. Indeed, her review of animal and human studies has led Rice (2000) to suggest parallels between effects of PCB exposure and ADHD. In all, then, the animal studies are quite suggestive or even compelling in the case of PCBs. Human studies clarify and amplify these issues, while adding further complexity.

Studies in Humans

We know that high-level PCB exposures can lead to behavioral problems and externalizing psychopathology (Lai et al., 2002). Aside from these relatively uncommon effects of high exposures, however, what about the far more common or even routine low-level exposures? At least three research programs have reported relevant data on offspring of women with exposure levels in the general population exposure range of 2–10 ppb.

First, a study at Wayne State University in Michigan that began in the 1980s looked at the offspring of a cohort of over 300 women, in which those who ate moderate to large amounts of Lake Michigan fish (a locus of substantial PCB contamination) were oversampled. The overall average PCB levels in this study were within the general population range, with blood serum levels at 5 ppb and umbilical cord levels at 2.5 ppb (Schwartz et al., 1983). The children were followed into the early teenage years. Initial evidence from this cohort suggested that affected functions in the developing children included intellectual development and attention (Jacobson & Jacobson, 1996), as well as visual discrimination and working memory (Jacobson, Jacobson, Padgett, Brumitt, & Billings, 1992), at ages 4 and 11 years. The latter study also provided evidence that prenatal exposures have the primary effect on early cognitive development. The Michigan study (Jacobson & Jacobson, 2002) replicated a prior report from the Netherlands (Patandin et al., 1999) that effects of PCBs on mental development at age 4 and verbal reasoning (from the Wechsler Intelligence Scale for Children—Revised Verbal IQ), auditory attention, and arithmetic ability at age 11 were moderated by whether or not children were breast-fed: Adverse effects on cognitive and behavioral development were largely carried by the group that was not breast-fed (or breast-fed for only a short time). Whether this effect was due to breast feeding per se, or whether breast feeding was a proxy for other protective factors (such as maternal IQ, SES, and so on) remains unclear. However, Jacobson and Jacobson (2002) examined ratings of the early home environment and of maternal verbal competency. They found that maternal verbal ability and in-home stimulation mediated the breast-feeding protective effect, suggesting that verbal or intellectual stimulation may have been the operative moderating mechanism that provided protection for these children.

Jacobson and Jacobson (2003) pursued these effects, including the moderator effect, in a more differentiated neuropsychological battery of measures at the age 11 follow-up. The battery, conceptualized roughly in line with the model outlined in Chapter 3 (although there are some differences between that model and theirs), included measures of selective attention (digit cancellation), vigilance (CPT), working memory and set shifting (WCST), and short-term and working memory (Sternberg task, digit span backward). In the sample as a whole, effects were seen on selective attention and output speed, which were attributed to poor response organization (since pure reaction time was not impaired on most tasks). However, effects were almost entirely carried by the non-breast-fed group, with weaknesses on commission errors on the CPT (see Chapter 4) and set shifting (indexed by perseverative errors on the WCST), as well as in arithmetic and in the aforementioned response organization (perhaps related to activation, as defined in Chapter 5). In all, effects on executive functioning were noteworthy. It was notable that sustained attention (vigilance) and visual–spatial functioning were spared in this sample. Furthermore, there was no association with examiner-rated activity level. The children with higher PCB exposures were rated by mothers as less hyperactive, and were less likely to be prescribed methylphenidate. Thus it appeared that PCB exposure might affect the executive functions that are also observed to be affected in ADHD, but that it did not lead to the hyperactive behaviors characterizing the ADHD syndrome.

Second, a North Carolina study that also began in the early 1980s followed a cohort of over 700 children from birth until the children were 5 years of age. Their mothers, the cohort of women recruited into the study, had no known excessive exposure to PCBs and had blood exposure levels estimated within the typical range (at that time) of about 5 ppb. Yet levels of background PCB exposure in breast milk (used here as in index of *in utero* exposure) were correlated with weakened motor reflex development neonatally and slower psychomotor development at ages 12, 18, and 24 months (Rogan et al., 1986; Gladen et al., 1988; Gladen & Rogan, 1991). A subsequent study in the Netherlands also found effects on cognitive and motor development at levels well below 5 ppb (Koopman-Esseboom et al., 1996).

These studies were extremely thorough in considering and ruling out via covariance a large number of potential confounds or alternative explanations of findings, including (but not limited to) SES, maternal age and education level, delivery complications, birthweight, alcohol use and smoking before and during the pregnancy, maternal blood lead concentrations, and qualities of the early home environment. Thus these findings were very well controlled and make clear that the effects observed cannot be explained other than as effects of PCB exposure.

Additional cohorts subsequently have been investigated in New York, Massachusetts, Germany, and elsewhere. No findings from those studies have overturned the basic pattern of findings showing that background-level PCB exposures have a negative effect on cognitive performance (for a review, see Schantz, Widholm, & Rice, 2003).

In the Oswego, New York cohort, recent work has looked more closely at response inhibition. Stewart et al. (2003) administered a CPT to this cohort of children at age 4 years ($n = 197$) and obtained structural MRI brain images at age 6 years for 60 children. PCB exposure was related to more commission errors on the CPT, with excess errors particularly in the latter portions of the task (consistent with activation problems). Size of the corpus callosum moderated this effect: Children with PCB exposure and smaller corpus callosum had the most commission errors. This effect again suggests that there are important moderators, perhaps related to early intellectual stimulation, of the impact of PCBs on response control. Once again, control of potential confounds was extensive, providing firmer support for the specificity of effects to PCBs.

More recent samples tend to have lower exposure levels, since PCBs were banned in industrialized countries many years ago. A newer sample from the Netherlands has an average exposure level between 2 and 5 ppb. In that sample, early exposure levels to PCB-class compounds predicted problems in executive functioning at age 9 years, again after controls for prenatal alcohol and cigarette use and for birthweight (Vreugdenhil, Mulder, Emmen, & Weisglad-Kuperus, 2004). As noted above, the Dutch study also revealed a moderator effect of breast feeding (perhaps a proxy for a range of protective effects in early socialization). Children who were formula-fed (which was correlated with lower family income and lower parental intellectual ability) showed dramatic negative effects of PCB exposure at age 42 months (a 6-point drop in Kaufman Ability Scale reasoning scores). In contrast, children who were breast-fed (which was correlated with a range of protective factors) showed minimal to no association between PCB level and cognitive consequences (Pastandin et al., 1999).

As the present review suggests, and as concluded in a comprehensive review by Schantz et al. (2003), the weight of epidemiological evidence shows effects on neuropsychological development in early childhood. Clearly, however, more has to be learned about what types of cognitive operations are affected in which children, and which toxins are to blame. For example, an important discovery has been that these low-level effects occur only in a subgroup of children who have preexisting liability to neuropsychological problems, in the form of either genetic or psychosocial risk factors. Furthermore, these effects may be specific to particular domains of cognitive or neuropsychological functioning. Although the nature of this specificity of effects remains to be clarified, the picture that has emerged thus far is of effects on response inhibition, executive functioning in general, and possibly reinforcement response and arithmetic ability. Other cognitive functions, such as spatial ability and nonverbal reasoning, appear to be spared (quite distinct from the picture for alcohol effects, for instance). Direct efforts to link these exposures to ADHD have been few; however, preliminary data suggest that PCBs at low levels do not lead to hyperactivity per se in children, but to problems in executive functioning that might fit the inattentive–disorganized as well as impulsive symptoms of ADHD.

Next Steps: Capitalizing on Knowledge about PCBs to Understand ADHD

In summary, growing evidence in human and animal studies suggests that low-level, background exposures to PCBs and related contaminants may disrupt development of two key sets of psychological mechanisms that are also disrupted in ADHD: higher-order executive functions such as working memory, and reinforcement responses. At the same time, some cognitive functions are not affected in either ADHD or PCB-exposure (e.g., attentional orienting). Not all studies are equally clear in their findings, however. Age of assessment may be a critical moderator of the degree of developmental effect observed. Moreover, in-home stimulation, breast feeding, or some other correlate of those measures appears to moderate and protect against low-level PCB effects on development. A major next step needed in this line of work is to look at ADHD symptoms and additional executive and cognitive measures in relation to background levels of exposure.

The other major next step, in relation to the argument in this book, is to begin to examine individual differences in vulnerability to low-grade background exposures. Thus, rather than only an exposure or dose-related "main effect" of PCBs, we are most interested in individual variation at similar exposure levels. Such effects would support a model in which children with vulnerable genotypes (perhaps including liability to ADHD) are more likely to exhibit poor functioning on measures of key cognitive and regulatory abilities at average background exposure levels. Most of the studies in this area have not asked this question, although initial findings related to moderation by brain structure (Stewart et al., 2003) and environmental stimulation (Jacobson & Jacobson, 2002; Walkawiak et al., 2001) are suggestive. Yet both of those moderators could be proxies for genotype. No study to date has looked at genotype in relation to response to PCB exposure—a logical and powerful aspect of this next step in research.

Therefore, it is plausible that varying background-level PCB exposures in early development could play a role in subtle cognitive dysfunctions found in catecholamine systems in children with ADHD who are genetically vulnerable to such effects, even as moderate to high heritability is reported in twins in the United States, Europe, and Australia. They qualify under our experiential criteria here as common or even ubiquitous effects that are probably shared among siblings, and so could contribute to risk for ADHD both via nonshared environment effects (in cases of relatively high-average exposure—e.g., 10–15 ppb in maternal tissue) and in conjunction with genotype–environment interactions. The demonstration of moderators of outcome heightens the interest in looking at such interactions. Such effects warrant investigation under a high-risk/high-payoff program of research investment. Such research can clarify causes and open up possibilities (which would probably have to occur at the policy level) for prevention of early developmental risk, with possible implications for ADHD.

CLINICAL IMPLICATIONS

The clinical implications of these major yet still somewhat speculative etiological possibilities are potentially vast. However, it is important for clinicians to recognize that none of the mechanisms discussed in this chapter have yet reached the phase of established clinical interventions (Rojas & Chan, 2005). Although such interventions as dietary supplementation may be considered in some instances, the medical risks of such interventions must be born in mind (see Arnold, 2002). For example, supplementation with dietary fatty acids could upset an already intact balance, so medical evaluation is critical. Consideration of this option may be more clearly warranted in children with eczema, thirst, allergies, or other atopic reactions—though still only with appropriate medical supervision. Some parents are interested in zinc supplements, which may be useful in cases of deficiency; again, however, misplaced supplementation could lead to excess zinc levels and medical complications, so medical monitoring is necessary. Though these interventions may be worth trying when appropriate indicators are in place, these treatments are not yet established as efficacious in ADHD.

Along the same lines, trial of an oligoantigenic (few-foods) diet may be considered, especially in children with atopic reactions (allergies, asthma). Such a trial has relatively few risks, although medical supervision is necessary to ensure adequate nutrition. Once more, parents should be advised that the treatment is not established, and the risks of delaying established treatments should be weighed. Clinicians may wish to monitor these literatures, because these types of interventions may become better established in the next few years, at least for defined subgroups of children.

The evidence that television viewing can lead to ADHD is too scanty at present to warrant any intervention recommendations on that front. If better-controlled replications begin to emerge, this evidence may become more noteworthy. On the other hand, there is clear justification in the research literature for advising parents that children's viewing of violent television programs and playing of violent video games should be supervised and sharply limited, especially if the children are at risk for developing aggressive behaviors (e.g., they exhibit strong oppositional tendencies at an early age). Furthermore—in light of the known rapidity of neural development in the first 24 months of life, as well as the lack of information about electronic media's effects during that period—parents can be reminded of the American Academy of Pediatrics guidelines, which advise against television viewing for children under the age of 2 years.

An important message in this chapter is that POPs (here described by the shorthand for the best-studied subclass, PCBs) may contribute to ADHD via prenatal, perinatal, and/or immediate postnatal exposures. With regard to clinical guidance concerning PCB exposures, controversy has ensued about breast feeding; professionals have made heated statements regarding the responsibility or irresponsibility of advising women either to be sure to breast-feed or to breast-feed cautiously. I do not enter into that controversy here, because so many complex health considerations are involved that have not even been touched on herein. However, it is notable that some studies found either breast feeding or its close correlates (e.g., stimulation in the home) to be protective against cognitive effects of low-level PCB exposure. At the same time, it remains somewhat unclear whether the primary damaging exposures to PCBs occur *in utero* or postnatally, but the strongest human findings so far suggest that effects on neuropsychological functioning are carried by prenatal exposure (Jacobson & Jacobson, 2002, 2003).

What *are* clear and noncontroversial, however, are public health guidelines on fish consumption. These advise pregnant and nursing women to limit intake of predator fish; lists of such fish are available from the EPA (see note 7 to Chapter 10). Even though effects of PCBs on ADHD are still uncertain, other health effects of these contaminants during dietary intake, along with risks of mercury exposure, render these guidelines prudent.

In sum, the clinical implications of this chapter include continued study and consideration of so-called "alternative" treatments for ADHD, as well as careful and appropriate psychoeducational, social work, and nursing counseling of parents before, during, and after pregnancy and during the early developmental years. For families seeking counseling about ADHD during school age, these alternative treatments can be discussed, especially if a child may belong to a relevant subgroup (e.g., the subgroup with marked allergy symptoms or atopy). However, as noted earlier, appropriate cautions should be borne in mind—including the potential risks of delaying well-established treatments for ADHD. Public health implications may be greater, and are considered in this book's concluding chapters. Common questions with which clinicians are faced, or that parents and educators may have, are listed in Table 11.1, along with the answers emanating from the literature reviewed in this chapter.

SUMMARY AND CONCLUSION

This chapter has highlighted three areas in which experiential effects could be fully consistent with high heritability of liability in ADHD. Each of these three putative risk domains—aspects of Western diet, tele-

TABLE 11.1. Frequently Asked Questions about ADHD and Common Experiential Risk Factors

Question	Answer
Does too much television cause ADHD?	There is insufficient evidence to say, but violent TV can worsen aggression in vulnerable youngsters.
Should I limit TV for my toddler?	Yes, especially if the child is under 2 years of age.
Does sugar cause ADHD?	No. But antibiotic–sugar interactions are still being investigated.
Will a healthier diet improve my child's ADHD?	Unknown.
Should I try an elimination diet for my child?	Only under medical supervision.
Should I add zinc supplements?	Possibly, but only under medical supervision.
Does pollution cause ADHD?	It might contribute. More definitive studies are now needed.

vision/other electronic media, and the environmental contaminants here labeled as PCBs—share the following characteristics:

1. They are essentially ubiquitous experiential effects on children in Western, industrialized societies and in nearly all societies in which ADHD has ever been studied. Thus they are likely to have shared effects (on both siblings in a family). This makes them candidates for hidden genotype–environment interactions in susceptible children, as described in Chapter 9.

2. They have plausible, if still speculative, mechanism linkages to neural and other developmental processes involved in ADHD—in particular, executive neuropsychological functions and catecholamine neurotransmitter systems.

3. Animal studies (in the case of key dietary factors and of PCBs) support a causal effect on either inattention or hyperactivity, and (in the case of PCBs) on several cognitive functions similar to those involved in ADHD—working memory, response inhibition, and reinforcement learning.

4. Pilot or initial correlational studies in humans provide support for possible links to ADHD and/or the neuropsychological mecha-

nisms I have posited as central in ADHD, even at routine exposure levels.

5. Many questions about their role continue to be asked in Western societies.

Each of these risk domains has another important characteristic. If a link to ADHD were established, that link would constitute a major breakthrough in public health understanding of children's ADHD in Western society. The ramifications for prevention and intervention would be direct and dramatic. Thus this chapter argues that these three candidate domains of experiential causal effects in ADHD, although they are at various stages of initial exploration, may justify more intensive high-risk/high-payoff study. The chances of finding a major breakthrough may be rated as uncertain, but the potential magnitude of payoff would be dramatic. The locus of such a breakthrough must be based, however, on a careful search for genotype–environment (gene × exposure) interactions.

Each of these risk domains also has important limitations as a potential explanation for ADHD. Most glaring is their nonspecificity. Each is associated with other effects on child development—sometimes, as in the case of dietary fatty acids, with an almost implausible array of alleged effects. Research to advance these as risk factors for ADHD must therefore carefully consider comorbidity and moderators of effect, as well as specific elements of the risk variable that may be causative. For instance, in the case of television, the effect of content on aggression is quite clear, so the effects on attention (if any) may occur by other mechanisms as yet undescribed.

One reason why PCBs stand out as promising is that effects have some degree of specificity to functions subserved by frontal–striatal neural networks (e.g., working memory, reinforcement learning), whereas other functions such as selective attention that are spared in ADHD are also apparently spared in PCB exposure. However, links to the hyperactive behavior seen in ADHD-C and ADHD-PHI are weak for PCBs. Instead, they appear most likely to affect inattention (in ADHD-PI) or inattention and disorganization (in ADHD-C). They therefore may act in concert with other causal streams if they contribute to ADHD.

In contrast to this intriguing specificity in neuropsychological effects of PCB exposure, dietary effects are likely to be more diffuse. Video games' and television's effects are far clearer on aggression (and perhaps on learning) than on attention or the other neuropsychological systems implicated in ADHD.

This chapter has highlighted these speculative risk factors because they have been so often underemphasized in the ADHD research literature. Each, however, now boasts a small initial literature. They should continue at the appropriate level of investment. At present, high-risk/high-payoff aggressive funding is warranted to pursue genotype–exposure interactions in relation to PCBs and related chemicals. Additional, though smaller, exploratory studies of omega-3 dietary deficiencies, dietary pesticide exposures, and electronic media exposures are warranted. Caffeine, sugar, and amino acid deficiencies are probably not promising directions for major research investment in ADHD.

PART IV

INTEGRATION

CHAPTER 12

Multiple Pathways
Reconsidered

OVERVIEW OF ADHD ETIOLOGY AND MECHANISM

To integrate the different domains discussed in this book, I suggest a conceptual integration that takes into account (1) what is known and what remains to be identified about the origins and prevention of ADHD; (2) what is known about within-child mechanisms (dysfunctions) that may be targets of clinical assessment and intervention; and (3) a model of multiple pathways to ADHD that may move us toward more formal, testable models of etiologies and causal heterogeneity. A substantial knowledge base is now available to guide the next generation of research and to help us move toward new discoveries. This knowledge base can also be used to suggest the most promising high-risk/high-payoff strategies for identifying preventable pathways to ADHD.

After the initial chapters laying out key issues and frameworks, Part II of this book (especially Chapters 4–7) has documented the breakdown of various neuropsychological mechanisms in ADHD. These are within-child dysfunctions observed at the group level. They are not present in all children with ADHD, and no one dysfunction can account for the entire spectrum of children so classified. At the same time, they characterize groups of children with the disorder, and thus they constitute our best-developed foundation for beginning to move toward diagnostic subtyping of children in relation to within-child dysfunction.

Part III of this book (especially Chapters 9–11) has noted that genetic influences play a substantial, but not an exclusive, role in the development of ADHD. The most important finding from behavioral genetic research is that shared environment effects (i.e., events that happen to all children in a family, such as experiencing the parents' divorce or having an alcoholic parent) are negligible in ADHD—a striking contrast to the state of affairs for aggression, which is influenced by shared environment. The examination of possible etiologies for ADHD has addressed two kinds of experiential influences: (1) those specific etiologies that could account for nonshared environment effects (relatively uncommon events that might happen to one child in a family, such as LBW or maternal smoking during pregnancy); and (2) those common experiential influences that could, via genotype–environment interactions, activate liability in the vulnerable child. Interactions of those shared environment effects with genotype would inflate the heritability term in twin studies.

Thus we can consider at least two initial pathways to ADHD:

1. A pathway of primary inheritance (extreme temperament), potentially mediated by genotype–environment correlations and maintained by socialization effects during development. There are probably several "subpaths" within this main pathway, however. For example, we might expect the following two routes (see Sonuga-Barke, 2005):

a. A pathway via weak "top-down" cortical control systems (effortful control), by way of extreme temperament. Such children would be expected to have prominent symptoms of inattention and disorganization, might also be impulsive, and might be expected to have executive functioning problems on neuropsychological assessment or to exhibit life problems consistent with poor executive functioning (e.g., poor temporal organization, poor maintenance of goals and objectives). They therefore might have either ADHD-C or ADHD-PI.

b. A pathway via "bottom-up" subcortical regulatory systems that are involved in reactive response (limbic reactivity), motor control (basal ganglia), and temporal information processing (cerebellum). These children would have prominent hyperactivity and impulsivity (they might have ADHD-C, in other words), and would be expected to have difficulty tolerating delayed rewards.

2. A pathway in which genetic liability is activated by experiential stressors on the developing neural system. The several candidate triggers reviewed in Chapters 10 and 11 are possibilities here, but these

need to be consolidated, because they doubtless covary. At the same time, allowance must be made for relatively uncommon versus very common exposures or risk factors. Therefore, we might expect the following "subpaths" within this general pathway:

    a. A pathway via uncommon triggers (either contributing to the nonshared environment effect, if they operate as nonshared environment terms either directly or via interaction with genotype, or contributing to the heritability term, if they tend to be familial or operate as shared environment). LBW—itself a marker of a dense clustering of risk factors that affect early health—is one final common pathway in this vein. It overlaps with prenatal cigarette exposure, low SES, and associated perinatal and prenatal difficulties. Some instances of prenatal alcohol exposure fall on this pathway; it may also include early lead exposure. These children would be expected to have hyperactivity (e.g., ADHD-C), along with reduced IQ (compared to their relatives), motor control problems, and possibly visual–spatial weakness. ADHD in this pathway may be viewed as falling at the mild end of a spectrum that includes mental retardation, cerebral palsy, and other neurological conditions at its more severely disordered end.

    b. A pathway via genotype–environment interactions involving common experiential events. These common events would be aspects of the shared environment (in fact, they would be experienced by virtually all children in the population), but the magnitude of their influence genotype–environment interactions is unknown. In twin studies, these effects would be hidden in the heritability term and would inflate heritability estimates (Purcell, 2002), as explained in Chapter 9. One intriguing hypothesis concerns exposure to specific toxins, particularly PCBs or other POPs, which may disrupt dopaminergic systems early in development and so may mimic the primarily genetic pathways described above. Children on this pathway would be expected to have significant executive functioning problems as well as reward response difficulties. These difficulties could result in ADHD-PI or, in combination with other risks, in ADHD-C with executive dysfunction.

    c. Speculatively, other pathways of this type could exist. One example is that widespread dietary inadequacies in the population may affect a subset of children (again, via genotype–environment interaction) who are vulnerable. This subgroup would be expected to have associated physical signs and symptoms (e.g., eczema, allergies, sleep problems, perhaps gastrointestinal problems).

These pathways may represent final endpoints of processes that can begin differently, illustrating the equifinality as well as the multifinality that probably occurs in ADHD. In Chapter 9, I have estimated the heritability of ADHD at 60–70% after adjusting for various biases and confounds. For purposes of this discussion, I use an estimate of 65% for heritability of liability to ADHD.

Also noted in Chapter 9 is that shared environment main effects (e.g., direct effects of experiences such as family discord, ineffective parenting, and other factors that influence all children in a family) are negligible in ADHD. Rather, these effects tend to aggravate aggressive and antisocial behaviors, but are not powerful causes of ADHD. When such familywide effects occur in relation to ADHD, they tend to be "driven" by a child's extreme impulsivity or activity level. They therefore are most simply viewed as reflecting the influence of heritable effects in ADHD development via geneotype–environment correlation. From this perspective, family process correlates of ADHD may contribute to maintaining the symptom profile over time (Campbell, 2002), but are rarely if ever the originating causes of the disorder.

Chapter 10 has discussed several of the best candidates for explaining the nonshared environment effect in ADHD (which I estimate as accounting for 25–35% of the variance in ADHD symptoms). These risks include LBW (really a marker of or final common pathway for a dense clustering of risk factors in disadvantaged families, as noted above). Prenatal cigarette and alcohol use are also noted as potential separate risks in their own right, along with lead exposure and potentially other, less well-documented heavy-metal exposures. All of these risks may tend to co-occur and concentrate in families undergoing extreme adversity. Yet enough studies have been able to disentangle some of these effects to indicate that some specific associations with ADHD appear to exist, though estimating their magnitude is difficult. These types of effects could function as nonshared environment effects if they specifically affect one child in a family (e.g., a mother drinks during one pregnancy, but not during the next). However, they could also afflict all children in a high-risk family and thus function as shared environment effects (e.g., all children in a house are exposed to dust that contains lead). The most important feature of these risk factors for our purposes is that they are relatively uncommon in the population, so that they affect only a minority of cases of ADHD—even if they operate via genotype–environment interactions. Of course, if these effects prove to be more common (e.g. effects of very low-level lead exposures between 1 and 10 ppb), then they may fall on a pathway that is more common and may play a larger role.

Figure 12.1 schematizes this state of affairs, indicating a large segment of heritable effects and a small portion of environmental effects that are known, as well as some unknown nonshared environment effects—perhaps including other toxin exposures (e.g., low-level lead effects, which are omitted from the figure in favor of the better-established high-level lead effects), child trauma, maternal stress during pregnancy, and other psychosocial risks that are to this point not well established but remain plausible hypotheses for affecting a subset of cases. The suggested percentage of attributable risk in Figure 12.1 for various causes are not established, but appear to be reasonable guesses based on the literature reviewed in Chapters 10 and 11. Note that effects of common risk agents (e.g., PCB exposure) are also excluded from the environmental effects in Figure 12.1. This is because such effects are shared environment effects—they affect all children in a family, or in some instances, nearly all children in a society. As main effects, such shared environment effects on ADHD are known to be small. If those effects are important, it is via their interaction with genotype. In that case, effects are hidden in the disorder's heritability.

Figure 12.1 therefore indicates that the heritable variation in ADHD liability is the largest single source of attributable risk for ADHD. Yet it reflects not one but at least three important processes. The first process may be called a genetic "main effect." It can be viewed for the moment as that state of affairs in which a child simply has an extreme temperament. In Chapter 8, I have proposed several possible temperament pathways to ADHD, including a highly reactive

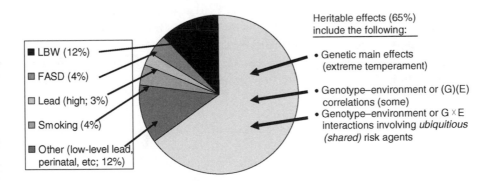

FIGURE 12.1. Schematic depiction of likely etiological influences on emergence of ADHD. LBW, low birthweight; lead (high), exposure to lead levels of 10 mcg/dl or higher; FASD, fetal alcohol spectrum disorders.

reward response ("approach") system, or a poorly developed effortful control ("constraint") system. Significant neurobiological markers can be applied to understanding such pathways.

Although driven by temperament, these pathways may be mediated, amplified, canalized, or otherwise influenced and expressed via socialization interactions during early development. In other words, a child with an extreme temperament is more difficult for parents, and so elicits different reactions from parents—a process that continues in a cascade of effects over time. If parents are unable to adapt their caregiving adequately to the child's unusual needs, then breakdowns in the socialization process may maintain and amplify the potential for the child to develop a disorder. Thus the figure represents a second element "hidden" in the heritable segment of the figure—namely, a subset of genotype–environment correlations of the sort just described.

A key question concerns whether the genotype for children with extreme temperament is distinct from the genotype for children who suffer environmental insults as main effects on their disorder. For example, Swanson et al. (2001a) have argued that the group suffering neurological insults is distinct genetically from the group with an extreme genotype. Jacobson and Jacobson (2003) have suggested a distinction between the neuropsychological profile of idiopathic ADHD and the profiles for children exposed to low-level lead, alcohol, and PCB contamination, respectively. Such ideas can contribute to subtyping based on etiological pathways.

Finally, the third element on the right-hand side of Figure 12.1 refers to genotype–environment interactions with common risk agents. These effects mimic heritable effects in twin studies, as explained in Chapter 9. These are environmental risks that are very common (affecting most children), but to which vulnerable children respond badly, perhaps leading to disorder. When the experiential risk factor is very common, then the main source of variation in relation to its effects is genetic variation between people in the population. I note in Chapter 9 that this was the case with TB in the United States early in the 20th century. Even though TB was known by then to be caused by a bacterium, its heritability was substantial; in other words, twin studies of TB detected heritability of *liability* to disorder. What was inherited was the vulnerability, predisposition, or susceptibility to the disorder.

An analogous process is possible in the case of ADHD—liability activated by particular environmental triggers. However, to fit existing knowledge, these triggers must be common in the population. Children may inherit a susceptibility to develop this disorder. Ubiquitous experiential events cause the disorder to emerge in some children, whereas other youngsters are invulnerable to it. The greatest potential payoff for high-risk/high-payoff research and public health investment in discovering *preventable* causes of ADHD lies here.

Table 12.1 summarizes these pathways again, offering readers a narrative view of this multipathway perspective. In Table 12.1 and Figure 12.1, I include my best guesses as to the percentages of cases of ADHD that might be attributable to particular etiologies. As should be apparent from Chapter 10, these figures have some empirical basis, but they remain too dependent on guesswork to be considered more than plausible hypotheses. Good epidemiological data about the population correlates of ADHD "caseness" and specific etiological subgroups simply do not yet exist.

With regard to Parts II and III of Table 12.1, we have no information about what percentage of ADHD cases may be related to interactions with ubiquitous risk agents. It is doubtful that the latter number is zero. If most of those effects are above a threshold of exposure, they would in fact be aspects of nonshared environment (and belong in Part I of Table 12.1 and on the left side of Figure 12.1). But it is more likely, based on the work reviewed in Chapter 11, that they are often in the genotype–environment interaction realm and belong in Part III of Table 12.1. It would be a major breakthrough to identify vulnerable

---

TABLE 12.1. Etiological Pathways to ADHD

I. Nonshared environment effects
   A. Lead exposure (main effect or G × E interaction) → arousal systems impaired → ADHD (3–5%)
   B. Low birthweight secondary to poor nutrition, cigarettes or other causes → multiple systems impaired → ADHD + motor and other difficulties (10–15%)
   C. Alcohol exposure without LBW → visual and motor systems also affected (4–5%)
   D. Severe trauma, multiple-trauma history in family, or maternal prenatal stress (unknown %)

II. Genetic main effects via temperament
   A. → (G)(E) correlations, effects on socialization
   B. → Different genetic type from the others?

III. G × E interaction effects involving ubiquitous risk agents
   A. PCBs → hormonal disruption → abnormal dopaminergic development
   B. Dietary deficiencies → vulnerable genotype → atopic reactions, sleep problems, ADHD

genotypes in relation to such a powerful experiential potentiator, and thus to know the percentage of cases attributable to such a mechanism.

These various etiological pathways presumably must exert their effect by passing through an internal mechanism in the child, which then can be measurable as "dysfunctional." Perhaps some percentage of cases in Figure 12.1 or Table 12.1 are attributable to marital/couple conflict, to exuberant temperament, or to other adaptational problems. If so, they should not be associated with neuropsychological deficit, neuroimaging difference, or long-term impairment when the child leaves the difficult situation.

Requiring explanation, however, is the vast array of neuropsychological findings associated with ADHD as detailed in Chapters 4–7. As detailed there, extensive cognitive weaknesses are reliably associated with ADHD at the group level. Where are these neuropsychological problems coming from? What causes these internal mechanisms to perform so poorly?

Needed, therefore, are empirical linkages of the neuropsychological pathways described in Chapters 4–7, the temperament pathways summarized in Chapter 8, and the etiological pathways described in Chapters 10–11 and here. The beginnings of such mappings are in place, but they remain crude, incomplete, and probably erroneous in many respects. Yet the clues are available: Dietary reactions should be associated with sleep disturbance, and possibly therefore with arousal or activation problems. Lead toxicity should be associated with spatial and motor problems, and possibly thus with hyperactivity and eventual antisocial behavior. Alcohol exposure should be associated with visual–spatial processing problems and problems in encoding and learning. PCB exposure should be linked with problems in executive functioning, including difficulties with working memory, response inhibition, and reinforcement response. LBW and teratogenic exposures should often co-occur with motor control problems. But virtually no studies have examined together (1) etiological agents or triggers, (2) neurocognitive functioning, and (3) behavioral clinical assessment of ADHD.

The preceding chapters also reveal that these associations are sufficiently nonspecific that we should be suspicious of whether we will actually find such 1:1 associations between etiology and neurocognitive performance. In fact, it is premature to attempt to make those 1:1 linkages or to evaluate their feasibility, because pieces of the descriptive research program on ADHD neurocognitive mechanisms are still missing.

The most important piece still missing is the individual-differences work on ADHD neuropsychology outlined in Chapter 8. Needed is careful descriptive work that puts multiple neuropsychological theories together in the same samples, to pursue the sorts of sample parsing illustrated in Chapter 8 (see also Nigg et al., 2005b). How many children with ADHD exceed a reasonable clinical threshold for failure on executive response inhibition *and* arousal *and* reinforcement learning? How many have a deficit in only one area? What is normative with regard to health on all of these measures? This type of question should form the center of upcoming neuropsychological research on ADHD. Once we understand this phenotypic structure—and doing so will require application of factor analysis, cluster analysis, and cutoff point analyses of the sorts that currently undergird the DSM-IV-TR clinical symptom cutoff points—we can move toward linking these "types" with etiologies.

For now, we are left with the uncertainty as to whether etiologies are specific to an etiological pathway (one neurocognitive domain), or whether they have nonspecific effects on combinations of these distributed neural systems. With this uncertainty before us, I outline key directions for the national research agenda into the etiology of ADHD.

RECOMMENDED HIGH-RISK/HIGH-PAYOFF RESEARCH INVESTMENT DIRECTIONS

We can use this framework to identify promising directions for high-risk/high-payoff etiological research. Potential areas of investigation can be evaluated for the degree to which they are ready for major public investment in an effort to make major new breakthroughs in understanding ADHD. Promising candidate *intrinsic* (within-child) mechanisms have been evaluated and described in Chapters 4–7; promising *extrinsic* causal etiologies have been evaluated in Chapters 10–11, in the context of the need to map multiple pathways as described in Chapter 8.

Fundamental Concerns

The studies recommended must, across the board, attend to fundamental concerns that should not warrant detailed review but that cannot be overlooked. First, they must consider clinical comorbidity carefully. As outlined in Chapter 8, comorbidity may all by itself provide a powerful clue to etiological pathways and to differences in neurocognitive mechanisms. Many etiological effects are nonspecific; some may be dosed. For example, LBW may at a severe "dose" lead to cerebral palsy, but at a milder "dose" may lead to ADHD. Lead exposure may also have dosed effects, with ADHD and learning problems at the mild end of a continuum.

Second, all studies must consider the definition of the ADHD phenotype. The ADHD subtypes in DSM-IV-TR may have different etiologies. ADHD-PHI may not be familial at all and may lack validity in school-age children (as opposed to preschoolers; Willcutt et al., 2001). Etiologies associated relatively more strongly with inattention than with hyperactivity (as may be the case in some studies of PCBs) also have to be considered. Likewise, the definition of HKD in ICD-10 may have a more homogenous etiological profile than the broader definition of ADHD in DSM-IV-TR (Swanson et al., 2004). Evaluation of these multiple phenotype definitions in the same samples is an obvious initial step in clarifying which phenotypes may belong with which etiologies.

Third, studies must grapple with the conundrum of IQ: Is it a correlative marker of the ADHD "insult," part of a causal pathway, or a spurious explanation for findings of normative variation? This is not to say that IQ should always simply be covaried; needed instead is thoughtful consideration of how it fits in. IQ is limited as an explanatory variable because it does not represent a discrete neural network or even a specific cognitive architecture. Rather, it is a multiply determined index of functioning that includes such nonspecific elements as speed of processing, cultural opportunity, and amount of intellectual stimulation. Perhaps impairments in working memory directly interfere with IQ (Kane & Engle, 2002). Alternatively, ADHD may result in reduced IQ (e.g., chronic poor attention leads to poor learning). A third possibility is that low IQ is an ancillary symptom of the same syndrome; in other words, the same insult that causes attention problems also impairs cognitive functions supporting IQ. This could be the case with LBW, lead exposure, and fetal alcohol spectrum disorders. In each of these scenarios, covarying IQ will obscure, not clarify, matters when researchers are examining an etiological agent's effect. However, IQ is well studied, has important clinical implications, and its extensive correlates are well defined in the literature. Ignoring its role entirely is simply not an option if we are to achieve a satisfactory, clinically meaningful understanding of ADHD.

Fourth, potential gender differences in etiology must be evaluated. Nearly all of the etiological mechanism reviewed in this book could have differential effects on boys versus girls. Hints of this differential effect are apparent for LBW, prenatal cigarette exposure, and other risks, with boys more vulnerable than girls. It has long been known that boys are more vulnerable than girls to a wide range of early pre- and perinatal insults. The protective or risk mechanisms contributing to those differential effects may prove to be important clues. For example, hormonal effects are important in early neural organization. They may be involved in protecting against some insults, or may be a route of effect for others (the latter is one possibility for the effects of PCBs).

Fifth, studies should consider assessment of possible psychosocial adversity (Counts et al., 2005). Many of the risk factors here are correlated with that adversity, whereas others are moderated, amplified, or buffered by psychosocial context, as illustrated in Chapter 11. Are these causal mechanisms mediators of adversity's influence?

Finally, studies of environmental risks must be integrated with molecular genetic designs. The linchpin of the line of thought advocated in this book concerns mapping genetic liability to risk potentiators in ADHD. I return to this final and crucial point at the conclusion of the chapter. Now, here are the directions I believe are most vital for research investment over the coming decade.

Intrinsic (Within-Child) Mechanisms

The field of neuropsychological examination of ADHD is now sufficiently mature that key areas are ready for more aggressive integrative work. Yet some basic groundwork is still needed in other areas.

1. *Neuropsychological measurement.* Measurement reliability and validity must continue to improve and be evaluated. As noted in the "Clinical Implications" sections of Chapters 4–7, reliability of measurement (or the lack thereof) remains a key limitation in applying new findings in the clinic. Relations among measures of these different domains require evaluation in normative and genetically informative samples, to determine whether the latent phenotypic and genotypic structures of the functional measures correspond to their hypothesized neural structures, whether they reflect one or more latent factors cutting across measures, and whether they are distinct from or overlap with latent measures of intelligence, g, or IQ (Kane & Engle, 2002).

2. *Neuropsychological integration.* Work on the relative weighting of different neuropsychological theories in predicting ADHD symptoms and ADHD caseness is needed. Such work would examine measures from different theoretical traditions (arousal vs. executive functioning

vs. motivation or reward response vs. temporal information processing) to see how they jointly relate to ADHD symptoms. Such work has not been done because it is so costly. The burden on children of completing extensive testing, and the large number of participants needed, prevent a short-term payoff. These samples must be accumulated gradually. Recent efforts by the field to assure that basic core batteries are administered across multiple sites may provide some help in this regard (Faraone, 2003). Furthermore, conclusions from such studies require caution with regard to the level of analysis of a measure. That is, molar trait or behavioral observation measures will correlate with one another more strongly than they will with molecular measures (e.g., reaction time), yet these correlations may fail to clarify relations among the constructs being measured.

3. *Neuropsychological heterogeneity.* Efforts that will lead toward accurate classification of children into phenotypes based on neuropsychological performance are needed. This work will also be slow and difficult, but it is essential. We need to know how many children with ADHD can reasonably have their symptoms attributed to problems with executive functioning, arousal, activation, or reward delay. The data presented in Chapter 8 (see also Nigg et al., 2005b) suggest that we may find something like the following: 30% of children with ADHD have deficits only in executive functioning (or a key component of it, such as response inhibition); 30% have a deficit only in reward responding; 20% have a deficit in both; and 20% have a deficit in neither. But this type of supposition needs far more empirical challenge and examination than it has so far received. Although a priori group designs may be helpful here, personological analytic techniques (designed to group types of individuals rather than to group variables) are available and so far have been little used on this problem. These include such methods as cluster analyses, Q-factor analyses, and other case assignment techniques. Also, inescapable is the need for longitudinal studies. Too little is known about how stable the ADHD DSM-IV-TR subtypes are over time (Lahey et al., 2005), much less about how stable a neuropsychological finding in a particular child with ADHD would be over time. Short-term longitudinal studies spanning weeks to months or a few years will be illuminating with regard to the eventual clinical usefulness of classifying children on neuropsychological grounds for clinical decision making. Overall, the effort to classify and subgroup the ADHD phenotype must begin to include putative cognitive or other within-child mechanisms, and not only behavioral endpoint descriptors.

Extrinsic Causal Mechanisms

Targets for Further Preliminary Exploration

Several specific etiological mechanisms are intriguing but insufficiently supported to justify a major research investment at this time. Instead, these mechanisms should be given a modest investment, which can allow investigators to try to obtain more supportive initial data with which to evaluate the worth of a larger public investment. In this category are the following, with mentions of which types of experimental or observational studies are most needed at present.

1. *Television and other electronic media.* Two kinds of preliminary studies are still needed to address the popular but poorly studied topic of electronic media's effects on ADHD. First, additional *experimental* studies that link television viewing or other media use causally with behavioral symptoms (overactivity, inattention) or cognitive functioning (poorly focused attention, low alertness) are needed. Second, *correlational* studies of television viewing/other media use and ADHD symptoms (as well as cognitive functioning) are needed that include adequate control for parental ADHD, or else include a genetically informative design. If both these types of initial studies yield positive results, more intensive investigation of this area may be warranted.

2. *Manganese in gasoline and soy-based infant formula.* More basic correlational data on the effects of manganese are needed, to evaluate whether there is an association with ADHD that is not due to ADHD's overlap with other disorders or to other spurious cause.

3. *Dietary additives and allergies.* Continued basic correlational and experimental studies are needed to determine whether the effects of dietary additives and allergies are replicable, and to begin to assess effect sizes. Animal studies may also be useful to evaluate causality. If this work continues to gain support in experimental and correlational designs, more large-scale testing may be warranted. The number of well-controlled studies to show an effect remains too small to allow strong conclusions as yet. This line of work is potentially important, however, due to both its potential to identify a clinically meaningful subtype and its obvious intervention implications.

4. *Dietary shortages of omega-3 fatty acids.* Many studies of omega-3 fatty acids to date have looked at learning disabilities or have used small or nonrepresentative samples, making it difficult to assess the applicability of the work to ADHD per se. Studies are needed that establish whether or not these dietary characteristics are related to

ADHD, apart from ADHD's overlap with learning disabilities. On the other hand, animal and human work on this topic to date has been promising. The physical symptoms that should accompany this effect would give promise for identifying a meaningful clinical subtype, and should also enable this hypothesis to be either clearly refuted or supported in a relatively short time. If such studies are positive, this line of work may soon be ready for more intensive investment.

5. *Mercury toxicity*. Correlations of low-level mercury exposures with ADHD symptoms apart from cognitive or motor problems warrant evaluation. Improved epidemiological data to evaluate how many children may be at risk due to mercury exposure are needed. Specificity to ADHD versus other types of neurodevelopmental problems needs to be further investigated in epidemiological studies. It is to be hoped that with mercury's established harmful effects on neural development, children's exposures will be sharply reduced by wise national policy, which should lessen the urgency of this set of questions in the future.

6. *Pre- and perinatal stress*. Little is known about how stress hormone activation *in utero* may influence later ADHD symptoms. Exploratory work is needed to evaluate this hypothesis in a preliminary form. This line of argument holds promise for linking ADHD symptoms to ecological stressors, such as family conflict, violence, and other contexts in the family.

Targets for Aggressive High-Risk/High-Payoff Strategies

A few lines of work on extrinsic mechanisms are sufficiently mature to warrant a large high-risk/high-payoff effort, to determine whether they may account for significant percentages of ADHD cases or variance and provide breakthrough opportunities for prevention.

1. *Low level lead exposures*. The long history of research on lead's effects leaves little doubt that lead can contribute to hyperactivity at high doses, and evidence that it can contribute to lowered IQ and poor attention, even in very low exposure ranges is now impossible to ignore. A correlation with ADHD symptoms at low exposure levels has been tested in only a small number of studies and needs to be confirmed. Needed are sufficiently large-scale studies to evaluate the likelihood of developing clinical ADHD at exposures in the of range 1–10 ppb. Also needed are individual-differences studies that could determine whether these associations may be nonlinear, and whether partic-

ular subgroups of children—perhaps those with particular genotypes—are susceptible to ADHD in the presence of these low-level lead exposures.

2. *Low-level POP exposures.* POPs (including PCBs) are difficult to study, because the critical prenatal exposure level can only be accurately assessed in prospective cohort designs beginning at birth or sooner; yet such samples typically will include only a small number of children with frank ADHD. Thus small but important effects or interactions may be missed due to insufficient power. The large number of potential compounds to study, and their potential variation in the population over time as some are banned and replaced by others, further complicate work in this area. The most relevant compounds in the environment may change from decade to decade as certain chemicals are phased out, banned, or replaced, and are gradually dispersed and reduced in the environment. However, studies using standard assays of the most common compounds have been successful. Animal work in this area is supportive of causal effects of early exposures on cognitive functions (e.g., working memory) that are subserved in humans by prefrontal–subcortical circuits. This cognitive profile is a reasonable model for the profile seen in ADHD. Although animal models of hyperactivity have also been related to PCB exposures, low-level exposures in humans have not been related to hyperactivity. However, they have been related to other behavior problems, and to inattention and impulsivity on neuropsychological tests (Jacobson & Jacobson, 2003). A key question here now concerns genotype–POP/PCB interactions. Do some children with low-level POP exposures develop either in ADHD-PI or ADHD-C? If so, what are their genotypes, and what are their neuropsychological profiles? Is lowered IQ a marker for this type of genetic risk, or is the ADHD pathway distinct from the low-IQ pathway?

3. *Overlap of LBW, lead, alcohol, nicotine, and other risk factors.* We know or suspect now that each of these individual factors increases the risk of ADHD at least slightly. We also are beginning to see the distinct neuropsychological signature of these events, which may enable meaningful etiological pathways to begin to be described when ADHD occurs. However, we do not yet know the magnitude of their individual and joint contribution to attributable risk. Measuring these effects in the population might enable investigators to reach a point at which they can say with some confidence that given percentages of cases are attributable to these causal triggers. Ultimately, this work would set the stage for clinical identification of those cases (e.g., ADHD, with motor delays, and an identified neurocognitive or neural marker of the causal

risk). Each subset of cases would then be approaching the point at which the behavioral disorder could be understood as an etiologically valid disease construct, with pathophysiology to be worked out in more detail related to those probabilistic causal triggers. This work would require specific neuropsychological, neuroimaging, and genetic studies of children exposed to these experiential risks. Ideal designs would feature (a) genetically informative samples (e.g. twins) and assessment of parental ADHD and antisocial personality disorder; (b) measures of specific environmental influences (e.g., LBW, prenatal alcohol exposure); and (c) molecular genetic data. Such designs could evaluate how much of shared environment is explained by these etiologies. They could then go on to evaluate genetic differences in children exposed to the causal factor (e.g., LBW) between those who do and do not develop ADHD. Finally, they would be in a position to evaluate whether genotype–environment interactions are occurring to an important degree. With a high-risk/high-payoff investment, it may be feasible to fully characterize a major set of etiological pathways to the condition.

Genotype–Environment Interplay

The real power in concerted study of common risk factors—such as low-level exposures to POPs or to lead—lies in identifying potential interactions with vulnerable genotype. Conversely, the greatest power in molecular genetic research lies in unmasking environmental effects operating on certain genotypes. The important role of such genotype–environment interplay is increasingly emphasized in conceptual models of antisocial behavior (Moffitt, 2005; Moffitt, Caspi, & Rutter, 2005) and developmental psychophathology generally (Rutter, 2005), but has not been much discussed as yet in ADHD. A key to this approach, as emphasized by Moffitt (2005), is identifying the relevant experiential triggers for the disorder or condition being investigated. This book's last few chapters have sought to do just that for ADHD. As those chapters have stressed, the important population effects observed in some instances are likely to include large effects in subgroups, and small or negligible effects in other groups. These effects may be moderated by other experiences, but also by genotype.

Genotype–environment interactions (one type of interplay, and themselves in some instances now referred to by the more versatile term of "interplay" rather than the statistical term "interactions") are of unknown magnitude in ADHD. In particular instances, their importance may be either negligible or extensive. The growing interest in considering these interactions, or interplay more generally, has emanated from recent breakthroughs using molecular approaches for other disorders. These molecular findings have overturned earlier suppositions that genotype–environment interactions are rare, as I have noted briefly in Chapter 9.

For example, Caspi et al. (2003) found that individuals with one or two copies of the short allele of the serotonin transporter gene (5HTTLPR) were more likely to develop depression in response to stressful events. Eley et al. (2004) replicated this result in adolescents, observing an interaction between 5HTTLPR and environmental risk for females (but not males) in predicting depression. In the first study to extend this type of finding to children, Kaufman et al. (2004) found a three-way interaction among 5HTTLPR, history of maltreatment, and availability of social support in predicting depression in children. Kendler et al. (2005) replicated Caspi et al.'s (2003) depression finding, and showed that the interaction was important for low-level (common) stressors. In relation to antisocial behavior, Caspi et al. (2002) found that individuals with particular alleles of a functional polymorphism in the gene encoding the neurotransmitter-metabolizing enzyme monoamine oxidase A (MAOA) developed antisocial behavior in response to maltreatment, whereas those without the risk allele on this gene did not.

Figure 12.2 illustrates in schematic terms the interaction Kaufman et al. (2004) observed among genotype, maltreatment, and support in predicting child depression The nature of such interactions has been that if children (or adults) have a "safe" genotype, they are relatively invulnerable to developing depression. However, if they have a "risk" genotype, they are vulnerable to the effects of experiential insult in triggering depression. To put this another way, for the vulnerable subgroup, the effects of the experiential trigger are much larger than for the population as a whole. A subgroup with a "risk" genotype and one experiential trigger will be even more vulnerable to a second such trigger. This is illustrated in Figure 12.2, where it can be seen that the simple effect of maltreatment on depression in the low-support group with two copies of the short allele was bigger than in the other groups.

Analogous work on genotype, environmental contaminants, and neuropsychological and behavioral outcomes in children is needed in relation to ADHD. Such work will be able to determine which children are most vulnerable to those insults that have effects at the population level. As has now been discovered with maltreatment, stress, and depression, and with early stimulation and LBW as well as early stimu-

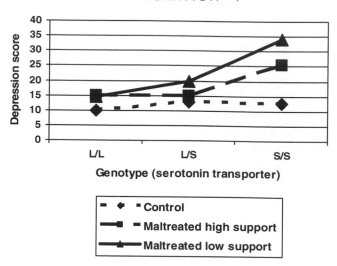

FIGURE 12.2. Interaction of genotype with two environmental factors (history of maltreatment and availability of social support) in predicting depression in children. Adapted from Kaufman et al. (2004). Copyright 2004 by the National Academy of Sciences. Adapted by permission.

lation and PCB exposure, effect magnitudes for environmental toxins and other early insults are likely to be much larger for vulnerable or susceptible individuals than for the population as a whole. Further identifying and characterizing such interactions and linking them with genotype would greatly advance our ability to describe pathways to ADHD.

Cultural Relativism and Causal Factors in ADHD: A Comment

A remark on social and international context is warranted, for the sake of both perspective and an integrated understanding. In the United States, Canada, Western Europe, Australia, and New Zealand, where most of the research on ADHD has been conducted, we have been fortunate that extreme population trauma (e.g., war on our soil) has been minimal in the past two generations, except for pockets of extreme violence or disadvantage. ADHD in these nations therefore can be meaningfully analyzed with regard to the individual differences and other subtle effects described in this book. In this context, where these population effects can be meaningfully analyzed, these efforts ideally will lead to prevention of a significant percentage of cases of ADHD and to better lives for many children. In other words, the research programs proposed here are designed to enhance the public health of nations and communities that have escaped the devastating social destruction of war, chronic terrorism, or armed conflict, with the resulting collapse of social structures. Families and children in too many parts of the world are exposed to such brutal deprivation or are in such poor physical health that psychopathological labels, not to mention studies of neuropsychological mechanisms, may seem grossly inadequate to describe their needs.

Research on the best means of helping children in those settings would require alternative models that have not been discussed here. In such settings, there may be value to understanding how traumas lead to neuropsychological and psychological changes that can be manifested as entrenched behavioral syndromes (e.g., aggression, ADHD) or as cognitive problems in learning, executive functioning, arousal regulation, and motivation. The goal of such efforts would be to improve clinical interventions for traumatized populations. Not insignificantly, when nations are recovering from chronic war or dislocation, their children may be exposed to very high levels of the risk factors discussed in this book. For example, in many nations, children are exposed to lead at far higher levels than in the United States (Fewtrell et al., 2004). As regions recovering from major dislocation gain or regain a public health infrastructure (e.g., Eastern Europe, Africa, parts of south Asia), reducing those exposures may dramatically improve children's mental and physical health and development.

Popular Theories Excluded from these Recommendations

Some readers may wonder why other sociological mechanisms have not been accorded more weight in these recommendations. For example, what about the busy pace of life, the high expectations, the two-parent working households, the inadequate schools, and other sociological forces that could be contributing to ADHD? Certainly one can find plenty of these kinds of suggestions in the popular books on ADHD today. Some of these concepts may touch on important ecological moderators of ADHD outcomes. For example, school systems with inadequate resources to teach children who have high activity levels may be powerful moderators of academic success for those children.

These types of sociological phenomena are not emphasized here for several reasons. First, the aim of this book is to evaluate our ability to validate ADHD as a disorder. The analysis presented in this book includes extensive evidence that such validation may be near at hand for major subgroups of children with ADHD. Potentially powerful explanatory mechanisms require immediate examination. We owe it to those children to understand the specific etiologies contributing to their problems, because that understanding will open up ever more effective prevention options.

Second, many of the factors omitted from consideration here (e.g., pace of life, no stay-at-home parent) would fall into the shared environment domain—which available evidence suggests is a negligible contributor to ADHD, unless such factors can be shown to exhibit powerful genotype–environment interactions.

Third, as we clarify specific etiologies, we should then be in a position to identify how many children with ADHD do not have a meaningful neurological dysfunction or genetic–experiential etiology. Some of those children might have high standing on a temperament trait that, in a sufficiently supportive context, would not warrant a disorder label. These adaptive cases of ADHD should then be the focus of studies concerning effects of school environment and the like on ADHD. Classification may ultimately exclude those children from the disorder designation. However, the range of neuropsychological problems described in Chapters 4–7 suggests that the percentage of children with ADHD in this adaptive group may be small.

Other readers may wonder why more emphasis has not been given in this book to the need for biological, neuroimaging, or molecular genetic advances, such as the work on haplotype mapping that I have highlighted as an important area of research in Chapter 9. Genetic progress is essential to the success of the programs I am suggesting here, because those programs will ultimately succeed when genotypes are paired with the experiential risk factors. However, because molecular genetic and neuroimaging work receives adequate emphasis in the field at present, this book has not belabored their advantages.

Cross-Cutting Issues: Nonspecificity and the Definition of the Phenotype in ADHD

I have noted at several points that the definition and boundaries of the ADHD phenotype require careful consideration in etiological research. In other words, what is the best way to define the disorder so as to capture etiological mechanisms? Should a narrow definition be used, such as in ICD-10, or a broad definition, such as in DSM-IV-TR? Should the DSM-IV-TR subtypes be studied together or treated as separate conditions? Alternatively, should subtypes be substantially reformulated on the basis of newer, latent-class analyses (Neuman et al., 1999, 2005; Rasmussen et al., 2004)? Although I bypass this latter question until more data are in hand, basic issues involved in phenotype definition warrant brief recapitulation here.

The first issue concerns nonspecificity. The overlap of etiological outcomes in ADHD and other conditions is important to recognize. All of the risk factors described here could lead to ADHD, or alternatively to learning disabilities, or in some instances to more severe conditions such as cerebral palsy or autism. This spectrum of effects is important to understand. Timing of the effect during neural development, dosage of the effect, or interaction with genotype could be the key moderator determining which outcome emanates from a given risk exposure. Research designs that integrate the study of ADHD with other outcomes have to be brought into dialogue with studies that focus on the etiology of ADHD to clarify this point.

The second issue concerns the relation of ADHD to overlapping (i.e., frequently co-occurring) psychiatric disorders, including mood disorders (depression and perhaps some instances of bipolar disorder, according to recent debates in the literature) and antisocial behaviors (aggressive behavior). I have noted in passing that the causal contributors to aggressive/antisocial behavior are somewhat distinct from those contributing to hyperactivity and/or attention problems. However, these conditions are still closely related. It appears likely that one major pathway entails an early etiological contribution to hyperactivity, with family and socialization moderating whether that early risk culminates in an antisocial/aggressive pathway or in a more benign hyperactive and/or inattentive pathway. It is in this respect that studies integrating family process and social context with etiologies of hyperactivity may have the biggest payoff.

These two issues (specificity and comorbidity) raise the question of whether the categorical DSM-IV-TR approach is most suitable for identifying etiological mechanisms in ADHD. As discussed in Chapter 2, empirically based models that focus on dimensional symptom clusters (Achenbach, Howell, Quay, & Conners, 1991) warrant more consideration here. Increasingly discussed in relation to potential changes in DSM-V is the possibility of a hierarchical conception of mental disorders (Krueger, 1999). This approach suggests that etiological agents should be examined both at the level of lower-order clusters or factors (e.g., ADHD subtypes, aggression or CD subtypes) and at the level of higher-order factors that may share common etiologies (e.g., externalizing behavior problems). Recognition that some causal agents may influence a higher-order shared factor, as opposed to a specific disorder, can resolve some of the confusion that otherwise results from failure to adequately consider either specificity or comorbidity in relation to these etiological effects, or from assuming a distinct categorical structure without shared elements across disorders.

The third issue concerns the ADHD phenotype itself, which, as just noted, can be defined relatively narrowly (ICD-10) or broadly (DSM-IV-TR). Evaluating the strength of the etiological "signal" with these subgroups is an ongoing challenge in redefining the phenotype. Few studies have examined multiple phenotypes at the same time. Subsequent steps should map the phenotypes that emerge in relation to specific etiological pathways. The "value" component of the disorder concept (Chapter 2 has indicated that a "value" component and a "fact" component are involved in some conceptions of disorder or disease) is unavoidable here. Scientists and clinicians always face the conundrum of making the disorder definition either too inclusive (and thus labeling too many "false positives"—labeling with a disorder children who really do not have a dysfunction that should justify a disorder label) or insufficiently inclusive (and thus failing to identify children who really are impaired and need health care services). A differentiated picture of ADHD based on within-child mechanisms and ultimately on etiological pathways (in addition to clinical behavioral descriptions) will ultimately help clarify matters. However, even that picture will never fully eliminate this inherent values decision, which must be made every day in clinical practice and in every era of taxonomic definition.

SUMMARY AND CONCLUSION

The ADHD field is poised at a moment of tremendous opportunity. Within-child neuropsychological correlates have now been described in detail, and these measurements continue to improve every year. Ready to be integrated with these advances are a vital array of etiological mechanisms that are increasingly well understood at a subtle level. Able to enrich this understanding further are unprecedented measurement tools that can assay genotype as well as neural structure and acti-

vation patterns. This rich array of descriptors, etiologies, and measures, if appropriately directed and utilized, has the potential to explain
the 30–35% of ADHD variance that is due to main effects of experience (probably in large part the effects of early neural injuries or
insults). A conclusive mapping of the majority of that variance would in
itself set the field on a course toward major breakthroughs. At least one
subgroup with a fully characterized etiology, pathophysiology, course,
and treatment, and perhaps more, might be identified. Even a single
such subgroup would require detailed genetic study to understand
individual differences in course, outcome, and intervention response.
However, targeted secondary and tertiary preventive interventions
could then be aimed at these at-risk youngsters.

Another etiological pathway is related to genetic effects, but via
genotype–environment interplay involving very common causal experiential risks. The role of such risks is often overlooked in the field today,
because of general lack of recognition that such effects are hidden in
the heritability term (which is large) and not in the environmental
terms (which are small) in twin studies of ADHD. Therefore, one major
goal of this book is to direct the attention of the field toward this overlooked opportunity to make potential breakthrough discoveries. I have
classified low-level lead and POP exposures (such as PCBs) as two areas
ripe for aggressive investment in high-risk/high-payoff research efforts.
The latter, in particular, appears poised to generate major discoveries—
even at the risk of coming up empty-handed. It is a risk well worth taking on the basis of the data available today.

All these areas of work, but especially work on low-level toxin
exposures, will only pay off in decisive breakthroughs if paired with
careful molecular genetic strategies. We already know that the main
effects of these agents in the population are real but modest. Perhaps
these main effects alone could explain some portion of ADHD cases.
But the real explanatory power will come when we identify which children carry liability genes that make them susceptible to more severe
responses to these toxic triggers. Those children may constitute only a
small portion of the population, once the molecular profiles are fully
understood; nevertheless, they may account for a sizable portion of the
ADHD cases in Western industrial society.

Genes, however, are not the only moderators to be tracked. Recall,
for example, that extra maternal warmth could blunt the harmful
effects of LBW in leading to ADHD (Tully et al., 2004), or that extra
stimulation of infants might prevent many of the outcomes associated

with low-level PCB exposure (Jacobson & Jacobson, 2002). Families besieged by multiple stressors and/or those with poor health care are likely to be the least able to sustain these protective actions for their at-risk youngsters. Society may be able to help with well-targeted supportive interventions if these at-risk cases can begin to be reliably identified and the magnitude of their risk reliably quantified. In the end, integrating genetic and experiential risks with genetic and experiential protections will be needed to provide a complete picture of ADHD causality suitable for major preventive interventions.

CHAPTER 13

Conclusion

IS ADHD VALID?: REPRISE

Impulsivity, hyperactivity, and behavioral attention problems are major concerns in our society because they are powerful correlates of a range of social ills that (taken collectively) cost society billions of dollars per year, as well as immeasurable lost potential and individual distress. As a result, they have been a major focus of both scientific research and clinical intervention for the better part of the past century. This cluster of behaviors and their study and treatment are now intersecting with sociological forces in which behavioral problems are medicalized, and the wisdom of such medicalization is being debated. Such debate is salutary. It obliges the field to evaluate how valid our conception of the syndrome of ADHD may be as a disease entity.

This book describes and evaluates substantial evidence relevant to both the neuropsychological correlates of the syndrome that may qualify as internal dysfunctions (one element of an etiologically valid disorder construct). It has also laid out a number of etiologies that might explain these neuropsychological findings and thus help us elucidate the causal sequences leading to the development of ADHD.

These pathways are unlikely to be unitary or simple. Self-regulation— the set of effortful and automatic abilities that collectively enable behavior to be adapted effectively to its context—is supported by series of neural circuits and their associated psychological capacities that are vulnerable to breakdown via any number of insults or developmental deviations. These abilities include a prefrontally mediated effortful control system, a subcortically mediated reactive control system, language abilities, and numerous reflexive adjustments in attention and motor control. Dopaminergic, noradrenergic, and other neural pathways support all of these ability systems. As clinicians and researchers, we often see overlapping problems in these systems and pathways. Moreover, the development of these abilities hinges on an "average expectable environment" that not only is free of neurotoxic interference in the unfolding of neural development, but provides adequate socialization support in the form of caregiver scaffolding, mirroring, and structure, so that self-control can be consolidated and organized during early development. An extreme temperament or an extremely disrupted ecology can provide alternate routes to the disruption of the synergy of process and development that becomes healthy self-regulation.

As a result of this general perspective and the data reviewed in this book, it should be concluded that at least two views of ADHD are unrealistically simplistic. First, the syndrome cannot be summarily dismissed as the product of an overly ambitious or misguided medical–industrial complex. Instead, it appears at least in a substantial number of cases to describe children who are victims of injury secondary to enormous social and personal miscalculations. In other words, children who have been exposed early in development to neural injury may consequently experience impaired self-regulation and a range of associated neuropsychological findings, emanating in ADHD as one part of the effect spectrum. All of these children may have executive, language, or motor impairments, and other findings of clinical importance, in addition to ADHD. Their history may include LBW, poor prenatal health, exposure to substances during fetal development, or undetected effects of lead or other toxin exposures.

Second, the syndrome cannot be satisfactorily understood as simply a genetic main effect. Too many experiential causal factors remain "at large" and insufficiently integrated into models of the disorder for us to rest easy with that explanation. For one thing, the nonshared environment effect—at about 30%—remains extremely important and may yet prove the most tractable domain for explaining the disorder's etiology in the near term (e.g., the next decade). For another, it remains far too possible that some significant portion of what appears as heritable variance reflects correlations between genetic liability and common (shared) experiential agents that potentiate the development of the disorder or weaken already vulnerable neural circuits as they are trying to develop.

Instead of these two simplistic views, what is needed is a differentiated picture of multiple specific etiological pathways that may characterize a valid disease entity in a susbstantial percentage (perhaps most) cases of the disorder as currently defined. Whereas it remains possible that we will find a subset of children with ADHD who simply do not have an internal dysfunction or deviation warranting the label of a disorder, that group will only be identified through a typological analysis of developmental pathways.

So how do we understand the validity of ADHD? Recall that this book opens with a distinction between clinical validity and etiological validity. The evidence on ADHD's clinical validity is sufficiently well established that I have not reviewed it in detail, but have only provided citations for interested readers. This means that the diagnostic criteria hold together statistically and do a relatively good job of identifying children who are impaired, at risk of poor outcomes, and likely to need assistance. Even so, those criteria will doubtless continue to be refined for that purpose as work on internal validity continues.

In contrast, I have noted that the etiological story, which would validate ADHD as a disorder in relation to a full explanation of causes and dysfunctions, is incomplete and is thus the focus of this volume. This incompleteness is the result of (1) poor sensitivity and specificity of group neurological findings in identifying individual cases, and (2) incomplete understanding of how neuropsychological dysfunctions are related to one another and to specific etiologies. Ultimately, what is needed is a specification of the particular etiological pathways that exist, what dysfunctions they cause that lead to impairment, and which children are validly assigned that designation. I have attempted in Chapters 4–7 to describe and organize the several classes of neuropsychological dysfunction that appear to be involved in ADHD at the *group* level. My major recommendation for the next step in this research—outlined in Chapter 8 and briefly summarized again in Chapter 12—is that it proceed to the difficult but important analysis of individual differences. Which children, and how many children, have a specific dysfunction? Continued confirmation of dysfunctions at the group level will now contribute relatively little of an incremental nature to this picture.

But this next step is only Step 1. Even if we identify a group of 30–40% of children with ADHD who have, say, a clear executive dysfunction, we still will not know whether this dysfunction is simply a correlate or is part of a causal pathway. To establish it as part of the cause, and then understand the causal cascade, we need to identify the extrinsic causal potentiators. This will not be as simple as identifying genotypes. In many instances, these genotypes are interacting with uncommon environmental triggers (nonshared environment) or with common risk agents that are attacking the entire population (and, in that case, contributing to apparent heritability). Specifying the individual children whose symptoms and impairment can be linked to specific potentiators and neuropsychological weaknesses, and describing how these children can be clinically identified, would largely complete the etiological picture and provide etiological validity.

Breakthroughs will come in the identification of etiological subgroups. For example, we have seen that a very small subgroup (under 1%) is explained by an abnormal thyroid gene that causes resistance to thyroid hormone and leads to ADHD. A larger subgroup (perhaps 12%) is probably explained by LBW—although LBW itself is a proxy for a range of risk and causal processes. Linking that to its own causes (poor prenatal care and nutrition, smoking), as well as to particular neuropsychological profiles in cases of ADHD (arousal, vigilance, motor problems), would bring us closer to completing the story for that subgroup.

However, the complete story would require integration with genotype, because only some children with LBW develop ADHD. Others have worse outcomes (e.g., cerebral palsy), and still others have better outcomes (few or no sequelae). It is also likely that genotype will further moderate these outcomes. Thus the complete mapping here is relatively straightforward in a conceptual sense, even though well-focused research will still take a decade or more to complete.

Remaining teratogenic influences are amenable to a similar research strategy. Once this strategy is carried out for the nonshared environment effects, it seems quite plausible that (1) at least one meaningful etiological subgroup will be validated (or perhaps more), and (2) new preventive and treatment interventions will become apparent. Under this scenario, in 10 or 15 years the field will be in a position in which 30% of ADHD cases have a known etiology and pathophysiology, and the remaining 70% remain idiopathic. The challenge then will be to explain the remainder. I have contended in this book that an unknown and possibly sizable portion of that remainder will be attributable to genotype–environment interplay involving ubiquitous risk agents; POPs (discusses here in relation to one well studied class: PCBs) constitute one speculative, but potentially high-payoff, candidate for such a risk agent.

DSM-V, DSM-VI, AND BEYOND

DSM-III (APA, 1980), DSM-III-R (APA, 1987), and DSM-IV/DSM-IV-TR (APA, 1994, 2000) all stayed at the behavioral or descriptive level in presenting diagnostic criteria for ADHD. In DSM-V, it would be useful for the appendices to allow for a research subtype of ADHD characterized by specific neuropsychological impairment (e.g., failure on normative executive function measures beyond the 95th percentile vs. national norms, accompanied by a full syndrome of ADHD behaviors). Validating such a subtype would require substantial work, but some formalization in DSM-V would enable this work to proceed in a more unified way across the entire public health research field. Of course, this subtype designation would be for research purposes only. It would remain premature to attempt to instantiate a neuropsychological ADHD subtype in clinical practice in DSM-V; rather, the need is to make systematic validation research possible. Eventually (perhaps in DSM-VI!), we may have a clinically validated subgroup, so that clinicians can formally diagnose "ADHD with executive functioning impairment" and make intervention recommendations accordingly. Treatment research as to whether such diagnosis moderates intervention outcome would of course be needed as part of that validation process.

It is ultimately to be hoped that mental disorders will begin to be classified in DSM-VI, or DSM-VII, according to etiological and developmental mechanisms along with behavioral phenotypes. These mappings and classifications may include neuropsychological features that are linked to neural circuits believed to have suffered suboptimal development leading to impairment. But they should go beyond that. "ADHD, with motor impairment, secondary to LBW and impairment of dopamine circuits" may be a possible diagnosis in some future decade. What will be of interest at that time is whether such a diagnosis will lead to more effective intervention than simply "ADHD." Even today, clinicians identify motor impairments, executive impairments, and so on, and make recommendations accordingly. But with a few exceptions (e.g., developmental coordination disorder), they lack agreed-upon and empirically validated criteria for doing so. The field will be in a better position to help children when such criteria exist and are anchored in known etiological pathways.

PREVENTION AND PUBLIC POLICY

Society has a huge stake in preventing ADHD and the worst outcomes that are associated with it. The worst outcomes are often associated with clinical comorbidity—language delays, cognitive delays, motor delays, and aggression. Many of those comorbid cases may be the direct results of the specific etiologies that have been emphasized herein. What would society stand to gain from preventing all sequelae of lead or mercury exposures? Of prenatal substance use? Of cigarette or alcohol toxicity? Of PCB exposures?

From the knowledge we already possess, we could predict that aggressive programs to provide adequate prenatal care to at-risk mothers or strong support to parents of at-risk infants might reduce the incidence not only of ADHD, but also of learning disabilities, other disorders, and eventual antisocial outcomes. These cost savings obviously could be great.

Aggressive further efforts to remove lead from children's environments will probably require the replacement of old housing stock (Needleman, 2004), which would be extremely expensive. But, as Needleman (2004) argues, it would probably pay for itself in public health and education savings, in that it would eliminate most of the remaining effects of early lead exposure. The effect on ADHD might be to reduce its incidence by 5–10%, but we would also see reductions in learning disabilities, mental retardation, antisocial outcomes, and other health costs.

This book has not examined the cost–benefit ratios of reducing such toxins as mercury. Yet, from the viewpoint of children's mental and physical health, reduction of mercury (which is well researched), manganese (which needs more investigation), and other toxic exposures should prove cost-effective in relation to health outcomes, even though it would entail high economic costs and changes in commercial activity (Koger et al., 2005). Doing so would require consideration of everything from alternative fuel sources (coal burning that emits mercury; manganese as a gasoline additive) to dietary changes (continued and more effective public health warnings about fish consumption; further evaluation of soy formula products fed to infants). Such considerations are obviously well outside the scope of this book. More evidence in relation to ADHD is needed to evaluate the likely impact of these types of efforts on the ADHD syndrome, but those public health investments are likely to pay off in myriad ways—not just in relation to ADHD.

The story of PCBs specifically, and POPs more generally, in child learning and health problems is now taking shape and appears likely to be significant. The production of many of these substances has already been banned, so an imagined prevention effort would require identifying children with risky genotypes and assessing their PCB or other POP exposures. Environmental interventions such as increasing in-home stimulation may enable prevention of cognitive decline and attention deficits in some cases, providing opportunity for secondary prevention. Implementing this vision would require coordinated planning and awaits further etiological research validation. In the meantime, continued efforts to monitor and publicize the effects of major dietary intakes (e.g., predator fish) can reduce both mercury and PCB/POP exposures.

In sum, whereas a major portion of the ADHD phenomenon is likely to be attributable to extreme temperament (largely heritable variation), it is likely that a significant secondary contribution to attention, learning, and other developmental problems in children has resulted from short-sighted and ill-considered injection into their environments of a vast range of chemicals with unknown effects over a long period of time. The price paid by society for lead and mercury exposures in children has already been unacceptable; it doubtless exceeds, certainly for the affected families, any imagined economic gain from the use of those metals. The price to be paid for the usage of PCBs and other contaminants may take decades to emerge. However, given that the loss of human potential resulting from such exposures may well be incalculable, it is unclear how one would meaningfully weight the "cost–benefit ratio" of injuring millions of children as we have, in effect, chosen to do in our society. In the past, such dangerous treatment of child development may have been excused by ignorance. But in the future, we should be able to draw lessons from this unfortunate legacy.

The core risk to children with regard to this entire toxicological line of risk factors, then, extends well beyond mental health care to the arena of public health policy. As illustrated by the example of lead and manganese, in which one toxic metal additive to gasoline (lead) was replaced by another (manganese) that may prove to be toxic also, simply eliminating proven toxins without considering the overall approach to use of such substances may prove fruitless. If we replace the old toxins with new ones, and then wait to discover the new toxicological effects, we can scarcely claim progress. Such an approach results in a waste of public health scientific time and resources, as well as of children's lives.

Bluntly put, potentially toxic substances should not be released into children's environments and developing nervous systems until they are proven safe. That "policy" would be a reversal of our past policy, which in effect has been to release potential toxins in large volume, hope that no harmful effects will occur, and then withdraw them after great harm has eventually been proved. This is an ineffective method of protecting children's health or of maximizing the health and well-being of society—and it is certainly a poor method of preventing unexpected mental health problems and costly developmental delays in children. In effect, our society's children have been subjects in a series of dangerous experiments, in which we find out what percentage of them will be injured or disabled by a given substance (Weiss, 2000). Yet responsible ethical guidelines—such as acknowledgment of who benefits and who may be harmed, voluntary participation, and the like—have not governed these experiments (see Koger et al., 2005). Any commitment to prevention of ADHD and associated conditions must be considered half-hearted unless it is accompanied by a commitment to such a "precautionary principle" in the release of new chemical compounds into children's environments.

This precautionary approach to protecting children's health has been undertaken in other nations. Sweden has implemented such a principle in relation to release of chemicals into children's environments; the Swedish focus is on suspected rather than proven harm as a criterion for restricting or regulating release (Koger et al., 2005). The Canadian Institute of Child Health has also recently issued a position statement advocating that a precautionary principle be implemented with regard to use of potentially toxic chemicals in Canada (this statement can be accessed at www.cich.ca).. In particular, the institute suggests that nonessential use of pesticides be banned when there is any possibility of exposure to children—for example, not applying pesticides or herbicides for purely cosmetic purposes to the grounds of a school. Similar positions warrant discussion in the United States and carry strong ethical weight.

On the other hand, the role of LBW in the development of ADHD is in one sense a "good outcome." With medical advances in neonatology, children who would have had severe mental retardation or cerebral palsy, or who would not have survived at all, are now able to lead relatively healthy lives. Nevertheless, many of them are impaired by ADHD. The goal for these children should be adequate intervention so as to reduce the chances of ADHD (e.g., early parenting guidance), as well as to reduce the chances of antisocial and other very negative outcomes for which they are at elevated risk.

FINAL SUMMATION

In the end, ADHD reflects multiple developmental pathways and causal processes, which we are now poised to map in specific rather than generic terms. It is not only an adaptation, although in some cases it may be. Often it is a result of disruption during development of sensitive neural systems needed for self-regulation. Various early risks during development affect a minority of these children via main effects of neural injury; those effects are often preventable, and policies should be altered based on present knowledge to enhance such prevention. A significant percentage of cases may represent extreme temperaments interacting with a society demanding tight conformity to indoor, desk-type work in childhood. Finally, an unknown percentage of cases may reflect the confluence or interaction of vulnerable constitution (genetic liability) and environmental risks (e.g., contaminants or teratogens). Studies identifying and mapping those interactions are our primary opportunities for discovering major new prevention avenues, and are the best places to invest public research dollars.

Some observers ask: How did ADHD evolve? Where were these children in the past? (See Jensen et al., 1997b, for a thoughtful discussion.) We can identify several possible answers at this point. Many of these children (e.g., those with LBW) did not survive in the past. Others, in the past, were in fact healthy because relevant triggering or amplifying causes (e.g., lead poisoning, alcohol use) had not yet been introduced into their prenatal or early postnatal environments. Still others (e.g., those with extreme temperaments) were able to adapt in a more agrarian economic structure that enabled them to avoid formal schooling and work in occupations that did not demand complex executive functioning or require confinement many hours per day in a static indoor environment. Finally, others were impaired in the past as well, though by different forms: They developed alcoholism, gambling addictions, or other disabilities that simply went untreated in prior eras. We do not know how many children with ADHD were at one time children with merely exuberant temperaments who adapted well in other contexts, but cannot do so in today's context. However, the significant neuropsychological problems often associated with the condition argue against this last group's being a large one.

Such evolutionary questions, however, assume that genetic main effects are the most important influences in ADHD. This may be so; however, I have argued here that the significant neuropsychological weaknesses seen in ADHD may well be related to a variety of early insults. The untapped potential to examine genotype–environment interactions involving common risk agents deserves more scrutiny in both conceptual and empirical work at this stage. The emerging excitement in the field about both genotype–environment interactions and correlations (Rutter & Silberg, 2002) is congruent with my recommendations, and entails an alternative conception of evolutionary effects. The most urgent public health questions facing the field of ADHD research involve examining these complex etiological pathways that involve joint effects of within-child and contextual factors in development. I recommend that research on those etiologies we are poised to understand be brought to fruition, and that a more specific map of etiological pathways be developed. Doing so will create a more satisfying context for pertinent future analysis about how a rapidly changing society may have altered children's capacity to adapt to its also rapidly changing demands.

Notes

CHAPTER 2

1. One could ask how much harm is enough to establish a diagnosis for a particular child, but that discussion (and the potential infinite regress it implies) is outside the scope of this book.
2. Note that the issue here is not whether the brain is involved in behavior; by definition, all behavior involves the brain. The issue is whether the primary explanation for the disorder is an abnormality of neural development.

CHAPTER 3

1. My presentation here follows closely several of the most widely accepted renderings of these hypothesized circuits (in particular, see Alexander, Crutcher, & DeLong, 1991; Alexander, DeLong, & Strick, 1986; Casey, Durston, & Fossella, 2001; Cummings, 1993; Kandell, Schwartz, & Jessell, 1991; Middleton & Strick, 2002). Most commentators accept a formulation of five parallel cortical–subcortical loops as presented by Alexander et al. (1986), but as many as seven such loops have been hypothesized (Middleton & Strick, 2002).
2. I omit the amygdala here for simplicity.
3. Dispute continues as to the degree of segregation of function within these loops. The approach of Alexander et al. (1986) was to conceptualize these loop functions as relatively segregated. That view has been questioned by subsequent proposals involving partially open loops that may cross-modulate more extensively (see Robins & Rogers, 1998). I therefore view these distinct functional properties as potentially heuristic, but not as confirmed properties. Two circuits are not depicted in Figure 3.2. The first runs from premotor and motor cortices to the putamen and on to the thalamus; it is a dopaminergic circuit involved in motor coordination and

response. An ocular–motor circuit is involved in control of eye movements and is potentially relevant to some ADHD findings described later.

CHAPTER 4

1. Note that other neural models of thes circuits are specifying them futher. For instance, a more refined formulation is to frame these abilities in relation to a dorsal and ventral attention network, as described by Corbetta and Shulman (2002). The dorsal network is a bilateral system involving intraparietal cortex and superior frontal cortex. It handles goal-directed attentional orienting and focusing. The ventral system is heavily right-lateralized, and involves the right temporoparietal junction and regions of right inferior frontal cortex, including the inferior frontal gyrus and middle frontal gyrus. It is involved in spontaneous attention capture. In this formulation, the ventral system probably also includes alerting functions described here as part of a vigilance network. Thus, further refinement of the neural networks at issue here will be important. For our purposes, however, the three-network model is most heuristic, because it enables us to cleanly distinguish (1) strategic attentional allocation (which involves frontal activity for maintaining task set, and dorsal parietal activity for attentional shift), (2) automatic attentional orienting (which involves aspects of both dorsal and ventral circuit), and (3) alerting (which involves aspects of the ventral circuit as well as additional subcortical structures as described in the text).
2. d is an effect size statistic; see Chapter 3 for an explanation.

CHAPTER 5

1. Although Pribram and McGuinness (1975) viewed this idea as similar to Gray's (1982) "approach" system, Gray emphasized motivation (cues for immediate or near-term reward) as the incentive context; I cover that perspective separately in Chapter 6.
2. Often these closely related processes are, for all practical purposes lumped together. However, one can conceptual distinguish late selection or filtering of information and then even later decisions according to task relevance of some information, involving higher-order cognitive control. Nonetheless, most of the interference control studies of ADHD have used tasks that simply require ignoring of distractors that cannot be perceptually filtered, and so must be effortfully filtered. These measures include the Stroop task, the Erikson flanker task, and appropriately designed selective attention tasks.
3. A potentially important distinction is that between competing (within-task) and noncompeting (extra-task) distractors. Most theorists (e.g., Barkley, 1997) predict an ADHD deficit only on the former. As reviewed by Barkley (1997), the few studies of extra-task distractors (e.g., more noise in the

room while a child does the task) suggest that they do not differentially affect performance of children with ADHD. Some studies suggest that increasing some types of extra-task stimulation may enhance the performance of children with ADHD (see Zentall & Zentall, 1983, for a classic early review). Recall the earlier discussion of interventions to help alertness.

4. A motivational theory of the task would predict that anxious children would stop significantly faster than typical controls—a prediction not upheld when tested (Oosterlaan et al., 1998). Children with both ADHD and anxiety were in between children with pure ADHD and control children in inhibitory efficiency in one study (Pliszka, Borcherding, Spratley, Leon, & Irick, 1997), but not in another (Manassis et al., 2000), raising the possibility that anxiety may partially buffer an ADHD deficit on this task. It will be important to determine whether children with ADHD + anxiety have ADHD symptoms as severe as those of children with ADHD but without anxiety. Overall, evidence for the executive nature of this task is good, but a secondary effect of anxiety on task performance needs clarification.

5. I have noted in Chapter 2 that specificity is an issue in most tasks used to evaluate ADHD deficits. The stop task is among the most studied in this regard. I (Nigg, 1999) found that stop inhibition also correlated with reading ability, and Oosterlaan et al. (1998) noted smaller but significant inhibition deficits in CD. Purvis and Tannock (2000) also reported associations of Stop task performance with reading disorder, although ADHD symptoms were not covaried in that analysis. Even so, an association with reading disorder is not usually observed on other inhibition tasks (Bayliss & Roodenrys, 2000). Although ADHD and reading disorder are readily dissociated on other tasks (Nigg et al., 1998; Pennington, Groisser, & Welsh, 1993), it will be important to determine whether some feature of the stop task is activating a noninhibitory problem in reading disorder, or whether the reading disorder finding is due to subthreshold ADHD symptoms. It will be equally important to determine whether the smaller deficits associated with CD can be explained by subthreshold ADHD symptoms.

CHAPTER 6

1. Newman and Wallace (1993) also suggested other routes to impulsivity, notably anxious impulsivity—which would be associated with high rather than low arousal. It is conceivable that some cases of ADHD with high anxiety could emerge from this pathway, with ADHD symptoms being due to impulsive behavior during anxious states rather than due to a primary deficit in executive or other inhibitory systems. For example, recall from Barry et al (2003a) that a few children with ADHD seem to exhibit cortical overarousal rather than the more typical underarousal.

2. Newman and Wallace (1993) also proposed that a controlled process, which they termed "self-regulation," can arise when the response modulation process requires it. This controlled process can occur in two ways: as part of

pursuing a deliberate goal (e.g., being "on guard"); or, more commonly, after being triggered by automatic orienting of attention to cues for novelty, threat, or some other unexpected stimulus. Plans and goals are then invoked in a deliberate review of behavior. Within the framework of this book, self-regulation involves effortful control or executive processes.

CHAPTER 9

1. For polygenic conditions, the distribution of the many possible genotypes for those many genes probably approximates a normal or gaussian distribution. Therefore, most biometric models assume an underlying continuum of liability (vulnerability or susceptibility) out of which categorical disorders emerge (Falconer, 1967; McGuffin, Owen, O'Donovan, Thapar, & Gottesman, 1994). The decomposition of variance in a twin study thus explains variance in liability to the disorder. That this is so is demonstrated by the effects of genotype–environment interplay in the example of tuberculosis given later in this chapter.

2. Strictly speaking, all human beings share in common more than 99% of their genes; these are invariant genes that make us human. Human variation is under the influence of the minority of genes that can vary between individuals. It is those variable genes that are referred to in the shorthand here. That is, of those, 50% are shared by siblings and by fraternal twins.

3. Some biometric models also separately estimate dominance or epistatic effects, providing "broad sense" heritability; in those instances, the "narrow-sense" heritability is the additive genetic effects alone. For more discussion, see McGuffin et al. (1994).

4. Each chromosome is divided into a short arm (p, for petit) and a long arm (q), and then divided into three regions and subdivided, resulting in the nomenclature used in this paragraph.

5. This is not to say that the heritability estimates are incorrect, but that they must be correctly interpreted as reflecting heritability of liability. Also, note that what are called "genotype–environment" effects in quantitative studies may in many instances really be "phenotype–environment" effects (that is, caregivers respond to the child's phenotype, not the child's genotype). This is an important complexity being discussed increasingly in the literature, but I bypass it here in the interests of simplicity.

6. Separate from this argument, but perhaps also relevant, is the reminder that heritability does not apeak to effects that move entire populations' risk level. Environmental main effects on an entire population (e.g., poor or improved nutrition, widespread lead exposure) would not be detected in a twin study, which is designed to detect variation within a population. The possibility that behavioral problems in children may be worsening over time, as noted in Chapter 1, illustrates this point, as do rapid increases in average height in the developed world in the past century. Height is heritable, but improved nutrition has caused the entire population to be taller.

CHAPTER 10

1. Epidemiologists use several statistics to capture risk—and, unfortunately, different terminologies are used by different authors, leading to some confusion in the field (see Tu, 2003; Mason, Scott, Chapman, & Tu, 2000). Therefore, it is important to be explicit about how the terms are used in this book. The formulas used here are the same as those suggested by Fletcher, Fletcher, and Wagner (1996). Here, the "odds ratio" is the ratio of the odds of disorder in an exposed group to the odds in an unexposed group. It is utilized in case–control studies in which one selects participants based on their affected–unaffected status and looks backward to see if they had the risk factor (Tu, 2003). The "relative risk" (also called the "risk ratio") is the ratio of disorder in the exposed versus unexposed group; that is, it is based on a prospective or cohort design in which participants are selected based on exposure to the risk factor, and then followed to see who develops the disorder. In some situations, the risk ratio and odds ratio can be different, and the odds ratio can then overestimate risk. However, when base rates are low (which is the case for ADHD), these two values are relatively equivalent (thus if 15% of exposed children have ADHD and 5% of unexposed children have ADHD, then the relative risk is 3.1 and the odds ratio is 3.0). I review both case–control and prospective or cohort designs in these next two chapters, but to keep the text from being tedious (and because the effect estimates remain rather crude), I use the terms interchangeably unless the estimates would be quite different from one another. Note that an odds ratio of 1.00 indicates there is no effect of the risk factor (unlike a correlation coefficient), whereas an odds ratio of 1.50 indicates a 1.5:1 ratio, or a 50% increase in risk in the exposed group.

   "Attributable risk" is the rate of disease in an exposed group minus the rate in an unexposed group (so if the exposed group has 15% ADHD and the unexposed population 5%, the attributable risk is 10%). It is related to relative risk as follows: Attributable risk = rate of disease in unexposed population × (relative risk − 1). "Population attributable risk" is attributable risk × prevalence of the risk factor in the population. "Population attributable fraction" (abbreviated in the rest of this note as PAF) reflects how much of the incidence of a disorder (here, ADHD) is due to a given risk factor and is computed as population attributable risk divided by total incidence of the disorder. It is based on the relative risk, but in some instances I have estimated the relative risk as the odds ratio when relative risk was not available. For more details on computing these statistics, see Fletcher et al. (1996), or Tu (2003).

   A necessary caveat is that PAF is based on incidence (new cases) of disorder—but incidence is essentially unknown for ADHD. As discussed in Chapter 1, I rely on several simplifying assumptions and an incidence rate of 6% (similar to the prevalence rate) herein. One could argue, however, for a lower incidence estimate (1% or even 0.5%). It therefore is important to note the effects of a higher or lower incidence estimate on the estimates of

PAF in relation to the environmental risks discussed in these chapters. In most cases, we are working from reasonable estimates of relative risk derived from studies that assessed ADHD in the same manner in the exposed and unexposed populations. When this type of risk ratio is available, then errors in the estimated incidence of ADHD will not appreciably affect estimates of the PAF. For example, this chapter provides a PAF for LBW of 12.8% when ADHD incidence is 6%. If ADHD incidence is estimated at 1%, the PAF for LBW changes only slightly (to 12.9%). This is because even though the attributable risk is distorted by errors in incidence estimates, in the case of PAF it is divided by that same incidence. Note that this reassuring point does not hold when we are working from raw percentages in an affected population (without good control groups). This is the case with fetal alcohol spectrum disorders as discussed later. Here, if we overestimate ADHD incidence, we will underestimate the risk factor's impact on ADHD in the PAF. All in all, then, using the high estimate of 6% ADHD incidence is unlikely to lead to any overestimates of risk factor effects in these chapters, but may lead to underestimates in some instances (notably fetal alcohol spectrum disorders).

As a final caveat, note that I use simplified versions of these statistics in my illustrative calculations in this chapter to illustrate (a) the relative risk (or odds ratio) in exposed groups, and then to estimate on that basis, often speculatively, (b) the possible percentage of ADHD cases attributable to a given risk factor. These simplified statistics do not consider interactions and are presented without confidence intervals; the reader is cautioned therefore to view these figures as illustrative. They are meant to serve as broad-gauge estimates, not precise claims, about the magnitude of these effects.

2. In developing countries, most prematurity has unknown origins; in contrast IUGR is related to malaria, low caloric intake relative to physical work of the mother, and a range of other causes. Measurement of IUGR is difficult in the absence of prenatal care, so data on its extent are often lacking.

3. The ADHD–smoking pathway does not appear to be attributable to medication treatment in childhood (Faraone & Wilens, 2003; Loney, Kramer, & Salisbury, 2002). Rather, nicotine's beneficial short-term effects on alertness and attention may result in a self-medicating mechanism that leads adolescents and adults with ADHD to smoke (Dinn, Aycicegi, & Harris, 2004; Downey, Pomerleau, & Pomerleau, 1996; Krause et al., 2002; Potter & Newhouse, 2004; Whalen, Jamner, Henker, Gehricke, & King 2003).

4. A confound would be genotype–environment correlations: Perhaps children who are hyperactive due to genotype tend to be more active and so ingest more lead, causing an artifactual association with behavior problems. The available evidence suggests that this effect is not likely. David, Hoffman, Sverd, and Clark (1977) found that lead levels were elevated in children with hyperactivity with no known organic cause, but were not elevated in children with a known organic etiology to their hyperactivity. Those results suggest that the lead poisoning preceded the hyperactivity in the first group.

5. See also information on a page of the EPA website (www.epa.gov/lead): "In 1978, there were nearly three to four million children with elevated blood lead levels in the United States. By 2002, that number had dropped to 310,000 . . . and it continues to decline."

6. Of equal concern is that blood lead levels above 10 mcg/dl also remain a major concern among some groups of children. For example, whereas the CDC estimated in 1997 that 4.4% of children in the U.S. had blood lead levels over 10 mcg/dl, as reviewed by Koller, Brown, Spurgeon, and Levey (2004) these rates were 24% in New Orleans; 27% in Wuxi City, China; 78% in Johannesberg, South Africa; and 87% in Dhaka, Bangladesh. See Fewtrell et al. (2004) for worldwide levels of exposure.

7. For more information about mercury, its dispersal, and its effects, see the EPA's web page on it (www.epa.gov/mercury). For EPA advisories about mercury levels in U.S. caught fish, see www.epa.gov/mercury/advisories.htm; women of childbearing age should avoid eating these fish as a precaution (Weiss, 1994). (See also www.epa.gov/waterscience/fishadvice/factsheet.html)

CHAPTER 11

1. However, several other hypotheses related to vitamin and mineral deficiencies are extant today. For example, of interest to some readers might be the potential role of dietary deficiencies in amino acids. Amino acids have potential relevance to ADHD, because they include precursors to the catecholamine neurotransmitters implicated in ADHD in neuropsychological and neuroimaging studies. However, treatment studies have not been encouraging (see Arnold, 2002), so I do not review these ancillary topics further. See Arnold (2002) for introductory comments on several less well-developed theories of dietary influence on ADHD.

2. Video game use is not as ubiquitous, but importantly, many children play video games instead of watching television, so that surveys of TV viewing may underestimate children's total exposure to electronic media. Only 25% of children in Wright et al.'s (2001) survey played video games on the days sampled, but some children were playing at ages 0–2 and overall use across all ages averaged 374 minutes (6.2 hours) per week for boys and 264 minutes (4.4 hours) per week for girls overall. Boys were more likely than girls to play with video games.

3. Television viewing may also influence children's health in ways that very indirectly affect alertness and attention. For example, more television viewing may be associated with obesity, lack of exercise, and other health effects that indirectly influence attention. However, such effects are not of primary interest to us here (even though poor physical fitness may be a complicating problem for many children with ADHD). We are interested, rather, in evidence for a relatively direct influence of television on neurocognitive development in vulnerable individuals.

References

Abel, E. L. (1995). An update on incidence of FAS: FAS is not an equal opportunity birth defect. *Neurotoxicology and Teratology, 17,* 437–443.

Achenbach, T. M. (1991). *Manual for the Young Adult Self Report and Young Adult Behavior Checklist.* Burlington: University of Vermont, Department of Psychiatry.

Achenbach, T. M. (1998). Diagnosis, assessment, taxonomy, and case formulations. In T. H. Ollendick & M. Hersen (Eds.), *Handbook of child psychopathology* (3rd ed., pp. 63–87). New York: Plenum Press.

Achenbach, T. M. (2000). Assessment of psychopathology. In A. J. Sameroff, M. Lewis, & S. M. Miller (Eds.), *Handbook of developmental psychopathology* (2nd ed., pp. 41–56). New York: Kluwer Academic/Plenum.

Achenbach, T. M., Dumenci, L., & Rescorla, L. A. (2002). Is American student behavior getting worse?: Teacher ratings over an 18-year period. *School Psychology Review, 31,* 428–442.

Achenbach, T. M., & Howell, C. T. (1993). Are American children's problems getting worse?: A 13-year comparison. *Journal of the American Academy of Child and Adolescent Psychiatry, 32,* 1145–1154.

Achenbach, T. M., Howell, C. T., Quay, H. C., & Conners, C. C. (1991). National survey of problems and competencies among four- to sixteen-year-olds: Parents' reports for normative and clinical samples. *Monographs of the Society for Research in Child Development, 56*(3, Serial No. 225), v–120.

Ahadi, S. A., & Rothbart, M. K. (1994). Temperament, development, and the Big Five. In C. F. Halverson, G. A. Kohnstamm, & R. P. Martin (Eds.), *The developing structure of temperament and personality from infancy to adulthood* (pp. 189–207). Hillsdale, NJ: Erlbaum.

Ahlbom, J., Fredriksson, A., & Eriksson, P. (1995). Exposure to an organophosphate (DFP) during a defined period in neonatal life induces permanent changes in brain muscarinic receptors and behaviour in adult mice. *Brain Research, 677,* 13–19.

Airaksinen, E. M., Michelsson, K., & Jokela, V. (2004). The occurrence of inattention, hyperactivity, impulsivity and coexisting symptoms in a population study of 471 6-8-year old children based on the FTF (Five to Fifteen) questionnaire. *European Child and Adolescent Psychiatry, 13*(Suppl. 3), 23–30.

Alexander, G. E., Crutcher, M. D., & DeLong, M. R. (1991). Basal ganglia thalamocortical circuits: Parallel substrates for motor, oculomotor, prefrontal and limbic functions. *Progress in Brain Research, 85,* 119–145.

Alexander, G. E., DeLong, M. R., & Strick, P. L. (1986). Parallel organization of functionally segregated circuits linking basal ganglia and cortex. *Annual Review of Neuroscience, 9,* 357–381.

Ali, N. J., Pitson, D., & Stradling, J. R. (1993). Snoring, sleep disturbance, and behavior in 4–5 year olds. *Archives of Disease in Childhood, 68,* 360–366.

Altmann, E. M. (2004a). Advance preparation in task switching: What work is being done? *Psychological Science, 15,* 616–622.

Altmann, E. M. (2004b). The preparation effect in task switching: Carryover of SOA. *Memory and Cognition, 32,* 153–163.

Aman, C. J., Roberts, R. J., & Pennington, B. F. (1998). A neuropsychological examination of the underlying deficit in ADHD: The frontal lobe versus right parietal lobe theories. *Developmental Psychology, 34,* 956–969.

Amen, D. (2001). *Healing ADD: The breakthrough program that allows you to see and heal the six types of ADD.* New York: Putnam.

American Academy of Child and Adolescent Psychiatry, Workgroup on Quality Issues. (1997). Practice parameters for the assessment and treatment of children, adolescents, and adults with attention-deficit/hyperactivity disorder. *Journal of the American Academy of Child and Adolescent Psychiatry, 36,* 85S–121S.

American Academy of Pediatrics. (2000). Clinical practice guidelines: Diagnosis and evaluation of the child with attention-deficit/hyperactivity disorder. *Pediatrics, 105,* 1158–1170.

American Psychiatric Association (APA). (1980) *Diagnostic and statistical manual of mental disorders* (3rd ed.). Washington, DC: Author.

American Psychiatric Association (APA). (1987) *Diagnostic and statistical manual of mental disorders* (3rd ed., rev.). Washington, DC: Author.

American Psychiatric Association (APA). (1994). *Diagnostic and statistical manual of mental disorders* (4th ed.). Washington, DC: Author.

American Psychiatric Association (APA). (2000). *Diagnostic and statistical manual of mental disorders* (4th ed., text rev.). Washington, DC: Author.

Anderson, C. A. (2004). An update on the effects of playing violent video games. *Journal of Adolescence, 27,* 113–122.

Anderson, C. A., Berkowitz, L., Donnerstein, E., Huesmann, L. R., Johnson, J. D., Linz, D., et al. (2003). The influence of media violence on youth. *Psychological Science in the Public Interest, 4*(3), 81–110.

Anderson, C. A., & Bushman, B. J. (2001). Effects of violent video games on aggressive behavior, aggressive cognition, aggressive affect, physiological arousal, and prosocial behavior: A meta-analytic review of the scientific literature. *Psychological Science, 12,* 353–359.

Anderson, D. R., & Evans, M. K. (2001). Perils and potential of media for toddlers. *Zero to Three, 22*(2), 10–16.

Anderson, D. R., Huston, A. C., Schmitt, K. L., Linebarger, D. L., & Wright, J. C. (2001). Early television viewing and adolescent behavior. *Mongraphs of the Society for Research in Child Development, 66*(1, Serial No. 264), 1–146.

Anderson, M. C. (2003). Rethinking interference theory: Executive control and the mechanisms of forgetting. *Journal of Memory and Language, 49,* 415–445.

Anderson, M. C., & Green, C. (2001). Suppressing unwanted memories by executive control. *Nature, 410,* 366–369.

Anderson, M. C., Ochsner, K. N., Kuhl, B., Cooper, J., Robertson, E., Gabrieli, S. W., et al. (2004). Neural systems underlying the suppression of unwanted memories. *Science, 303,* 232–235.

Andreou, C., Karapetsas, A., Agapitou, P., & Gourgoulianis, K. (2003). Verbal intelligence and sleep disorders in children with ADHD. *Perceptual and Motor Skills, 96,* 1283–1288.

Angell, M. (2004). *The truth about drug companies: How they deceive us and what to do about it.* New York: Random House.

Angold, A., Costello, E. J., & Erkanli, A. (1999). Comorbidity. *Journal of Child Psychology and Psychiatry, 40,* 57–87.

Arnett, P. A., & Newman, J. P. (2000). Gray(s three-arousal model: An empirical investigation. *Personality and Individual Differences, 28,* 1171–1189.

Arnold, L. E. (2002). Treatment alternatives for attention deficit hyperactivity disorder. In P. S. Jensen & J. R. Cooper (Eds), *Attention deficit hyperactivity disorder: State of the science, best practices* (pp 13-1–13-29). Kingston, NJ: Civic Research Institute.

Arnold, L. G. (2001). Alternative treatments for adults with attention-deficit hyperactivity disorder (ADHD). *Annals of the New York Academy of Sciences, 931,* 310–341.

Arnsten, A. F. T. (2001). Dopaminergic and noradrenergic influences on cognitive functions mediated by prefrontal cortex. In M. V. Solanto, A. F. T. Arnsten, & F. X. Castellanos (Eds.), *Stimulant drugs and ADHD: Basic and clinical neuroscience* (pp. 185–208). New York: Oxford University Press.

Aron, A. R., Fletcher, P. C., Bullmore, E. T., Sahakian, B. J., & Robbins, T. W. (2003a). Stop signal inhibition disrupted by damage to right inferior frontal gyrus in humans. *Nature Neuroscience, 6,* 115–116.

Aron, A. R., Watkins, L., Sahakian, B. J., Monsell, S., Barker, R. A., & Robbins, T. W. (2003b). Task-set switching deficits in early-stage Huntington's disease: Implications for basal ganglia function. *Journal of Cognitive Neuroscience, 15,* 629–642.

Asherson, P., & the IMAGE Consortium. (2004). Attention-deficit hyperactivity disorder in the post-genomic era. *European Child and Adolescent Psychiatry, 13*(Suppl. 1), I50–I70.

Aylward, G. P. (2002). Cognitive and neuropsychological outcomes: More than IQ. *Mental Retardation and Developmental Disabilities Research Review, 8,* 234–240.

Baddeley, A. D. (2001). Is working memory still working? *American Psychologist, 56,* 851–864.

Baddeley, A. D., & Hitch, G. J. (1994). Developments in the concept of working memory. *Neuropsychology, 8,* 485–493.

Baddeley, A. D., & Logie, R. H. (1999). Working memory: The multiple component model. In A. Miyake & P. Shah (Eds.), *Models of working memory: Mechanisms of action maintenance and executive control* (pp. 28–61). New York: Cambridge University Press.

Baker, L., & Cantwell, D. P. (1992). Attention deficit disorder and speech/language problems. *Comprehensive Mental Health Care, 2*, 3–16.

Bakker, S. C., van der Meulen, E. M., Buitelaar, J. K., Sandkuijl, L. A., Pauls, D. L., Monsuur, A. J., et al. (2003). A whole-genome scan in 164 Dutch sib pairs with attention-deficit/hyperactivity disorder: Suggestive evidence for linkage on chromosomes 7p and 15q. *American Journal of Human Genetics, 72*, 1251–1260.

Ball, J. D., & Koloian, B. (1995). Sleep patterns among ADHD children. *Clinical Psychology Review, 15*, 681–691.

Banich, M. T. (1998). The missing link: The role of interhemispheric interaction in attentional processing. *Brain and Cognition, 36*, 128–157.

Banich, M. T., Passarotti, A. M., & Janes, D. (2000a). Interhemispheric interaction during childhood: I. Neurologically intact children. *Developmental Neuropsychology, 18*, 33–51.

Banich, M. T., Passarotti, A. M., White, D. A., Nortz, M. J., & Steiner, R. D. (2000b). Interhemispheric interaction during childhood: II. Children with early-treated phenylketonuria. *Developmental Neuropsychology, 18*, 53–71.

Bank, L., Marlowe, J. H., Reid, J. B., Patterson, G. R., & Weinrott, M. R. (1991). A comparative evaluation of parent-training interventions for families of chronic delinquents. *Journal of Abnormal Child Psychology, 19*, 15–33.

Barkley, R. A. (1997). Behavioral inhibition, sustained attention, and executive function: Constructing a unified theory of ADHD. *Psychological Bulletin, 121*, 65–94.

Barkley, R. A. (2006). *Attention-deficit hyperactivity disorder: A handbook for diagnosis and treatment* (3rd ed.). New York: Guilford Press.

Barkley, R. A., Cook, E. H., Jr., Diamond, A., Zametkin, A., Thapar, A., Teeter, A., et al. (2002). International consensus statement on ADHD. *Clinical Child and Family Psychology Review, 5*, 89–111.

Barkley, R. A., & Cunningham, C. (1979). The effects of methylphenidate on the mother–child interactions of hyperactive children. *Archives of General Psychiatry, 36*, 201–208.

Barkley, R. A., Edwards, G., Laneri, M., Fletcher, K., & Metevia, L. (2001a). Executive functioning, temporal discounting, and sense of time in adolescents with attention deficit hyperactivity disorder (ADHD) and oppositional defiant disorder (ODD). *Journal of Abnormal Child Psychology, 29*, 541–556.

Barkley, R. A., Grodzinsky, G., & DuPaul, G. J. (1992). Frontal lobe functions in attention deficit disorder with and without hyperactivity: A review and research report. *Journal of Abnormal Child Psychology, 20*, 163–188.

Barkley, R. A., Koplowitz, S., Anderson, T., & McMurray, M. B. (1997). Sense of time in children with ADHD: Effects of duration, distraction, and stimulant medication. *Journal of the International Neuropsychological Society, 3*, 359–369.

Barkley, R. A., Murphy, K. R., & Bush, T. (2001b). Time perception and repro duction in young adults with attention deficit hyperactivity disorder. *Neuropsychology, 15,* 351–360.

Barr, C. L., Xu, C., Kroft, J., Feng, Y., Wigg, K., Zai, G., et al. (2001). Haplotype study of three polymorphisms at the dopamine transporter locus confirm linkage to attention-deficit/hyperactivity disorder. *Biological Psychiatry, 49,* 333–339.

Barry, R. J., Clarke, A. R., & Johnstone, S. J. (2003a). A review of electrophysiology in attention-deficit/hyperactivity disorder: I. Qualitative and quantitative electroencephalography. *Clinical Neurophysiology, 114,* 171–183.

Barry, R. J., Clarke, A. R., & Johnstone, S. J. (2003b). A review of electrophysiology in attention-deficit/hyperactivity disorder: II. Event-related potentials. *Clinical Neurophysiology, 114,* 184–198.

Barsky, A. J., & Borus, J. F. (1995). Somaticization and medicalization in the era of managed care. *Journal of the American Medical Association, 274,* 1931–1934.

Baumgaertel, A., Wolraich, M. L., & Dietrich, M. (1995). Comparison of diagnostic criteria for attention deficit disorders in a German elementary school sample. *Journal of the American Academy of Child and Adolescent Psychiatry, 34,* 629–638.

Baxter, M. G., Bucci, D. J., Holland, P. C., & Gallagher, M. (1999). Impairments in conditioned stimulus processing and conditioned responding after combined selective removal of hippocampal and neocortical cholinergic input. *Behavioral Neuroscience, 113,* 486–495.

Bayliss, D. M., & Roodenrys, S. (2000). Executive processing and attention deficit hyperactivity disorder: An application of the supervisory attentional system. *Developmental Neuropsychology, 17,* 161–180.

Beauchaine, T. P. (2001). Vagal tone, development, and Gray's motivational theory: Toward an integrated model of autonomic nervous system functioning in psychopathology. *Development and Psychopathology, 13,* 183–214.

Bedard, A. C., Nichols, S., Barbosa, J. A., Schachar, R., Logan, G. D., & Tannock, R. (2002). The development of selective inhibitory control across the life span. *Developmental Neuropsychology, 21,* 93–111.

Bekaroglu, M., Aslan, Y., Gedik, Y., & Deger, O. (1996). Relationships between serum free fatty acids and zinc, and attention deficit hyperactivity disorder: A research note. *Journal of Child Psychology and Psychiatry, 37,* 225–227.

Bellinger, D., Hu, H., Titlebaum, L., & Needleman, H. L. (1994). Attentional correlates of dentin and bone lead levels in adolescents. *Archives of Environmental Health, 49,* 98–105.

Bellinger, D., & Needleman, H. L. (1994). The neurotoxicity of prenatal exposure to lead: Kinetics, mechanisms, and expressions. In H. L. Needleman & D. Bellinger (Eds.), *Prenatal exposure to toxicants* (pp. 89–111). Baltimore: Johns Hopkins University Press.

Benes, F. M. (2001). The development of prefrontal cortex: The maturation of neurotransmitter systems and their interactions. In C. A. Nelson & M. Luciana (Eds.), *Handbook of developmental cognitive neuroscience* (pp. 79–92). Cambridge, MA: MIT Press.

Ben-Pazi, H., Gross-Tsur, V., Bergman, H., & Shalev, R. S. (2003). Abnormal rhythmic motor response in children with attention-deficit-hyperactivity disorder. *Developmental Medicine and Child Neurology, 45,* 743–745.

Berger, A., & Posner, M. I. (2000). Pathologies of brain attentional networks. *Neuroscience and Biobehavioral Reviews, 24,* 3–5.

Berger, A., Sadeh, M., Tzur, G., Shuper, A., Kornreich, L., Inbar, D., et al. (2005). Task switching after cerebellar damage. *Neuropsychology, 19,* 362–370.

Berk, L. E. (1986). Relationship of elementary school children's private speech to behavioral accompaniment to task, attention, and task performance. *Developmental Psychology, 22,* 671–680.

Berman, T., Douglas, V., & Barr, R. (1999). Effects of methylphenidate on complex cognitive processing in attention-deficit hyperactivity disorder. *Journal of Abnormal Psychology, 108,* 90–105.

Bernard, S. M. (2003). Should the Centers for Disease Control and Prevention's childhood lead poisoning intervention level be lowered? *American Journal of Public Health, 93,* 1253–1260.

Bernard, S. M., & McGeehin, M. A. (2003). Prevelence of blood lead levels > or = 5 micro g/dl among US children 1 to 5 years of age and socioeconomic and demographic factors associated with blood lead levels of 5 to 10 micro g/dl, Third National Health and Nutrition Examination Survey, 1988–1994.

Berridge, C. W., & Waterhouse, B. D. (2003). The locus coeruleus–noradrenergic system: Modulation of behavioral state and state-dependent cognitive processes. *Brain Research Reviews, 42,* 33–84.

Biederman, J., Faraone, S. V., & Monuteaux, M. C. (2002). Differential effect of environmental adversity by gender: Rutter's index of adversity in a group of boys and girls with and without ADHD. *American Journal of Psychiatry, 159,* 1556–1562.

Biederman, J., Faraone, S. V., Weber, W., Russell, R. L., Rater, M., & Park, K. S. (1997). Correspondence between DSM-III-R and DSM-IV attention-deficit/hyperactivity disorder. *Journal of the American Academy of Child and Adolescent Psychiatry, 36,* 1682–1687.

Biederman, J., Hirshfeld-Becker, D. R., Rosenbaum, J. F., Herot, C., Friedman, D., Snidman, N., et al. (2001). Further evidence of association between behavioral inhibition and social anxiety in children. *American Journal of Psychiatry, 158,* 1673–1679.

Biederman, J., Milberger, S., Faraone, S. V., Guite, J., & Warburton, R. (1994). Associations between childhood asthma and ADHD: Issues of psychiatric comorbidity and familiality. *Journal of the American Academy of Child and Adolescent Psychiatry, 33,* 842–848.

Biederman, J., Monuteaux, M., Doyle, A. E., Seidman, L. J., Wilens, T. E., Ferrero, F., et al. (2004). Impact of executive function deficits and ADHD on academic outcomes in children. *Journal of Consulting and Clinical Psychology, 72*(5), 757–766.

Birbaumer, N., Veit, R., Lotze, M., Erb, M., Hermann, C., Grodd, W., et al. (2005). Deficient fear conditioning in psychopathy: A functional magnetic resonance imaging study. *Archives of General Psychiatry, 62,* 799–805.

Bird, H. R. (2002). The diagnostic classification, epidemiology, and cross-cultural validity of ADHD. In P. S. Jensen, & J. R. Cooper (Eds.), *Attention deficit hyperactivity disorder: State of the science-best practices* (pp. 2-1–2-16). Kingston, NJ: Civic Research Institute.

Birnbaum, S. G., Podell, D. M., & Arnsten, A. F. (2000). Noradrenergic alpha-2 receptor agonists reverse working memory deficits induced by the anxiogenic drug, FG7142, in rats. *Pharmacology, Biochemistry and Behavior, 67,* 397–403.

Blair, R. J. R. (2001). Neurocognitive models of aggression, the antisocial personality disorders, and psychopathy. *Journal of Neurology, Neurosurgery, and Psychiatry, 71,* 727–731.

Block, J. H., & Block, J. (1980). The role of ego-control and ego-resiliency in the organization of behavior. In W. A. Collins (Ed.), *Minnesota Symposium on Child Psychology: Vol. 13. Development of cognition, affect, and social relations* (pp. 39–100). Hillsdale NJ: Erlbaum.

Bonefeld-Jorgensen, E. C., Andersen, H. R., Rasmussen, T. H., & Vinggaard, A. M. (2001). Effect of highly bioaccumulated polychlorinated biphenyl congeners on estrogen and androgen receptor activity. *Toxicology, 158,* 141–153.

Bor, W., & Sanders, M. R. (2004). Correlates of self-reported coercive parenting of preschool-aged children at high risk for the development of conduct problems. *Australian and New Zealand Journal of Psychiatry, 38,* 738–745.

Bor, W., Sanders, M. R., & Markie-Dadds, C. (2002). The effects of the Triple P-Positive Parenting Program on preschool children with co-occurring disruptive behavior and attentional/hyperactive difficulties. *Journal of Abnormal Child Psychology, 30,* 571–587.

Borger, N., & van der Meere, J. (2000). Motor control and state regulation in children with ADHD: A cardiac response study. *Biological Psychology, 51,* 247–267.

Boris, M., & Mandel, F. S. (1994). Foods and additives are common causes of the attention deficit hyperactive disorder in children. *Annals of Allergy, 72,* 462–468.

Botting, N., Powls, A., Cooke, R. W., & Marlow, N. (1997). Attention deficit hyperactivity disorders and other psychiatric outcomes in very low birthweight children at 12 years. *Journal of Child Psychology and Psychiatry, 38,* 931–941.

Bouchard, T. J. (1994). Genes, environment, and personality. *Science, 264,* 1700–1701.

Boucugnani, L. L., & Jones, R. W. (1989). Behaviors analogous to frontal lobe dysfunction in children with attention deficit hyperactivity disorder. *Archives of Clinical Neuropsychology, 4,* 161–173.

Bradley, C. (1937). The behavior of children receiving Benzedrine. *American Journal of Psychiatry, 94,* 577–585.

Brandeis, D., van Leeuwen, T. H., Rubia, K., Vitacco, D., Steger, J., Pascual-Marqui, R. D., et al. (1998). Neuroelectric mapping reveals precursor of stop failures in children with attention deficits. *Behavioural Brain Research, 94,* 111–125.

Breakey, J. (1997). The role of diet and behavior in childhood. *Journal of Pediatrics and Child Health, 33*, 190–194.

Breslau, N., Brown, G. C., DelDotto, J. E., Kumar, S., Ezhuthachan, S., Andreski, P., et al. (1996). Psychiatric sequelae of low birth weight at 6 years of age. *Journal of Abnormal Child Psychology, 24*, 385–400.

Breslau, N., & Chilcoat, H. D. (2000). Psychiatric sequelae of low birthweight at 11 years of age. *Biological Psychiatry, 47*, 1005–1011.

Breslau, N., Klein, N., & Allen, L. (1988). Very low birthweight: Behavioral sequelae at nine years of age. *Journal of the American Academy of Child and Adolescent Psychiatry, 27*, 605–122.

Brockel, B. J., & Cory-Slechta, D. A. (1998). Lead, attention, and impulsive behavior: Changes in a fixed ratio waiting-for-reward paradigm. *Pharmacology, Biochemistry and Behavior, 60*, 545–552.

Broderick, P., & Benjamin, A.B. (2004). Caffeine and psychiatric symptoms: A review. *Journal of the Oklahoma State Medical Association, 97*, 5538–542.

Brook, J. S., Brook, D. W., & Whiteman, M. (2000). The influence of maternal smoking during pregnancy on toddlers' negativity. *Archives of Pediatrics and Adolescent Medicine, 154*, 381–385.

Brown, K. (2003). Psychopharmacology: The medication merry-go-round. *Science, 299*, 1646–1649.

Brown, L. N., & Vickers, J. N. (2004). Temporal judgements, hemispheric equivalence, and interhemispheric transfer in adolescents with attention deficit hyperactivity disorder. *Experimental Brain Research, 154*, 76–84.

Brown, T. E. (Ed.). (2000). *Attention-deficit disorders and comorbidities in children, adolescents, and adults.* Washington, DC: American Psychiatric Press.

Bruininks, R. H. (1978). *Bruininks–Oseretsky Test of Motor Proficiency: Examiner's Manual.* Circle Pines, MN: American Guidance Service.

Bruininks, R. H., & Bruininks, B. D. (2006). *Bruininks–Oseretsky Test of Motor Proficiency, Second Edition: Examiner's manual.* Circle Pines, MN: American Guidance Service.

Bu-Haroon, A., Eapen, V., & Bener, A. (1999). The prevalence of hyperactivity symptoms in the United Arab Emirates. *Nordic Journal of Psychiatry, 53*, 439–442.

Burden, M. J., Jacobson, S. W., Sokol, R. W., & Jacobson, J. L. (2005). Effects of prenatal alcohol exposure on attention and working memory at 7.5 years of age. *Alcoholism: Clinical and Experimental Research, 29*, 443–452.

Burke, J. D., Loeber, R., & Lahey, B. B. (2001). Which aspects of ADHD are associated with tobacco use in early adolescence? *Journal of Child Psychology and Psychiatry, 42*, 493–502.

Burt, S. A., Krueger, R. F., McGue, M., & Iacono, W. G. (2001). Sources of covariation among attention-deficit/hyperactivity disorder, oppositional defiant disorder, and conduct disorder: The importance of shared environment. *Journal of Abnormal Psychology, 110*, 516–525.

Burt, S. A., Krueger, R. F., McGue, M., & Iacono, W. G. (2003). Parent–child conflict and the comorbidity among childhood externalizing disorders. *Archives of General Psychiatry, 60*, 505–513.

Bush, G., Frazier, J. A., Rauch, S. L., Seidman, L. J., Whalen, P. J., Jenike, M. A., et al. (1999). Anterior cingulate cortex dysfunction in attention deficit/ hyperactivity disorder revealed by fMRI and the Counting Stroop. *Biological Psychiatry, 45*, 1542–1552.

Bushman, B. J., & Anderson, C. A. (2001). Media violence and the American public: Scientific facts versus media misinformation. *American Psychologist, 56*, 477–489.

Bushnell, P. J., & Rice, D. C. (1999). Behavioral assessments of learning and attention in rats exposed perinatally to 3,3',4,4',5–pentachlorobiphenyl (PCB 126). *Neurotoxicology and Teratology, 21*, 381–392.

Cabeza, R., & Nyberg, L. (1997). Imaging cognition: An empirical review of PET studies with normal subjects. *Journal of Cognitive Neuroscience, 9*, 1–26.

Cadoret, R. J., Yates, W. R., Troughton, E., Woodworth, G., & Stewart, M. A. (1995). Genetic–environmental interaction in the genesis of aggressivity and conduct disorders. *Archives of General Psychiatry, 52*, 916–924.

Calkins, S. D., & Fox, N. A. (2002). Self-regulatory processes in early personality development: A multilevel approach to the study of childhood social withdrawal and aggression. *Development and Psychopathology, 14*, 477–498.

Campbell, S. B. (2002). *Behavior problems in preschool children* (2nd ed.). New York: Guilford Press.

Canfield, R. L., Gendle, M. H., & Cory-Slechta, D. A. (2004). Impaired neuropsychological functioning in lead exposed children. *Developmental Neuropsychology, 26*, 513–540.

Canfield, R. L., Henderson, D. R., Cory-Slechta, D. A., Cox, C., Jusko, T. A., & Lanphear, B. P. (2003a). Intellectual impairment in children with blood lead concentrations below 10 microg per deciliter. *New England Journal of Medicine, 348*(16), 1517–1526.

Canfield, R. L., Kreher, D. A., Cornwell, C., & Henderson, C. R. (2003b). Low-level lead exposure, executive functioning, and learning in early childhood. *Neuropsychology, Development, and Cognition: Section C Child Neuropsychology, 9*, 35–53.

Cantwell, D. P. (1972). Psychiatric illness in the families of hyperactive children. *Archives of General Psychiatry, 27*, 414–417.

Capaldi, D. M., Pears, K. C., Patterson, G. R., & Owen, L. D. (2003). Continuity of parenting practices across generations in an at-risk sample: A prospective comparison of direct and mediated associations. *Journal of Abnormal Child Psychology, 31*, 127–142.

Carlson, C., & Mann, M. (2002). Sluggish cognitive tempo predicts a different pattern of impairment in the attention deficit hyperactivity disorder, predominantly inattentive type. *Journal of Clinical Child and Adolescent Psychology, 31*, 123–129.

Carlson, E. A., Jacobvitz, D., & Sroufe, L. A. (1995). A developmental investigation of inattentiveness and hyperactivity. *Child Development, 66*, 37–54.

Caron, C., & Rutter, M. (1991). Comorbidity in child psychopathology: Concepts, issues and research strategies. *Journal of Child Psychology and Psychiatry, 32*, 1063–1080.

Carr, L., Nigg, J. T., & Henderson, J. (2005). *Motor and cognitive inhibition in adults with ADHD*. Manuscript submitted for publication.

Carson, R. C. (1991). Dilemmas in the pathway of the DSM-IV. *Journal of Abnormal Psychology, 100,* 302–307.

Carte, E. C., Nigg, J. T., & Hinshaw, S. P. (1996). Neuropsychological functioning, motor speed, and language processing in boys with and without ADHD. *Journal of Abnormal Child Psychology, 24,* 481–498.

Carter, C. S., Krener, P., Chaderjian, M., Northcutt, C., & Wolfe, V. (1995). Abnormal processing of irrelevant information in attention deficit hyperactivity disorder. *Psychiatry Research, 56,* 59–70.

Casey, B. J., Castellanos, F. X., Giedd, J. N., & Marsh, W. L. (1997a). Implication of right frontostriatal circuitry in response inhibition and attention-deficit/hyperactivity disorder. *Journal of the American Academy of Child and Adolescent Psychiatry, 36,* 374–383.

Casey, B. J., Durston, S., & Fossella, J. A. (2001). Evidence for a mechanistic model of cognitive control. *Clinical Neuroscience Research, 1,* 267–282.

Casey, B. J., Tottenham, N., & Fossella, J. (2002). Clinical, imaging, lesion, and genetic approaches toward a model of cognitive control. *Developmental Psychobiology, 40,* 237–254.

Casey, B. J., Trainor, R. J., Orendi, J. L., Schubert, A. B., Nystrom, LE., Giedd, J. N., et al. (1997b). A developmental functional MRI study of prefrontal activation during performance of a go–no-go task. *Journal of Cognitive Neuroscience, 9,* 835–847.

Caspi, A., McClay, J., Moffitt, T. E., Mill, J., Martin, J., Craig, I. W., et al. (2002). Role of genotype in the cycle of violence in maltreated children. *Science, 297,* 851–854.

Caspi, A., Sugden, K., Moffitt, T. E., Taylor, A., Craig, I. W., Harrington, H., et al. (2003). Influence of life stress on depression: Moderation by a polymorphism in the 5-HTT gene. *Science, 301,* 386–389.

Castellanos, F. X. (2001). Neuroimaging studies of ADHD. In M. V. Solanto, A. F. T. Arnsten, & F. X. Castellanos (Eds.), *Stimulant drugs and ADHD: Basic and clinical neuroscience* (pp. 243–258). Oxford: Oxford University Press.

Castellanos, F. X., Lee, P. P., Sharp, W., Jeffries, N. O., Greenstein, D. K., Clasen, L. S., et al. (2002). Developmental trajectories of brain volume abnormalities in children and adolescents with attention-deficit/hyperactivity disorder. *Journal of the American Medical Association, 288,* 1740–1748.

Castellanos, F. X., Marvasti, F. F., Ducharme, J. L., Walter, J. M., Israel, M. E., Krain, A., et al. (2000). Executive function oculomotor tasks in girls with ADHD. *Journal of the American Academy of Child and Adolescent Psychiatry, 39,* 644–650.

Castellanos, F. X., & Rapoport, J. L. (2002). Effects of caffeine on development and behavior in infancy and childhood: A review of the published literature. *Food and Chemical Toxicology, 40,* 1235–1242.

Castellanos, F. X., Sharp, W. S., Gottesman, R. F., Greenstein, D. K., Giedd, J. N., & Rapoport, J. L. (2003). Anatomic brain abnormalities in monozygotic twins discordant for attention deficit hyperactivity disorder. *American Journal of Psychiatry, 160,* 1693–1696.

Castellanos, F. X., & Tannock, R. (2002). Neuroscience of attention-deficit/hyperactivity disorder: The search for endophenotypes. *Nature Reviews Neuroscience, 3,* 617–628.

Centers for Disease Control and Prevention (CDC). (2004a). Alcohol consumption among women who are pregnant or who might become pregnant—United States, 2002. *Morbidity and Mortality Weekly Report, 53*(50), 1178–1181.

Centers for Disease Control and Prevention (CDC). (2004b). Blood lead levels in residents of homes with elevated lead in tap water—District of Columbia, 2004. *Morbidity and Mortality Weekly Report, 53*(12), 268–270.

Centers for Disease Control and Prevention (CDC). (2004c). Smoking during pregnancy—United States, 1990–2002. *Morbidity and Mortality Weekly Report, 53*(39), 911–912.

Centonze, D., Gubellini, P., Bernardi, G., & Calabresi, P. (2001). Impaired excitatory transmission in the striatum of rats chronically intoxicated with manganese. *Experimental Neurology, 172*, 469–476.

Cepeda, N. J., Cepeda, M. L., & Kramer, A. F. (2000). Task switching and attention deficit hyperactivity disorder. *Journal of Abnormal Child Psychology, 28*, 213–226.

Chabot, R. J., & Serfontein, G. (1996). Quantitative electroencephalographic profiles of children with attention deficit disorder. *Biological Psychiatry, 40*, 951–963.

Chambless, D. L., & Ollendick, T. H. (2001). Empirically supported psychological interventions: Controversies and evidence. *Annual Review of Psychology, 52*, 685–716.

Chambless, D. L., Sanderson, W. C., Shoham, V., Bennett Johnson, S., Pope, K. S., Crits-Cristoph, P., et al. (1996). An update on empirically validated therapies. *The Clinical Psychologist, 49*, 5–18.

Chan, E., Zhan, C., & Homer, C. J. (2002). Health care use and costs for children with attention-deficit/hyperactivity disorder. *Archives of Pediatric and Adolescent Medicine, 156*, 504–511.

Chan, J., Edman, J. C., & Koltai, P. J. (2004). Obstructive sleep apnea in children. *American Family Physician, 69*, 1147–1154.

Chen, Y. C. J., Guo, Y. L., Hsu, C. C., & Rogan, W. J. (1992). Cognitive development of yu-cheng ("oil disease") children prenatally exposed to heat-degraded PCB's. *Journal of the American Medical Association, 268*, 3213–3218.

Chhabildas, N., Pennington, B. F., & Willcutt, E. G. (2001). A comparison of the neuropsychological profiles of the DSM-IV subtypes of ADHD. *Journal of Abnormal Child Psychology, 29*, 529–540.

Chiba, A. A., Bucci, D. J., Holland, P. C., & Gallagher, M. (1995). Basal forebrain cholinergic lesions disrupt increments but not decrements in conditioned stimulus processing. *Journal of Neuroscience, 15*, 7315–7322.

Chiodo, L. M., Jacobson, S. W., & Jacobson, J. L. (2004). Neurodevelopmental effects of postnatal lead exposure at very low levels. *Neurotoxicology and Teratology, 26*, 359–364.

Chomitz, V. R., Cheung, L. W. Y., & Lieberman, E. (1995). The role of lifestyle in preventing low birth weight. *The Future of Children, 5*(1), 121–138.

Christakis, D. A., Zimmerman, F. J., DiGiuseppe, D. L., & McCarty, C. A. (2004), Early television exposure and subsequent attentional problems in children. *Pediatrics, 113*, 917–918.

Chudley, A. E., Conry, J., Cook, J. L., Loock, C., Rosales, T., & LeBlanc, N. (2005). Fetal alcohol spectrum disorder: Canadian guidelines for diagnosis. *Canadian Medical Association Journal, 172*(5, Suppl.), S1–S21. (Available online at www.cmaj.ca/content/vol172/5_suppl/index.shtml)

Cicchetti, D. (2002). The impact of social experience on neurobiological systems: Illustration from a constructivist view of child maltreatment. *Cognitive Development, 17,* 1407–1428.

Cicchetti, D., & Dawson, G. (2002). Editorial: Multiple levels of analysis. *Development and Psychopathology, 14,* 417–420.

Cicchetti, D., & Lynch, M. (1995). Failures in the expectable environment and their impact on individual development: The case of child maltreatment. In D. Cicchetti & D. J. Cohen (Eds.), *Developmental psychopathology: Vol. 2. Risk, disorder, and adaptation* (pp. 32–71). New York: Wiley.

Cicchetti, D., & Rogosch, F. A. (2001). Diverse patterns of neuroendocrine activity in maltreated children. *Development and Psychopathology, 13,* 677–693.

Clark, L. A., Watson, D., & Mineka, S. (1994). Temperament, personality, and the mood and anxiety disorders. *Journal of Abnormal Psychology, 103,* 103–116.

Clarke, A., Barry, R., McCarthy, R., & Selikowitz, M. (2001a). EEG-defined subtypes of children with attention-deficit/hyperactivity disorder. *Clinical Neurophysiology, 112,* 2098–2105.

Clarke, A., Barry, R., McCarthy, R., & Selikowitz, M. (2001b). Excess beta in children with attention-deficit/hyperactivity disorder: An atypical electrophysiological group. *Psychiatry Research, 103,* 205–218.

Clarren, S. K., Astley, S. J., Bowden, D. M., Lai, H, Brent-Milam, A. H., Rudeen, P. K., et al. (1990). Neuroanatomic and neurochemical abnormalities in nonhuman primate infants exposed to weekly doses of ethanol during gestation. *Alcoholism: Clinical and Experimental Research, 14,* 674–683.

Clements, S. D., & Peters, J. E. (1962). Minimal brain dysfunction in the school-age child: Diagnosis and treatment. *Archives of General Psychiatry, 6,* 185–197.

Cnattingius, S. (2004). The epidemiology of smoking during pregnancy: Smoking prevalence, maternal characteristics, and pregnancy outcomes. *Nicotine and Tobacco Research, 6*(Suppl. 2), S125–S140.

Cohen, J. (1988). *Statistical power analysis for the behavioral sciences* (2nd ed.). Hillsdale, NJ: Erlbaum.

Cohen-Zion, M., & Ancoli-Israel, S. (2004). Sleep in children with attention-deficit hyperactivity disorder (ADHD): A review of naturalistic and stimulant intervention studies. *Sleep Medicine Reviews, 8*(5), 379–402.

Coles, C. D., Platzman, K. A., Lynch, M. E., & Freides, D. (2002). Auditory and visual sustained attention in adolescents prenatally exposed to alcohol. *Alcoholism: Clinical and Experimental Research, 26,* 263–271.

Coles, C. D., Platzman, K. A., Raskind-Hood, C. L., Brown, R. T., Falek, A., & Smith, I. E. (1997). A comparison of children affected by prenatal alcohol exposure and attention deficit hyperactivity disorder. *Alcoholism: Clinical and Experimental Research, 21,* 150–161.

Collipp, P. J., Chen, S. Y., & Maitinsky, S. (1983). Manganese in infant formulas and learning disability. *Annals of Nutrition and Metabolism, 27,* 488–494.

Congressional Public Health Summit. (2000, July 26). Joint statement on the impact of entertainment violence on children. Retrieved from www.aap.org/advocacy/releases/jstmtevc.htm.

Conners, C. K. (1980). *Food additives and hyperactive children.* New York: Plenum Press.

Conners, C. K., Epstein, J. N., March, J. S., Angold, A., Wells, K. C., Klaric, J., et al. (2001). Multimodal treatment of ADHD in the MTA: An alternative outcome analysis. *Journal of the American Academy of Child and Adolescent Psychiatry, 40,* 159–167.

Conners, C. K., & Jeff, J. L. (1999). *ADHD in adults and children: The latest assessment and treatment strategies.* Kansas City, MO: Compact Clinicals.

Conrad, P. (1992). Medicalization and social control. *Annual Review of Sociology, 18,* 209–232.

Cook, E. H., Stein, M. A., Krasowski, M. D., Cox, N. J., Olkon, D. M., Kieffer, J. E., et al. (1995). Asssociation of attention deficit disorder and the dopamine transporter gene. *American Journal of Human Genetics, 56,* 993–998.

Cooper, J. R. (2002). Availability of stimulant medications: Nature and extent of abuse and associated harm. In P. S. Jensen & J. R. Cooper (Eds.), *Attention deficit hyperactivity disorder: State of the science, best practices* (pp. 21-1–21-18). Kingston, NJ: Civic Research Institute.

Corbetta, M., & Shulman, G. L. (2002). Control of goal-directed and stimulus-driven attention in the brain. *Nature Reviews Neuroscience, 3,* 201–215.

Corkum, P., Tannock, R., & Moldofsky, H. (1998). Sleep disturbances in children with attention-deficit/hyperactivity disorder. *Journal of the American Academy of Child and Adolescent Psychiatry, 37,* 637–646.

Cory-Slechta, D. A. (2003). Lead-induced impairments in complex cognitive function: Offerings from experimental studies. *Child Neuropsychology, 9,* 54–75.

Counts, C. A., Nigg, J. T., Stawicki, J. A., Rappley, M. D., & Von Eye, A. (2005). Family adversity in DSM-IV ADHD combined and inattentive subtypes and associated disruptive behavior problems. *Journal of the American Academy of Child and Adolescent Psychiatry, 44,* 690–698.

Cowan, N. (1988). Evolving conceptions of memory storage, selective attention, and their mutual constraints within the human information processing system. *Psychological Bulletin, 104,* 163–191.

Cowan, N. (1995). *Attention and memory: An integrated framework.* New York: Oxford University Press.

Cowan, N. (1999). An embedded-process model of working memory. In A. Miyake & P. Shah (Eds.), *Models of working memory: Mechanisms of action maintenance and executive control* (pp. 62–101). New York: Cambridge University Press.

Cox, E. R., Motheral, B. R., Henderson, R. R., & Mager, D. (2003). Geographic variation in the prevalence of stimulant medication use among children 5 to 14 years old: Results from a commercially insured US sample. *Pediatrics, 111,* 237–243.

Crabtree, V.L. Ivanenko, A., & Gozal, D. (2003). Clinical and parental assessment of sleep in children with attention-deficit/hyperactivity disorder referred to a pediatric sleep medicine center. *Clinical Pediatrics, 42,* 807–813.

Crawford, M. A. (1992). Essential fatty acids and neurodevelopmental disorder. In N. G. Bazan (Ed.), *Neurobiology of essential fatty acids* (pp. 307–314). New York: Plenum Press.

Crockenberg, S., & Leerkes, E. (2003). Infant negative emotionality, caregiving, and family relationships. In A. Booth & N. Crouter (Eds.), *Children's influence on family dynamics: The neglected side of family relationships* (pp. 57–78). Mahwah, NJ: Erlbaum.

Crosbie, J., & Schachar, R. (2001). Deficient inhibition as a marker for familial ADHD. *American Journal of Psychiatry, 158,* 1884–1890.

Cummings, J. L. (1993). Frontal–subcortical circuits and human behavior. *Archives of Neurology, 50,* 873–880.

Curl, C. L., Fenske, R. A., & Elgethun, K. (2003). Organophosphorus pesticide exposure of urban and suburban preschool children with organic and conventional diets. *Environmental Health Perspectives, 111,* 377–382.

Dalebout, S., Nelson, N., Hletko, P., & Frentheway, B. (1991). Selective auditory attention and children with attention-deficit hyperactivity disorder: Effects of repeated measurement with and without methylphenidate. *Language, Speech, and Hearing Services in Schools, 22,* 219–227.

Daly, G., Hawi, Z., Fitzgerald, M., & Gill, M. (1999). Mapping susceptibility loci in attention deficit hyperactivity disorder: Preferential transmission of parental alleles at DAT1, DBH and DRD5 to affected children. *Molecular Psychiatry, 4,* 192–196.

Daly, M. J., Rioux, J. D., Schaffner, S. F., Hudson, T. J., & Lander, E. S. (2001). High-resolution haplotype structure in the human genome. *Nature Genetics, 29,* 229–232.

Danforth, J. S., Barkley, R. A., & Stokes, T. F. (1991). Observations of parent–child interactions with hyperactive children: Research and clinical implications. *Clinical Psychology Review, 11,* 703–727.

Das, J. P., Snyder, T. J., & Mishra, R. K. (1992). Assessment of attention: Teachers(rating scales and measures of selective attention. *Journal of Psychoeducational Assessment. 10,* 37–46.

Daugherty, T. K., & Quay, H. C. (1991). Response perseveration and delayed responding in childhood behavior disorders. *Journal of Child Psychology and Psychiatry, 32,* 453–461.

Daugherty, T. K., Quay, H. C., & Ramos, L. (1993). Response perseveration, inhibitory control, and central dopaminergic activity in childhood behavior disorders. *Journal of Genetic Psychology, 154,* 177–188.

David, O. J., Hoffman, S. P., Sverd, J., & Clark, J. (1977). Lead and hyperactivity: lead levels among hyperactive children. *Journal of Abnormal Child Psychology, 5,* 405–416.

Davidson, E., & Prior, M. (1978). Laterality and selective attention in hyperactive children. *Journal of Abnormal Child Psychology, 6,* 475–481.

DeFries, J. C., Filipek, P. A., Fulker, D. F., Olson, R. K., Pennington, B. F.,

Smith, S. D., et al. (1997). Colorado Learning Disabilities Research Center. *Learning Disabilities, 8,* 7–19.

DeFries, J. C., & Fulker, D. W. (1988). Multiple regression analysis of twin data: Etiology of deviant scores versus individual differences. *Acta Genetica Medicae et Gemellologiae, 37,* 105–216.

Delion, S., Chalon, S., Herault, J., Guilloteau, D., Besnard, J. C., & Durand, G. (1995). Chronic dietary ?-linolenic acid deficiency alters dopaminergic and serotonergic neurotransmission in rats. *Journal of Nutrition, 124,* 2466–2476.

Delis, D. C., Kaplan, E., & Kramer, J. H. (2001). *Delis–Kaplan Executive Function Battery.* San Antonio, TX: Psychological Corporation.

Dempster, F. N. (1993). Resistance to interference: Developmental changes in a basic processing mechanism. In M. L. Howe & R. Pasnak (Eds.), *Emerging themes in cognitive development: Vol. 1. Foundations* (pp. 3–27). New York: Springer-Verlag.

Denckla, M. B. (1985). Revised Neurological Examination for Subtle Signs. *Psychopharmacology Bulletin, 21,* 773–779.

Denckla, M. B., & Rudell, R. G. (1978). Anomalies of motor development in hyperactive boys. *Annals of Neurology, 3,* 231–233.

Depue, R. A., & Collins, P. F. (1999). Neurobiology of the structure of personality: Dopamine, facilitation of incentive motivation, and extraversion. *Behavioral and Brain Sciences, 22,* 491–569.

Depue, R. A., & Lenzenweger, M. F. (2005). A neurobehavioral dimensional model of personality disturbance. In M. F. Lenzenweger & J. F. Clarkin (Eds.), *Major theories of personality disorder* (2nd ed., pp. 391–454). New York: Guilford Press.

Depue, R. A., & Spoont, M. R. (1986). Conceptualizing a serotonin trait. *Annals of the New York Academy of Sciences, 487,* 47–62.

Derryberry, D., & Rothbart, M. K. (1988). Arousal, affect, and attention as components of temperament. *Journal of Personality and Social Psychology, 55,* 958–966.

Derryberry, D., & Rothbart, M. K. (1997). Reactive and effortful processes in the organization of temperament. *Development and Psychopathology, 9,* 633–652.

Derryberry, D., & Tucker, D. M. (1994). Motivating the focus of attention. In P. Niedenthal & S. Kiayama (Eds.), *The heart's eye: Emotional influences on perception and attention* (pp. 167–196). San Diego, CA: Academic Press.

Diamond, A. (2000). Close interrelation of motor development and cognitive development and of the cerebellum and prefrontal cortex. *Child Development, 71,* 44–56.

Dietrich, K. N., Ware, J. H., Salganik, M., Radcliffe, J., Rogan, W. J., Rhoads, G. G., Fay, M. E., Davoli, C. T., Denckla, M. B., Bornschein, R. L., Schwarz, D., Dockery, D. W., Adubato, S., Jones, R. L.; Treatment of Lead-Exposed Children Clinical Trial Group. (2004). Effect of chelation therapy on the neuropsychological and behavioral development of lead-exposed children after school entry. *Pediatrics, 114,* 19–26.

Digman, J. M. (1990). Personality structure: Emergence of the five-factor model. *Annual Review of Psychology, 41,* 417–440.

Digman, J. M. (1994). Child personality and temperament: Does the five-factor model embrace both domains? In C. F. Halverson, G. A. Kohnstamm, & R. P. Martin (Eds.), *The developing structure of temperament and personality from infancy to adulthood* (pp. 323–338). Hillsdale, NJ: Erlbaum.

Dinn, W. M., Aycicegi, A., & Harris, C. L. (2004). Cigarette smoking in a student sample: Neurocognitive and clinical correlates. *Addiction and Behavior, 29,* 107–126.

Dougherty, D. M., Mathias, C. W., Marsh, D. M., & Jagar, A. A. (2005). Laboratory behavioral measures of impulsivity. *Behavior Research Methods, 37,* 82–90.

Douglas, V. I. (1972). Stop, look, and listen: The problem of sustained attention and impulse control in hyperactive and normal children. *Canadian Journal of Behavioural Science, 4,* 259–282.

Douglas, V. I. (1988). Cognitive deficits in children with attention deficit disorder with hyperactivity. In L. M. Bloomingdale & J. Sergeant (Eds.), *Attention deficit disorder: Criteria, cognition, intervention* (pp. 65–81). New York: Pergamon Press.

Douglas, V. I. (1999). Cognitive control processes in ADHD. In H. C. Quay & A. E. Hogan (Eds.), *Handbook of disruptive behavior disorders* (pp. 105–138). New York: Kluwer Academuc/Plenum.

Downey, K. K., Pomerleau, C. S., & Pomerleau, O. F. (1996). Personality differences related to smoking and adult attention deficit hyperactivity disorder. *Journal of Substance Abuse, 8,* 129–135.

Doyle, A. E., Biederman, J., Seidman, L. J., Weber, W., & Faraone, S. V. (2000). Diagnostic efficiency of neuropsychological test scores for discriminating boys with and without attention deficit-hyperactivity disorder. *Journal of Consulting and Clinical Psychology, 68,* 477–488.

Drummond, C. R., Ahmad, S. A., & Rourke, B. P. (2005). Rules for the classification of younger children with nonverbal learning disabilities and basic phonological processing disabilities. *Archives of Clinical Neuropsychology, 20,* 171–182.

Dubey, D. R., O'Leary, S. G., & Kaufman, K. F. (1983). Training parents of hyperactive children in child management: a comparative outcome study. *Journal of Abnormal Child Psychology, 11,* 229–245.

Durston, S., Tottenham, N. T., Thomas, K. M., Davidson, M. C., Eigsti, I. M., Yang, Y., et al. (2003). Differential patterns of striatal activation in young children with and without ADHD. *Biological Psychiatry, 53,* 871–878.

Dykman, R. A., Ackerman, P. T., & Oglesby, D. M. (1992). Heart rate reactivity in attention deficit disorder subgroups. *Integrative Physiological and Behavioral Science, 27,* 228–245.

Eaves, L. J., & Erkanli, A. (2003). Markov Monte Carlo approaches to analysis of genetic and environmental components of human developmental change and G × E interaction. *Behavior Genetics, 33,* 279–299.

Eaves, L. J., Silberg, J. L., Meyer, J. M., Maes, H. H., Simonof, E., Pickles, A., et al. (1997). Genetics and developmental psychopathology: 2. The main effects of genes and environment of behavioral problems in the Virginia Twin Study of Adolescent Behavioral Development. *Journal of Child Psychology and Psychiatry, 38,* 965980.

Eisenberg, N., Cumberland, A., Spinrad, T. L., Fabes, R. A., Shepard, S., Reiser, M., et al. (2001). The relations of regulation and emotionality to children's externalizing and internalizing problem behavior. *Child Development, 72,* 1112–1134.

Eisenberg, N., & Morris, A. S. (2002). Children's emotion-related regulation. In R. V. Kail (Ed.), *Advances in child development and behavior* (Vol. 30, pp. 189–229). San Diego, CA: Academic Press.

Eisenberg, N., Sadovsky, A., Spinrad, T., Fabes, R. A., Losoya, S., Valiente, C., et al. (2005). The relations of problem behavior status to children's negative emotionality, effortful control, and impulsivity: Concurrent relations and prediction of change. *Developmental Psychology, 41,* 193–211.

Eley, T. C., Sugden, K., Corsico, A., Gregory, A. M., Sham, P., McGuffin, et al. (2004). Gene–environment interaction analysis of serotonin system markers with adolescent depression. *Molecular Psychiatry, 9,* 908–915.

Elia, J., Gulotta, C., Rose, S. R., Marin, G., & Rapoport, J. L. (1994). Thyroid function and attention-deficit hyperactivity disorder. *Journal of the American Academy of Child and Adolescent Psychiatry, 33,* 169–172.

Eliasson, A. C., Rosblad, B., & Forssberg, H. (2004). Disturbances in programming goal-directed arm movements in children with ADHD. *Developmental Medicine and Child Neurology, 46,* 19–27.

Engle, R. W. (2002). Working memory capacity as executive attention. *Current Directions in Psychological Science, 11*(1), 19–23.

Engle, R. W., Kane, M. J., & Touholski, S. W. (1999). Individual differences in working memory capacity and what they tell us about controlled attention, general fluid intelligence, and functions of the prefrontal cortex. In A. Miyake & P. Shah (Eds.), *Models of working memory: Mechanisms of action maintenance and executive control* (pp. 102–134). New York: Cambridge University Press.

Eppright, T. D., Vogel, S. J., Horwitz, F., & Tevendale, H. D. (1997). Results of blood lead screening in children referred for behavioral disorders. *Molecular Medicine, 94,* 295–297.

Erikson, C. W., & Hoffman, J. E. (1972). Temporal and spatial characteristics of selective encoding from visual displays. *Perception and Psychophysics, 12,* 201–204.

Eriksson, P., Ankarberg, E., Viberg, H., & Fredriksson, A. (2001). The developing cholinergic system as target for environmental toxicants, nicotine and polychlorinated biphenyls (PCBs): Implications for neurotoxicological processes in mice. *Neurotoxicology Research, 3,* 37–51.

Eriksson, P., & Fredriksson, A. (1991). Neurotoxic effects of two different pyrethroids, bioallethrin and deltamethrin, on immature and adult mice: Changes in behavioral and muscarinic receptor variables. *Toxicology and Applied Pharmacology, 108,* 78–85.

Ernst, M., Moolchan, E. T., & Robinson, M. L. (2001). Behavioral and neural consequences of prenatal exposure to nicotine. *Journal of the American Academy of Child and Adolescent Psychiatry, 40,* 630–641.

Ershoff, D. H., Ashford, T. H., & Goldenberg, R. L. (2004). Helping pregnant women quit smoking: An overview. *Nicotine and Tobacco Research, 6*(Suppl. 2), S101–S105.

Eysenck, H. J. (1955). Cortical inhibition, figural aftereffect, and theory of personality. *Journal of Abnormal and Social Psychology, 51,* 94–106.

Eysenck, H. J. (1967). *The biological basis of personality.* Springfield, IL: Thomas.

Eysenck, H. J., & Eysenck, M. W. (1985). *Personality and individual differences.* New York: Plenum Press.

Falconer, D. S. (1967). The inheritance of liability to diseases with variable age of onset, with particular reference to diabetes mellitus. *Annals of Human Genetics, 31,* 1–20.

Famularo, R., Kinscherff, R., & Fenton, T. (1992). Psychiatric diagnosis of maltreated children: Preliminary findings. *Journal of the American Academy of Child and Adolescent Psychiatry, 31,* 863–867.

Faraone, S. B. (2003). Report from the fourth international meeting of the attention deficit hyperactivity disorder molecular genetics network. *American Journal of Medical Genetics B. Neuropsychiatric Genetics, 121*(1), 55–59.

Faraone, S. V. (2000). Genetics of childhood disorders: XX. ADHD, Part 4: Is ADHD genetically heterogeneous? *Journal of the American Academy of Child and Adolescent Psychiatry, 39,* 1455–1457.

Faraone, S. V. (2001). Report from the second international meeting of the Attention Deficit Hyperactivity Disorder Molecular Genetics Network. *American Journal of Medical Genetics, 105,* 255–258.

Faraone, S. V. (2005). The scientific foundation for understanding attention-deficit/hyperactivity disorder as a valid psychiatric disorder. *European Journal of Child and Adolescent Psychiatry, 14,* 1–10.

Faraone, S. V., Biederman, J., & Friedman, D. (2000a). Validity of DSM-IV subtypes of attention-deficit/hyperactivity disorder: A family study perspective. *Journal of the American Academy of Child and Adolescent Psychiatry, 39,* 300–309.

Faraone, S. V., Biederman, J., Mick, E., Williamson, S., Wilens, T., Spencer, T., et al. (2000b). Family study of girls with attention deficit hyperactivity disorder. *American Journal of Psychiatry, 157,* 1077–1083.

Faraone, S. V., Doyle, A. E., Mick, E., & Biederman, J. (2001). Meta-analysis of the association between the 7–repeat allele of the dopamine D4 receptor gene and attention-deficit hyperactivity disorder. *American Journal of Psychiatry, 158,* 1052–1057.

Faraone, S. V., Perlis, R. H., Doyle, A. H., Smoller, J. W., Goralnick, J. J., Holmgren, M. A., & Sklar, P. (2005). Molecular genetics of attention-deficit/hyperactivity disorder. *Biological Psychiatry,57,* 1313–1323.

Faraone, S. V., & Wilens, T. (2003). Does stimulant treatment lead to substance-use disorders? *Journal of Clinical Psychiatry, 64*(Suppl. 11), 9–13.

Farrington, D. P., Loeber, R., & van Kammen, W. B. (1990). Long term criminal outcomes of hyperactivity–impulsivity–attention deficit and conduct problems in childhood. In L. Robins & M. Rutter (Eds.), *Straight and devious pathways from childhood to adulthood* (pp. 62–81). New York: Cambridge University Press.

Feingold, B. F. (1975). Hyperkinesis and learning disabilities linked to artificial food flavors and colors. *American Journal of Nursing, 75,* 797–803.

Ferguson, S. A. (2001). A review of rodent models of ADHD. In M. V. Solanto, A. F. T. Arnsten, & F. X. Castellanos (Eds.), *Stimulant drugs and ADHD:*

Basic and clinical neuroscience (pp. 209–220). New York: Oxford University Press.

Fergusson, D. M., Horwood, L. J., & Lynskey, M. T. (1993). Maternal smoking before and after pregnancy: Effects on behavioral outcomes in middle childhood. *Pediatrics, 92,* 815–822.

Ferini-Strambi, L., Fantini, M. L., & Castronovo, C. (2004). Epidemiology of obstructive sleep apnea syndrome. *Minerva Medica, 95*(3), 187–202.

Feussner, G. (2002). Diversion, trafficking, and abuse of methylphenidate. In P. S. Jensen & J. R. Cooper (Eds.), *Attention deficit hyperactivity disorder: State of the science-best practices* (pp. 20-1–20-20). Kingston, NJ: Civic Research Institute.

Fewtrell, L. J., Pruss-Ustun, A., Landrigan, P., & Ayuso-Mateos, J. L. (2004). Estimating the global burden of disease of mild mental retardation and cardiovascular disease from environmental lead exposure. *Environmental Research, 94,* 120–133.

Fine, P. E. M. (1981). Immunogenetics of susceptibility to leprosy, tuberculosis, and leishmaniasis: An epidemiological perspective. *International Journal of Leprosy and Other Mycobacterial Diseases, 49,* 437–454.

Fisher, S. E., Francks, C., McCracken, J. T., McGough, J. J., Marlow, A. J., MacPhie, I. L., et al. (2002). A genomewide scan for loci involved in attention-deficit/hyperactivity disorder. *American Journal of Human Genetics, 70,* 1183–1196.

Fletcher, R. H., Fletcher, S. W., & Wagner, E. H. (1996). *Clinical epidemiology: The essentials* (3rd ed.). Baltimore: Williams & Wilkins.

Forehand, R., Rogers, T., McMahon, R. J., Wells, K. C., & Griest, D. L. (1981). Teaching parents to modify child behavior problems: An examination of some follow-up data. *Journal of Pediatric Psychology, 6,* 313–322.

Foulder-Hughes, L. A., & Cooke, R. W. I. (2003). Motor, cognitive, and behavioral disorders in children born very preterm. *Developmental Medicine and Child Neurology, 45, 97–103.*

Fowles, D. C. (1980). The three arousal model: Implications of Gray(s two-factor learning theory for heart rate, electrodermal activity, and psychopathy. *Psychophysiology, 17,* 84–104.

Fowles, D. C. (1983). Motivational effects on heart rate and electrodermal activity: Implications for research on personality and psychopathology. *Journal of Research in Personality, 17,* 48–71.

Fowles, D. C. (1988). Psychophysiology and psychopathology: A motivational approach. *Psychophysiology, 25,* 373–391.

Frick, P. J., Lahey, B. B., Christ, M. A. G., Loeber, R., & Green, S. (1991). History of childhood behavior problems in biological relatives of boys with attention-deficit hyperactivity disorder and conduct disorder. *Journal of Clinical Child Psychology, 20,* 445–451.

Frick, P. J., Lilienfeld, S. O., Ellis, M., Loney, B., & Silverthorn, P. (1999). The association between anxiety and psychopathy dimensions in children. *Journal of Abnormal Child Psychology, 27,* 383–392.

Friedman, N. P., & Miyake, A. M. (2004). The relations among inhibition and interference control functions: A latent-variable analysis. *Journal of Experimental Psychology: General, 133*(1), 101–135.

Fung, M. T., Raine, A., Loeber, R., Lynam, D. R., Steinhauer, S. R., Venables, P. H., et al. (2005). Reduced electrodermal activity in psychopathy-prone adolescents. *Journal of Abnormal Psychology, 114,* 187–196.

Fuster, J. M. (1997). *The prefrontal cortex: Anatomy, physiology and neuropsychology of the frontal lobe* (3rd ed.). New York: Raven Press.

Gabriel, S. B., Schaffner, S. F., Nguyen, H., Moore, J. M., Roy, J., Blumenstiel, B., et al. (2002). The structure of haplotype blocks in the human genome. *Science, 296,* 2225–2229.

Gadow, K. D., Nolan, E. E., Litcher, L., Carlson, G. A., Panina, N., Colovakha, E., et al. (2000). Comparison of attention-deficit/hyperactivity disorder symptom subtypes in Ukranian schoolchildren. *Journal of the American Academy of Child and Adolescent Psychiatry, 39,* 1520–1527.

Gaines, A. D. (1992). From DSM-I to III-R: Voices of self, mastery and the other: A cultural constructivist reading of U. S. psychiatric classification. *Social Science and Medicine, 35,* 3–24.

Garber, J., & Hollon, S. D. (1991). What can specificity designs say about causality in psychopathology research? *Psychological Bulletin, 110,* 129–136.

Gaub, M., & Carlson, C. L. (1997). Gender differences in ADHD: A meta-analysis and critical review. *Journal of the American Academy of Child and Adolescent Psychiatry, 36,* 1036–1045.

Ge, X., Conger, R. D., Cadoret, R. J., Neiderhiser, J. M., et al. (1996). The developmental interface between nature and nurture: A mutual influence model of child antisocial behavior and parent behaviors. *Developmental Psychology, 32*(4), 574–589.

Geist, E. A., & Gibson, M. (2000). The effect of network and public television programs on four and five year olds ability to attend to educational tasks. *Journal of Instructional Psychology, 27,* 250–261.

Giedd, J. N., Blumenthal, J., Molloy, E., & Castellanos, F. X. (2001). Brain imaging of attention deficit/hyperactivity disorder. *Annals of the New York Academy of Sciences, 931,* 33–49.

Gill, M., Daly, G., Heron, S., Hawi, Z., & Fitzgerald, M. (1997). Confirmation of association between attention deficit hyperactivity disorder and a dopamine transporter polymorphism. *Molecular Psychiatry, 2,* 311–313.

Gillberg, C. (2003). Deficits in attention, motor control, and perception: A brief review. *Archives of Disease in Childhood, 88,* 904–910.

Gillberg, C., Carlstrom, G., Rasmussen, P., & Waldenstrom, E. (1983). Perceptual, motor and attentional deficits in seven-year-old children: Neurological screening aspects. *Acta Pediatrica Scandinavica, 72,* 119–124.

Gillberg, C., & Rasmussen, P. (1982). Perceptual motor and attentional deficits in seven-year-old children: Background factors. *Developmental Medicine and Child Neurology, 24,* 752–770.

Gillberg, C., Rasmussen, P., Carstrom, G., Svenson, B., & Waldenstrom, E. (1982). Perceptual, motor, and attentional deficits in six-year-old children: Epidemiological aspects. *Journal of Child Psychology and Psychiatry, 23,* 131–144.

Gladen, B. C., & Rogan, W. J. (1991). Effect of perinatal polychlorinated biphenyls and dichloroethane on later development. *Journal of Pediatrics, 119,* 58–63.

Gladen, B. C., Rogan, W. J., Hardy, P., Thullen, J., Tingelstad, J., & Tully, M. (1988). Development after exposure to polychlorinated biphenyls and dichloroethane transplacentally and through human milk. *Journal of Pediatrics, 113,* 991–995.

Glod, C. A., & Teicher, M. H. (1996). Relationship between early abuse, post-traumatic stress disorder, and activity levels in prepubertal children. *Journal of the American Academy of Child and Adolescent Psychiatry, 34,* 1384–1393.

Goldman, L. R. (1995a). Case studies of environmental risks to children. *The Future of Children, 5*(2), 27–33.

Goldman, L. R. (1995b). Children—unique and vulnerable: Environmental risk factors facing children and recommendations for response. *Environmental Health Perspectives, 106*(Suppl. 6), 13–18.

Goldsmith, H. H., Lemery, K. S., & Essex, M. J. (2004). Roles for temperament in the liability to psychopathology in childhood. In L. DiLalla (Ed.), *Behavior genetic principles: Development, personality, and psychopathology* (pp. 19–39). Washington, DC: American Psychological Association Press.

Goldstein, S., & Turner, D. (2001). The extent of drug therapy for ADHD among children in a large public school district. *Journal of Attention Disorders, 4,* 212–219.

Gomez, R., Harvey, J., Quick, C., Scharer, I., & Harris, G. (1999). DSM-IV AD/HD: Confirmatory factor models, prevalence, and gender and age differences based on parent and teacher ratings of Australian primary school children. *Journal of Child Psychology and Psychiatry, 40,* 265–274.

Gong, Z., & Evans, H. L. (1997). Effect of chelation with meso-dimercaptosuccinic acid (DMSA) before and after the appearance of lead-induced neurotoxicity in the rat. *Toxicology and Applied Pharmacology, 144,* 205–214.

Goodman, R., & Stevenson, J. (1989). A twin study of hyperactivity: I. An examination of hyperactivity scores and categories derived from Rutter teacher and parent questionnaires. *Journal of Child Psychology and Psychiatry, 30,* 671689.

Goodyear, P., & Hynd, G. W. (1992). Attention-deficit disorder with (ADD/H) and without (ADD/WO) hyperactivity: Behavioral and neuropsychological differentiation. *Journal of Clinical Child Psychology, 21,* 273–305.

Gordon, M. (1991). *Instruction manual for the Gordon Diagnostic System,* Model III-R. Dewitt, NY: Gordon Systems.

Gordon, M., Antshel, K., Faraone, S. V., Barkley, R., Lewandowski, L., Hudziak, J., et al. (2005). Symptoms versus impairment: The case for respecting DSM-IV's criterion D. *ADHD Report, 13*(4), 1–9.

Gorenstein, E. E., Mammato, C. A., & Sandy, J. M. (1989). Performance of inattentive–overactive children on selected measures of prefrontal-type function. *Journal of Clinical Psychology, 45,* 619–632.

Gorenstein, E. E., & Newman, J. P. (1980). Disinhibitory psychopathology: A new perspective and a model for research. *Psychological Review, 87,* 301–315.

Gosden, N. P., Kramp, P., Gabrielsen, G., & Sestoft, D. (2003). Prevalence of mental disorders among 15–17-year-old male adolescent remand prisoners in Denmark. *Acta Psychiatrica Scandinavica, 107,* 102–110.

Gottlieb, D. J., Vezina, R. M., Chase, C., Lesko, S. M., Heeren, T. C., Weese-Mayer, D. E., et al. (2003). Symptoms of sleep-disordered breathing in 5-year-old children are associated with sleepiness and problem behaviors. *Pediatrics, 112,* 870–877.

Grady, D. L., Chi, H. C., Ding, Y. C., Smith, M., Wang, E., Schuch, S., et al. (2003). High prevalence of rare dopamine receptor D4 alleles in children diagnosed with attention-deficit hyperactivity disorder. *Molecular Psychiatry, 8,* 536–545.

Graetz, B. W., Sawyer, M. G., Hazell, P. L., Arney, F., & Baghurst, P. (2001). Validity of DSM-IV ADHD subtypes in a nationally representative sample of Australian children and adolescents. *Journal of the American Academy of Child and Adolescent Psychiatry, 40,* 1410–1417.

Grandjean, P., Weihe, P., White, R. F., Debes, F., Araki, S., Yokoyama, K., et al. (1997). Cognitive deficit in 7-year-old children with prenatal exposure to methylmercury. *Neurotoxicology and Teratology, 19,* 417–428.

Gray, J. A. (1971). *The psychobiology of fear and stress.* Cambridge, UK: Cambridge University Press.

Gray, J. A. (1982). *The neuropsychology of anxiety: An enquiry into the functions of the septo-hippocampal system.* New York: Oxford University Press.

Gray, J. A. (1991). Neural systems, emotion, and personality. In J. Madden (Ed.), *Neurobiology of learning, emotion, and affect* (pp. 273–306). New York: Raven Press.

Gray, J. A., & McNaughton, N. (1996). The neuropsychology of anxiety: Reprise. In R. Zinbarg, R. J. McNally, D. H. Barlow, B. F. Chorpita, & J. Turovsky (Eds.), *Nebraska Symposium on Motivation: Vol 43. Perspectives on anxiety, panic, and fear* (pp. 61–134). Lincoln: University of Nebraska Press.

Greenberg, L. M., & Waldman, I. D. (1993). Developmental normative data on the Test of Variables of Attention (T.O.V.A.®). *Journal of Child Psychiatry and Psychology, 34*(6), 1019–1030.

Greenberg, M. T., Kusche, C. A., & Speltz, M. (1991). Emotional regulation, self-control, and psychopathology: The role of relationships in early childhood. In D. Cicchetti (Ed.), *Internalizing and externalizing expressions of dysfunction* (pp. 21–55). Hillsdale, NJ: Erlbaum.

Greenberg, M. T., Speltz, M. L., DeKlyen, M., & Jones, K. (2001). Correlates of clinic referral for early conduct problems: Variable- and person-oriented approaches. *Development and Psychopathology, 13,* 255–276.

Grodzinsky, G. M., & Barkley, R. A. (1999). Predictive power of frontal lobe tests in the diagnosis of attention-deficit hyperactivity disorder. *Clinical Neuropsychologist, 13,* 12–21.

Grodzinsky, G. M., & Diamond, R. (1992). Frontal lobe functioning in boys with attention deficit hyperactivity disorder. *Developmental Neuropsychology, 8,* 427–445.

Gruber, R., & Sadeh, A. (2004). Sleep and neurobehavioral functioning in boys with attention-deficit/hyperactivity disorder and no reported breathing problems. *Sleep: Journal of Sleep and Sleep Disorders Research, 27,* 267–273.

Grych, J. H., & Fincham, F. D. (1990). Marital conflict and children's adjustment: A cognitive-contextual framework. *Psychological Bulletin, 108,* 267–290.

Guitton, D., Buchtel, H. A., & Douglas, R. M. (1985). Frontal lobe lesions in man cause difficulties in suppressing reflexive glances and in generating goal-directed saccades. *Experimental Brain Research, 58,* 455–472.

Hack, M., Klein, N. K., & Taylor, H. G. (1995). Long term developmental outcomes of low birth weight infants. *The Future of Children, 5*(1), 176–196.

Haenlein, M., & Caul, W. F. (1987). Attention deficit disorder with hyperactivity: A specific hypothesis of reward dysfunction. *Journal of the American Academy of Child and Adolescent Psychiatry, 26,* 356–362.

Halperin, J., Wolf, L., Greenblatt, E., & Young, G. (1991). Subtype analysis of commission errors on the continuous performance test in children. *Developmental Neuropsychology, 7,* 207–217.

Hanes, D. P., Patterson, W. F., & Schall, J. D. (1998). The role of frontal eye field in countermanding saccades: Visual, movement and fixation activity. *Journal of Neurophysiology, 79,* 817–834.

Hanes, D. P., & Schall, J. D. (1995). Countermanding saccades in macaque. *Visual Neuroscience, 12,* 929–937.

Hankin, J. R., Sloan, J. J., Firestone, I. J., Ager, J. W., Sokol, R. J., & Martier, S. S. (1993). A time series analysis of the impact of the alcohol warning label on antenatal drinking. *Alcoholism: Clinical and Experimental Research, 17,* 284–289.

Hare, T., Tottenham, N., Davidson, M. C., Glover, G. H., & Casey, B. J. (2005). Contributions of striatal and amygdala activity in emotion regulation. *Biological Psychiatry, 57,* 624–632.

Harmon-Jones, E. (2003). Early career award: Clarifying the emotive functions of asymmetrical frontal cortical activity. *Psychophysiology, 40,* 838–848.

Harmon-Jones, E. (2004). Contributions from research on anger and cognitive dissonance to understanding the motivational functions of asymmetrical frontal brain activity. *Biological Psychology, 67,* 51–76.

Harnishfeger, K. K. (1995). The development of cognitive inhibition: Theories, definitions, and research evidence. In F. N. Dempster & C. J. Brainerd (Eds.), *Interference and inhibition in cognition* (pp. 175–204). San Diego, CA: Academic Press.

Hart, E. L., Lahey, B. B., Loeber, R., Applegate, B., & Frick, P. J. (1995). Developmental changes in attention-deficit hyperactivity disorder in boys: A four year longitudinal study. *Journal of Abnormal Child Psychology, 23,* 729–750.

Hartman, C. A., Hox, J., Mellenbergh, G. J., Boyle, M. H., Offord, D. R., Racine, Y., et al. (2001). DSM-IV internal construct validity: When a taxonomy meets data. *Journal of Child Psychology and Psychiatry, 42,* 817–836.

Hartung, C. M., Milich, R., Lynam, D. R., & Martin, C. A. (2002). Understanding the relations among gender, disinhibition, and disruptive behavior in adolescents. *Journal of Abnormal Psychology, 111,* 659–664.

Harvald, B., & Hauge, M. (1956). A catamnestic investigation of Danish twins: A preliminary report. *Danish Medical Bulletin, 3,* 150–156.

Hasher, L., & Zacks, R. T. (1988). Working memory, comprehension, and aging: A review and a new view. *Psychology of Learning and Motivation, 22,* 193–225.

Hauser, P., Zametkin, A. J., Martinez, P., Vitiello, B., Matochik, J. A., Mixson, A. J., et al. (1993). Attention deficit-hyperactivity disorder in people with generalized resistance to thyroid hormone. *New England Journal of Medicine, 328,* 997–1001.

Hawi, Z., Lowe, N., Kirley, A., Gruenhage, F., Nothen, M., Greenwood, T., et al. (2003). Linkage disequilibrium mapping at DAT1, DRD5 and DBH narrows the search for ADHD susceptibility alleles at these loci. *Molecular Psychiatry, 8,* 299–308.

Hay, D. A., Bennett, K. S., Levy, F., Sergeant, J. A., & Swanson, J. M. (in press). A twin study of ADHD rated by DSM-IV and the Strengths and Weaknesses of ADHD Symptoms and Normal Behaviors (SWAN) scale. *Biological Psychiatry.*

Healy, J. M. (1990). *Endangered minds: Why our children don't think.* New York: Simon & Schuster.

Hechtman, L., Abikoff, H., Klein, R. G., Greenfield, B., Etcovitch, J., Cousins, L., et al. (2004). Children with ADHD treated with long-term methylphenidate and multimodal psychosocial treatment: Impact on parental practices. *Journal of the American Academy of Child and Adolescent Psychiatry, 43,* 830–838.

Henderson, S. E., & Sugden, D. A. (1992). *Movement Assessment Battery for Children.* San Antonio, TX: Psychological Corporation.

Heudorf, U., Angerer, J., & Drexler, H. (2004). Current internal exposure to pesticides in children and adolescents in Germany: Urinary levels of metabolites of pyrethroid and organophosphorus insecticides. *International Archives of Occupational and Environmental Health, 77,* 67–72.

Hill, S. Y., Lowers, L., Locke-Wellman, J., & Shen, S. A. (2000). Maternal smoking and drinking during pregnancy and the risk for child and adolescent psychiatric disorders. *Journal of Studies on Alcohol, 61,* 661–668.

Hinshaw, S. P. (1987). On the distinction between attentional deficits/hyperactivity and conduct problems/aggression in child psychopathology. *Psychological Bulletin, 101,* 443–463.

Hinshaw, S. P. (1999). Psychosocial intervention for childhood ADHD: Etiologic and developmental themes, comorbidity, and integration with pharmacotherapy. In D. Cicchetti & S. L. Toth (Eds.), *Rochester Symposium on Developmental Psychopathology: Vol. 9. Developmental approaches to prevention and intervention* (pp. 221–270). Rochester, NY: University of Rochester Press.

Hinshaw, S. P. (2001). Is the inattentive type of ADHD a separate disorder? *Clinical Psychology: Science and Practice, 8,* 498–501.

Hinshaw, S. P. (2002a). Is ADHD an impairing condition in childhood and adolescence? In P. S. Jensen & J. R. Cooper (Eds.), *Attention-deficit hyperactivity disorder: State of the science, best practices* (pp. 5-1–5-21). Kingston, NJ: Civic Research Institute.

Hinshaw, S. P. (2002b). Preadolescent girls with attention-deficit/hyperactivity disorder: I. Background characteristics, comorbidity, cognitive and social functioning, and parenting practices. *Journal of Consulting and Clinical Psychology, 70,* 1086–1098.

Hinshaw, S. P., Carte, E. T., Sami, N., Treuting, J. J., & Zupan, B. A. (2002). Preadolescent girls with attention-deficit/hyperactivity disorder: II. Neuropsychological performance in relation to subtypes and individual classification. *Journal of Consulting and Clinical Psychology, 70,* 1099–1111.

Hinshaw, S. P., Owens, E. B., Wells, K. C., Kraemer, H. C., Abikoff, H. B., Arnold, L. E., et al. (2000). Family processes and treatment outcome in the MTA: Negative/ineffective parenting practices in relation to multimodal treatment. *Journal of Abnormal Child Psychology, 28,* 555–568.

Hirsch, A. (1886). *Handbook of geographical and historical pathology* (Vol. 3, 2nd ed.). London: New Sydenham Society.

Holena, E., Nafstad, I., Skaare, J. U., Bernhoff, A., Engen, P., & Sagvolden, T. (1995). Behavioral effects of pre- and postnatal exposure to individual polychlorinated biphenyl cogeners in rats. *Environmental Toxicology and Chemistry, 14,* 967–976.

Holena, E., Nafstad, I., Skaare, J. U., & Sagvolden, T. (1998). Behavioral hyperactivity in rats following postnatal exposure to sub-toxic doses of polychlorinated biphenyl cogeners 153 and 126. *Behavioural Brain Research, 94,* 213–224.

Hollich, G. J., Hirsh-Pasek, K., & Golinkoff, R. M. (2000). Breaking the language barrier: An emergenist coalition model for the origins of word learning. *Monographs of the Society for Research in Child Development, 65*(3), 1–135.

Hollingsworth, D. E., McAuliffe, S. P., & Knowlton, B. J. (2001). Temporal allocation of visual attention in adult attention deficit hyperactivity disorder. *Journal of Cognitive Neuroscience, 13,* 298–305.

Holman, R. T. (1998). The slow discovery of the importance of ?3 essential fatty acids in human health. *Journal of Nutrition, 128,* 427S-433S.

Hooper, M. L., & Chang, P. (1998). Comparison of demands of sustained attentional events between public and private children's television programs. *Perceptual and Motor Skills, 86*(2), 431–434.

Horrobin, D. (2003, February 12). Not in the genes: Enthusiasts for genomics have corrupted scientific endeavor and undermined hope of medical progress. Retrieved from www.guardian.co.uk/comment/story/0,3604,893790,00.html

Horrobin, D. F., Glen, A. I. M., & Hudson, C. J. (1995). Possible relevance of phospholipid abnormalities and genetic interactions in psychiatric disorders: The relationship between dyslexia and schizophrenia. *Medical Hypotheses, 45,* 605–613.

Houghton, S., Douglas, G., West, J., Whiting, K., Wall, M., Langsford, S., et al. (1999). Differential patterns of executive function in children with attention-deficit hyperactivity disorder according to gender and subtype. *Journal of Child Neurology, 14,* 801–805.

Hoyert, D. L., Mathews, T. J., Menacker, F., Strobino, D. M., & Guyer, B. (2006). Annual summary of vital statistics: 2004. *Pediatrics, 117,* 168–183.

Hoyme, H. E., May, P. A., Kalberg, W. O., Kodituwakku, P., Gossage, J. P., Trujillo, P. M., et al. (2005). A practical clinical approach to diagnosis of fetal alcohol spectrum disorders: Clarification of the 1996 Institute of Medicine Criteria. *Pediatrics, 115*, 39–47.

Huang-Pollock, C. L., Carr, T. H., & Nigg, J. T. (2002). Development of selective attention: Perceptual load influences early versus late attentional selection in children and adults. *Developmental Psychology, 38*, 363–375.

Huang-Pollock, C. L., & Nigg, J. T. (2003). Searching for the attention deficit in attention deficit hyperactivity disorder: The case of visuospatial orienting. *Clinical Psychology Review, 23*, 801–830.

Huang-Pollock, C. L., Nigg, J. T., & Carr, T. H. (2005). Selective attention in ADHD using a perceptual load paradigm. *Journal of Child Psychology and Psychiatry, 46*, 1211–1218.

Huang-Pollock, C. L., Nigg, J. T., Henderson, J. M., & Carr, T. H. (2000, June). *Covert attention in children with ADHD.* Poster presented at the annual meeting of the Association for Psychological Science, Miami, FL.

Huston, A. C., & Wright, J. C. (1998). Mass media and children's development. In W. Damon (Series Ed.) & I. Sigel & K. A. Renninger (Vol. Eds.), *Handbook of child psychology: Vol. 4. Child psychology in practice* (5th ed., pp. 999–1058). New York: Wiley.

Iaboni, F., Douglas, V. I., & Baker, A. G. (1995). Effects of reward and response costs on inhibition in ADHD children. *Journal of Abnormal Psychology, 104*, 232–240.

Iaboni, F., Douglas, V. I., & Ditto, B. (1997). Psychophysiological response of ADHD children to reward and extinction. *Psychophysiology, 34*, 116–123.

Icenogle, L. M., Christopher, N. C., Blackwelder, W. P., Caldwell, D. P., Qiao, D., Seidler, F. J., et al. (2004). Behavioral alterations in adolescent and adult rats caused by a brief subtoxic exposure to chlorpyrifos during neurulation. *Neurotoxicology and Teratology, 26*, 95–101.

Ivry, R. B. (1997). Cerebellar timing systems. *International Review of Neurobiology, 41*, 555–573.

Ivry, R. B. (2003). Cerebellar involvement in clumsiness and other developmental disorders. *Neural Plasticity, 10*, 141–153.

Ivry, R. B., & Keele, S. W. (1989). Timing functions of the cerebellum. *Journal of Cognitive Neuroscience, 1*, 136–152.

Jacobson, J. L., & Jacobson, S. W. (1996). Intellectual impairment in children exposed to polychlorinated biphenyls *in utero. New England Journal of Medicine, 335*, 783–789.

Jacobson, J. L., & Jacobson, S. W. (2002). Breast-feeding and gender as moderators of teratogenic effects on cognitive development. *Neurotoxicology and Teratology, 24*, 249–358.

Jacobson, J. L., & Jacobson, S. W. (2003). Prenatal exposure to polychlorinated biphenyls and attention at school age. *Journal of Pediatrics, 143*, 780–788.

Jacobson, J. L., Jacobson, S. W., Padgett, R. J., Brumitt, G. A., & Billings, R. L. (1992). Effects of prenatal PCB exposure on cognitive processing efficiency and sustained attention. *Developmental Psychology, 28*, 297–306.

Jacobson, J. L., Jacobson, S. W., Sokol, R. J., & Ager, J. W. (1998). Relation of maternal age and pattern of pregnancy drinking to functionally significant cognitive deficit in infancy. *Alcoholism: Clinical and Experimental Research, 22*, 345–351.

Jacobson, S. W., Chiodo, L. M., Jacobson, J. L., & Sokol, R. J. (2002). Validity of maternal report of alcohol, cocaine, and smoking during pregnancy in relation to infant neurobehavioral outcome. *Pediatrics, 109*, 815–825.

Jacobson, S. W., Jacobson, J. L., Sokol, R. J., Chiodo, L. M., & Corobana, R. (2004). Maternal age, alcohol abuse history, and quality of parenting as moderators of the effects of prenatal alcohol exposure on 7. 5 year intellectual function. *Alcohol Clinical and Experimental Research, 28*, 1732–1745.

Jacobvitz, D., Hazen, N., Curran, M., & Hitchens, K. (2004). Observations of early triadic family interactions: Boundary disturbances in the family predict symptoms of depression, anxiety, and attention-deficit/hyperactivity disorder in middle childhood. *Development and Psychopathology, 16*, 577–592.

James, A., & Taylor, E. (1990). Sex differences in the hyperkinetic syndrome of childhood. *Journal of Child Psychology and Psychiatry, 31*, 437–446.

Jennings, R. J., van der Molen, M. W., Pelham, W., Debski, K. B., & Hoza, B. (1997). Inhibition in boys with attention deficit hyperactivity disorder as indexed by heart rate change. *Developmental Psychology, 33*, 308–318.

Jensen, P. S., & Cooper, J. R. (2002). *Attention deficit hyperactivity disorder: State of the science, best practices.* Kingston, NJ: Civic Research Institute.

Jensen, P. S., Hinshaw, S. P., Kraemer, H. C., Lenora, N., Newcorn, J. H., Abikoff, H. B., et al. (2001). ADHD comorbidity findings from the MTA study: Comparing comorbid subgroups. *Journal of the American Academy of Child and Adolescent Psychiatry, 40*, 147–158.

Jensen, P. S., Kettle, L., Roper, M. T., Sloan, M. T., Dulcan, M. K., Hoven, C., et al. (1999). Are stimulants overprescribed?: Treatment of ADHD in four U.S. communities. *Journal of the American Academy of Child and Adolescent Psychiatry, 38*, 797–804.

Jensen, P. S., Martin, D., & Cantwell, D. (1997a). Comorbidity in ADHD: Implications for research, practice, and DSM-IV. *Journal of the American Academy of Child and Adolescent Psychiatry, 36*, 1065–1079.

Jensen, P. S., Mrazek, D., Knapp, P. K., Steinberg, L., Pfeffer, C., Schowalter, J., et al. (1997b). Evolution and revolution in child psychiatry: ADHD as a disorder of adaptation. *Journal of the American Academy of Child and Adolescent Psychiatry, 36*, 1672–1678.

Jester, J. M., Nigg, J. T., Adams, K., Fitzgerald, H. E., Puttler, L. I., Wong, M. M., et al. (2005). Inattention/hyperactivity and aggression from early childhood to adolescence: Heterogeneity of trajectories and differential influence of family environment characteristics. *Development and Psychopathology, 17*, 99–125.

Johansen, E. B., Aase, H., Meyer, A., & Sagvolden, T. (2002). Attention deficit/hyperactivity disorder behavior explained by dysfunctional reinforcement and extinction processes. *Behavioural Brain Research, 130*, 37–45.

John, O. P., & Srivastava, S. (1999). The Big Five trait taxonomy: History, measurement, and theoretical perspectives. In L. A. Pervin & O. P. John

(Eds.), *Handbook of personality: Theory and research* (2nd ed., pp. 102138). New York: Guilford Press.

Johnson, S. F., McCarter, R. J., & Ferencz, C. (1987). Changes in alcohol, cigarette, and recreational drug use during pregnancy: Implications for intervention. *American Journal of Epidemiology, 126,* 701.

Johnston, C. (2002). Impact of attention deficit hyperactivity disorder on social and vocational functioning in adults. In P. S. Jensen & J. R. Cooper (Eds.), *Attention deficit hyperactivity disorder: State of the science, best practices* (pp. 6-1-6-21). Kingston, NJ: Civic Research Institute.

Johnston, C., & Mash, E. J. (2001). Families of children with attention-deficit/hyperactivity disorder: Review and recommendations for future research. *Clinical Child and Family Psychology Review, 4*(3), 183–207.

Johnstone, S. J., Tardif, H. P., Barry, R. J., & Sands, T. (2001). Nasal bilevel positive airway pressure therapy in children with a sleep-related breathing disorder and attention-deficit hyperactivity disorder: Effects on electrophysiological measures of brain function. *Sleep Medicine, 2*(5), 407–416.

Jonides, J., Lacey, S. C., & Nee, D. E. (2005). Processes of working memory in mind and brain. *Current Directions in Psychological Science, 14*(1), 2–5.

Jonkman, L., Kemmer, C., Verbaten, M., van Engeland, H., Kenemans, J., Camfferman, G., et al. (1999). Perceptual and response interference in children with attention-deficit hyperactivity disorder and the effects of methylphenidate. *Psychophysiology, 36,* 419–429.

Kadesjo, B., & Gillberg, C. (1998). Attention deficits and clumsiness in Swedish 7-year-old children. *Developmental Medicine and Child Neurology, 40,* 796–811.

Kagan, J. (1997). Temperament and the reactions to the unfamiliar. *Child Development, 68,* 139–143.

Kagan, J. (2003). Behavioral inhibition as a temperamental category. In R. J. Davidson, K. R. Scherer, & H. H. Goldsmith (Eds.), *Handbook of affective sciences* (pp. 320–331). New York: Oxford University Press.

Kagan, J., Reznick, J. S., & Gibbons, J. (1989). Inhibited and uninhibited types of children. *Child Development, 60,* 838–845.

Kagan, J., & Snidman, N. (2004). *The long shadow of temperament.* Cambridge, MA: Harvard University Press.

Kahn, R. S., Khoury, J., Nichols, W. C., & Lanphear, B. P. (2003). Role of dopamine transporter genotype and maternal prenatal smoking in childhood hyperactive–impulsive, inattentive, and oppositional behaviors. *Journal of Pediatrics, 143,* 104–110.

Kahneman, D., & Henik, A. (1981). Perceptual organization and attention. In K. Kubovy & J. R. Pomerantz (Eds.), *Perceptual organization* (pp. 181–211). Hillsdale, NJ: Erlbaum.

Kaiser Family Foundation. (1999). *Kids and media and the new millennium.* Menlo Park, CA: Author. (Available at www.kff.org)

Kaiser Family Foundation. (2003). *Zero to Six: Electronic Media in the Lives of Infants, Toddlers, and Preschoolers.* Menlo Park, CA: Author. (Available at www.kff.org)

Kallman, F. J., & Reisner, D. (1943). Twin studies on the significance of genetic factors in tuberculosis. *Annual Review of Tuberculosis, 47,* 549–574.

Kamrin, M. A. (1997). *Pesticide profiles: Toxicity, environmental impact, and fate.* Boca Raton, FL: CRC/Lewis.

Kandell, E. R., Schwartz, J. H., & Jessell, T. M. (1991). *Principles of neural science* (3rd ed.). Norwalk, CT: Appleton & Lange.

Kane, M. J., & Engle, R. W. (2001). Working memory capacity and the control of attention: The contributions of goal neglect, response competition, and task set to Stroop interference. *Journal of Experimental Psychology: General, 132,* 47–70.

Kane, M. J., & Engle, R. W. (2002). The role of prefrontal cortex in working memory capacity, executive attention, and general fluid intelligence: An individual differences perspective. *Psychonomic Bulletin and Review, 9,* 637–671.

Kane, M. J., Hambrick, D. Z., Tuholski, S. W., Wilhelm, O., Payne, T. W., & Engle, R. W. (2004). The generality of working memory capacity: A latent-variable approach to verbal and visuospatial memory span and reasoning. *Journal of Experimental Psychology: General, 133,* 189–217.

Karatekin, C., & Asarnow, R. F. (1998). Working memory in childhood-onset schizophrenia and attention-deficit/hyperactivity disorder. *Psychiatry Research, 80,* 165–176.

Karatekin, C., Markiewics, S. W., & Siegel, M. A. (2003). A preliminary study of motor problems in children with attention-deficit/hyperactivity disorder. *Perceptual and Motor Skills, 97,* 1267–1280.

Kass, S. J., Wallace, J. C., & Vodanovich, S. J. (2003). Boredom proneness and sleep disorders as predictors of adult attention deficit scores. *Journal of Attention Disorders, 7,* 83–91.

Kassirer, J. (2004). *On the take: How big business is corrupting American medicine.* New York: Oxford University Press.

Kaufman, J., Yang, B. Z., Douglas-Palumberi, H., Houshyar, S., Lipschitz, D., Krystal, J. H., et al. (2004). Social supports and serotonin transporter gene moderate depression in maltreated children. *Proceedings of the National Academy of Sciences USA, 101,* 17316–17321.

Kavale, K. A., & Forness, S. R. (1983). Hyperactivity and diet treatment: A meta-analysis of the Feingold hypothesis. *Journal of Learning Disabilities, 16,* 324–330.

Kelleher, K. J. (2002). Use of services and costs for youth with ADHD and related conditions. In P. S. Jensen & J. R. Cooper (Eds.), *Attention deficit hyperactivity disorder: State of the science, best practices* (pp. 27-1–27-12). Kingston, NJ: Civic Research Institute.

Kemp, S. L., Kirk, U., & Korkman, M. (2001). *Essentials of NEPSY assessment.* New York: Wiley.

Kendell, R. E. (1986). What are mental disorders? In A. M. Freedman, R. Brotman, I. Silverman, & D. Hutson (Eds.), *Issues in psychiatric classification: Science, practice, and social policy* (p. 23–45). New York: Human Sciences Press.

Kendler, K. S., Kuhn, J. W., Vittum, J., Prescott, C. A., & Riley, B. (2005). The interaction of stressful life events and a serotonin transporter polymorphism in the prediction of episodes of major depression. *Archives of General Psychiatry, 62,* 529–535.

Kimberg, D. Y., & Farah, M. J. (1998). Is there an inhibitory module in the prefrontal cortex? Working memory and the mechanisms underlying cognitive control. In S. Monsell & J. Driver (Eds.), *Attention and performance: Vol. 18. Control of cognitive processes* (pp. 740–751). Cambridge, MA: MIT Press.

Kirk, V. G., & Bohn, S. (2004). Periodic limb movements in children: Prevalence in a referred population. *Sleep, 27,* 313–315.

Kirmayer, L. J. (1988). Mind and body as metaphors: Hidden values in biomedicine. In M. Lock & D. Gordon (Eds.), *Biomedicine examined* (pp. 57–92). Dordrecht, The Netherlands: Kluwer.

Kirmayer, L. J., & Young. A. (1999). Culture and context in the evolutionary concept of mental disorder. *Journal of Abnormal Psychology, 108,* 446–452.

Kirov, R., Kinkelbur, J., Heipke, S., Kostanecka-Endress, T., Westhoff, M., Cohrs, S., et al. (2004). Is there a specific polysomnographic sleep pattern in children with attention deficit/hyperactivity disorder? *Journal of Sleep Research, 13,* 87–93.

Klasen, H. (2000). A name, what's in a name?: The medicalization of hyperactivity, revisited. *Harvard Review of Psychiatry, 7,* 334–344.

Klein, D. F. (1978). A proposed definition of mental illness. In R. Spitzer & D. F. Klein (Eds.), *Critical issues in psychiatric diagnosis* (pp. 41–71). New York: Raven Press.

Klein, D. F. (1999). Harmful dysfunction, disorder, disease, illness, and evolution. *Journal of Abnormal Psychology, 108,* 421–429.

Klein, R. G. (2002). Alcohol, stimulants, nicotine, and other drugs in ADHD. In P. S. Jensen & J. R. Cooper (Eds.), *Attention deficit hyperactivity disorder: State of the science, best practices* (pp. 16-1–16-17). Kingston, NJ: Civic Research Institute.

Klinberg, T., Forssberg, H., & Westerberg, H. (2002). Training of working memory in children with ADHD. *Journal of Clinical and Experimental Neuropsychology, 24,* 781–791.

Klorman, R., Hazel-Fernandez, L. A., Shaywitz, S. E., Fletcher, J. M., Marchione, K. E., Holahan, J. M., et al. (1999). Executive functioning deficits in attention-deficit/hyperactivity disorder are independent of oppositional defiant or reading disorder. *Journal of the American Academy of Child and Adolescent Psychiatry, 38,* 1148–1155.

Knight, C. A., Knight, I., Mitchell, D. C., & Zepp, J. E. (2004). Beverage caffeine intake in U.S. consumers and subpopulations of interest: Estimates from the Share of Intake Panel survey. *Food and Chemical Toxicology, 42,* 1923–1930.

Kochanska, G., Murray, K., & Coy, K. C. (1997). Inhibitory control as a contributor to conscience in childhood: From toddler to early school age. *Child Development, 68,* 263–277.

Kochanska, G., Murray, K., & Harlan, E. T. (2000). Effortful control in early childhood: Continuity and change, antecedents, and implications for social development. *Developmental Psychology, 36,* 220–232.

Kociancic, T., Reed, M. D., & Findling, R. L. (2004). Evaluation of risks associated with short- and long-term psychostimulant therapy for treatment of ADHD in children. *Expert Opinion on Drug Safety, 3,* 93–100.

Kodituwakku, P. W., Handmaker, N. S., Cutler, S. K., Weathersby, E. K., & Handmaker, S. D. (1995). Specific impairments in self-regulation in children exposed to alcohol prenatally. *Alcoholism: Clinical and Experimental Research, 19,* 1558–1564.

Kodl, M. M., & Wakschlag, L. S. (2004). Does a childhood history of externalizing problems predict smoking during pregnancy? *Addiction and Behavior, 29,* 273–279.

Koger, S. M., Schettler, T., & Weiss, B. (2005). Environmental toxicants and developmental disabilities. *American Psychologist, 60,* 243–255.

Kolb, B., & Whishaw, I. Q. (1990). *Fundamentals of human neuropsychology* (3rd ed). New York: Freeman.

Koller, K., Brown, T., Spurgeon, A., & Levey, L. (2004). Recent developments in low-level lead exposure and intellectual impairment in children. *Environmental Health Perspectives, 112,* 987–994.

Konishi, S., Nakajima, K., Uchida, I., Kikyo, H., Kameyama, M., & Miyashita, Y. (1999). Common inhibitory mechanism in human inferior prefrontal cortex revealed by event-related functional MRI. *Brain, 122,* 981–991.

Konofal, E., Lecendreux, M., Bouvard, M. P., & Mouren-Simeoni, M. C. (2001). High levels of nocturnal activity in children with attention-deficit hyperactivity disorder: A video analysis. *Psychiatry and Clinical Neurosciences, 55,* 97–103.

Koopman-Esseboom, C., Weisglas-Kuperus, N., De Ridder, M. A. J., Van der Paauw, C. G., Tuinstra, L. G., & Sauer, P. J. (1996). Effects of polychlorinated biphenyl/dioxin exposure and feeding type on infants' mental and psychomotor development. *Pediatrics, 97,* 700–706.

Koren, G., Nulman, I., Chudley, A. E., & Loocke, C. (2003). Fetal alcohol spectrum disorder. *Canadian Medical Association Journal, 169,* 1181–1185.

Korkman, M., Kirk, U., & Kemp, S. L. (1998). *NEPSY: A developmental neuropsychological assessment.* San Antonio, TX: Psychological Corporation.

Koschack, J., Kunert, H. J., Derichs, G., Weniger, G., & Irle, E. (2003). Impaired and enhanced attentional function in children with attention deficit/hyperactivity disorder. *Psychological Medicine, 33,* 481–489.

Kotimaa, A. J., Moilanen, I., Taanila, A., Ebeling, H., Smalley, S. L., McGough, J. J., et al. (2003). Maternal smoking and hyperactivity in 8-year-old children. *Journal of the American Academy of Child and Adolescent Psychiatry, 42,* 826–833.

Kramer, S. (1987). Determinants of low birth weight: Methodological assessment and meta-analysis. *Bulletin of the World Health Organization, 65,* 663–737.

Kramer, S., Goulet, L., Lydon, J., Seguin, L., McNamara, H., Dassa, C., et al. (2001). Socio-economic disparities in preterm birth: Causal pathways and mechanisms. *Paediatric and Perinatal Epidemiology, 15*(Suppl. 2), 104–123.

Krause, K. H., Dresel, S. H., Krause, J., Kung, H. F., Tatsch, K., & Ackenheil, M. (2002). Stimulant-like action of nicotine on striatal dopamine transporter in the brain of adults with attention deficit hyperactivity disorder. *International Journal of Neuropsychopharmacology, 5,* 111–113.

Kreppner, J. M., O'Connor, T. G., Rutter, M., Beckett, C., Castle, J., Croft, C., et al. (2001). Can inattention/overactivity be an institutional deprivation syndrome? *Journal of Abnormal Child Psychology, 29*, 513–528.

Kristjansson, E. A., Fried, P. A., & Watkinson, B. (1989). Maternal smoking during pregnancy affects children's vigilance performance. *Drug and Alcohol Dependence, 24*, 11–19.

Krueger, R. F. (1999). The structure of common mental disorders. *Archives of General Psychiatry, 56*, 921–926.

Lachman, R., Lachman, J. L., & Butterfield, E. C. (1979). *Cognitive psychology and information processing: An introduction.* Hillsdale, NJ: Erlbaum.

Lahey, B. B. (2001). Should the combined and predominantly inattentive types of ADHD be considered distinct and unrelated disorders?: Not now, at least. *Clinical Psychology: Science and Practice, 8*, 494–497.

Lahey, B. B., Loeber, R., Hart, E. L., Frick, P. J., Applegate, B., Zhang, Q., et al. (1995). Four year longitudinal study of conduct disorder in boys: Patterns and predictors of persistence. *Journal of Abnormal Psychology, 104*, 83–93.

Lahey, B. B., Miller, T. L., Gordon, R. A., & Riley, A. W. (1999). Developmental epidemiology of the disruptive behavior disorders. In H. C. Quay & A. E. Hogan (Eds.), *Handbook of disruptive behavior disorders* (pp. 23–48). New York: Kluwer Academic/Plenum Press.

Lahey, B. B., Pelham, W. E., Loney, J., Lee, S. S., & Willcutt, E. (2005). Instability of the DSM-IV subtypes of ADHD from preschool through elementary school. *Archives of General Psychiatry, 62*, 896–902.

Lahey, B. B., Pelham, W. E., Stein, M. A., Loney, J., Trapani, C., Nugent, K., et al. (1998). Validity of DSM-IV attention-deficit/hyperactivity disorder for younger children. *Journal of the American Academy of Child and Adolescent Psychiatry, 37*, 695–702.

Lahey, B. B., Piacentini, J. C., McBurnett, K., Stone, P., Hartdagen, S., & Hynd, G. (1988). Psychopathology in the parents of children with conduct disorder and hyperactivity. *Journal of the American Academy of Child and Adolescent Psychiatry, 27*, 163–170.

Lahey, B. B., & Willcutt, E. G. (2002). Validity of the diagnosis and dimensions of attention deficit hyperactivity disorder. In P. S. Jensen & J. R. Cooper (Eds.), *Attention deficit hyperactivity disorder: State of the science, best practices* (pp. 1-1–1-23). Kingston, NJ: Civic Research Institute.

LaHoste, G. J., Swanson, J. M., Wigal, S. B., Glabe, C., King, N., & Kennedy, J. L. (1996). Dopamine D4 receptor gene polymorphism is associated with attention deficit hyperactivity disorder. *Molecular Psychiatry, 1*, 121–124.

Lai, T., Liu, X., Guo, Y. L., Yu, M. L., Hsu, C. C., & Rogan, W. J. (2002). A cohort study of behavioral problems and intelligence in children with high prenatal polychlorinated biphenyl exposure. *Archives of General Psychiatry, 59*, 1061–1066.

Landgren, M., Kjellman, B., & Gillberg, C. (1998). Attention deficit disorder with developmental coordination disorders. *Archives of Disease in Childhood, 79*, 207–212.

Langley, K., Marshall, L., van den Bree, M., Hollie, T., Owen, M., O'Donovan, M. O., et al. (2004). Association of the dopamine D4 receptor gene 7-

repeat allele with neuropsychological test performance of children with ADHD. *American Journal of Psychiatry, 161,* 133–138.

Lanphear, B. P., Dietrich, K., Auinger, P., & Cox, C. (2000). Cognitive deficits associated with blood lead concentrations <10 microg/dL in US children and adolescents. *Public Health Reports, 115,* 521–529.

Larson, R. W., & Varma, S. (1998). How children and adolescents spend time across the world: Work, play, and developmental opportunities. *Psychological Bulletin, 125,* 701–736.

Laufer, M. W., & Denhoff, E. (1957) Hyperkinetic behavior syndrome in children. *Journal of Pediatrics, 50,* 463–473.

Lavie, N. (1995). Perceptual load as a necessary condition for selective attention. *Journal of Experimental Psychology: Human Perception and Performance, 21,* 451–468.

Lavie, N., & Tsal, Y. (1994). Perceptual load as a major determinant of the locus of selection in visual attention. *Perception and Psychophysics, 56,* 183–197.

Lawson, D. C., Turic, D., Langley, K., Pay, H. M., Govan, C. F., Norton, N., et al. (2003). Association analysis of monoamine oxidase A and attention deficit hyperactivity disorder. *American Journal of Medical Genetics: Part B. Neuropsychiatric Genetic, 116B,* 84–89.

Lazzaro, I., Gordon, E., Li, W., Lim, C. L., Plahn, M., Whitmont, S., et al. (1999). Simultaneous EEG and EDA measures in adolescent attention deficit hyperactivity disorder. *International Journal of Psychophysiology, 34,* 123–134.

LeBourgeois, M. K., Avis, K., Mixon, M., Olmi, J., & Harsh, J. (2004). Snoring, sleep quality, and sleepiness across attention-deficit/hyperactivity disorder subtypes. *Sleep, 27,* 520–525.

Leerkes, E. M., & Crockenberg, S. C. (2002). The development of maternal self-efficacy and its impact on maternal behavior. *Infancy, 3,* 227–247.

LeFever, G. B., Dawson, K. V., & Morrow, A. L. (1999). The extent of drug therapy for attention deficit-hyperactivity disorder among children in public schools. *American Journal of Public Health, 89,* 1359–1364.

Lemery, K. S., Goldsmith, H. H., Klinnert, M. D., & Mrazek, D. A. (1999). Developmental models of infant and childhood temperament. *Developmental Psychology, 35,* 189–204.

Lerner, J. V., & Lerner, R. M. (1994). Exploration of the goodness of fit model in early adolescence. In W. B. Carey & S. C. McDevitt (Eds.), *Individual differences as risk factors for the mental health of children: A Festschrift for Stella Chess and Alexander Thomas* (pp. 161–169). New York: Brunner/Mazel.

Leung, P. W. L., & Connolly, K. J. (1996). Distractibility in hyperactive and conduct disordered children. *Journal of Child Psychology and Psychiatry, 37,* 305–312.

Leung, P. W. L., Luk, S. L., Ho, T. P., Taylor, E., Mak, F. L., & Bacon-Shone, J. (1996). The diagnosis and prevalence of hyperactivity in Chinese schoolboys. *British Journal of Psychiatry, 168,* 486–496.

Levin, E. D., Conners, C. K., Sparrow, E., Hinton, S. C., Erhardt, D., Meck, W. H., et al. (1996). Nicotine effects on adults with attention-deficit/hyperactivity disorder. *Psychopharmacology. 123,* 55–63.

Leviton, A. (1992). Behavioral correlates of caffeine consumption by children. *Clinical Pediatrics, 31,* 742–750.

Levy, F., Hay, D. A., McStephen, M., Wood, C., & Waldman, I. (1997). Attention-deficit hyperactivity disorder: A category or a continuum? Genetic analysis of a large-scale twin study. *Journal of the American Academy of Child and Adolescent Psychiatry, 36,* 737–744.

Levy, F., & Hay, D. A. (Eds.). (2001). *Attention, genes, and attention deficit hyperactivity disorder.* Philadelphia: Psychology Press.

Levy, F., McStephen, M., & Hay, D. A. (2001). The diagnostic genetics of ADHD symptoms and subtypes. In F. Levy and D. Hay (Eds.). *Attention, Genes, and ADHD* (pp. 35–57). Philadelphia: Taylor & Francis.

Lezak, M. D., Howieson, D. B., & Loring, D. W. (2004). *Neuropsychological assessment* (4th ed.). New York: Oxford University Press.

Lilienfeld, S. O., & Marino, L. (1995). Mental disorder as a Roschian concept: A critique of Wakefield's "harmful dysfunction" analysis. *Journal of Abnormal Psychology, 104,* 411–420.

Lilienfeld, S. O., & Marino, L. (1999). Essentialism revisited: Evolutionary theory and the concept of mental disorder. *Journal of Abnormal Psychology, 108,* 400–411.

Linnet, K. M., Dalsgaard, S., Obel, C., Wisborg, K., Henriksen, T. B., Rodriguez, A., et al. (2003). Maternal lifestyle factors in pregnancy risk of attention deficit hyperactivity disorder and associated behaviors: Review of the current evidence. *American Journal of Psychiatry, 160,* 1028–1040.

Little, B. R. (1999). Personality and motivation: Personal action and the conative evolution. In L. A. Pervin & O. P. John (Eds.), *Handbook of personality: Theory and research* (2nd ed., pp. 501–524). New York: Guilford Press.

Liu, X., Kurita, H., Guo, C., Tachimori, H., Ze, J., & Okawa, M. (2000). Behavioral and emotional problems in Chinese children: Teacher reports for ages 6 to 11. *Journal of Child Psychology and Psychiatry, 41,* 253–260.

Logan, G. D. (1994). A user's guide to the stop signal paradigm. In D. Dagenbach & T. Carr (Eds.), *Inhibition in language, memory, and attention* (pp. 189–239). San Diego, CA: Academic Press.

Logan, G. D., & Cowan, W. B. (1984). On the ability to inhibit thought and action: A theory of an act of control. *Psychological Review, 91,* 295–327.

Logan, G. D., Schachar, R. J., & Tannock, R. (1997). Impulsivity and inhibitory control. *Psychological Science, 8,* 60–64.

Loney, J., Kramer, J. R., & Salisbury, H. (2002). Medicated vs. unmedicated ADHD children: Adult involvement with legal and illegal drugs. In P. S. Jensen & J. R. Cooper (Eds.), *Attention deficit hyperactivity disorder: State of the science, best practices* (pp. 17-1–17-6). Kingston, NJ: Civic Research Institute.

Longnecker, M. P., Rogan, W. J., & Lucier, G. (1997). The human health effects of DDT (dichlorodiphenyl-trichloroethane) and PCBs (polychlorinated biphenyls) and an overview of organochlorines in public health. *Annual Review of Public Health, 18,* 211–244.

Longnecker, M. P., Wolff, M. S., Gladen, B., Brock J. W., Grandjean P., Jacobson, J. L., et al. (2003). Comparison of polychlorinated biphenyl levels across studies of human neurodevelopment. *Environmental Health Perspectives, 111,* 65–70.

Loo, S. K., Specter, E., Smolen, A., Hopfer, C., Teale, P. D., & Reite, M. L. (2003). Functional effects of the DAT1 polymorphism on EEG measures in ADHD. *Journal of the American Academy of Child and Adolescent Psychiatry, 42,* 986–993.

Losier, B. J., McGrath, P. J., & Klein, R. M. (1996). Error patterns on the continuous performance test in non-medicated and medicated samples of children with and without ADHD: A meta-analytic review. *Journal of Child Psychology and Psychiatry, 37,* 971–988.

Lufi, D., Cohen, A., & Parish-Plass, J. (1990). Identifying attention deficit hyperactive disorder with the WISC-R and the Stroop color and word test. *Psychology in the Schools, 27,* 28–34.

Luman, M., Oosterlaan, J., & Sergeant, J. A. (2005). The impact of reinforcement contingencies on AD/HD: A review and theoretical appraisal. *Clinical Psychology Review, 25,* 183–213.

Lynam, D. R. (1997). Pursuing the psychopath: Capturing the fledgling psychopath in a nomological net. *Journal of Abnormal Psychology, 106,* 425–438.

Lynam, D. R. (1998). Early identification of the fledgling psychopath: Locating the psychopathic child in the current nomenclature. *Journal of Abnormal Psychology, 107,* 566–575.

Lynam, D. R. (2002). Fledgling psychopathy: A view from personality theory. *Law and Human Behavior, 26,* 255–259.

Lynskey, M. T., & Fergusson, D. M. (1995). Childhood conduct problems, attention deficit behaviors, and adolescent alcohol, tobacco, and illicit drug use. *Journal of Abnormal Child Psychology, 23,* 281–302.

Lyon, G. R., & Krasnegor, N. A. (1996). *Attention, memory and executive function.* Baltimore: Brookes.

MacCoon, D. G., Wallace, J. F., & Newman, J. P. (2004). Self-regulation: The context-appropriate allocation of attentional capacity to dominant and non-dominant cues. In R. F. Baumeister & K. D. Vohs (Eds.). *Handbook of self-regulation* (pp. 422–444). New York: Guilford Press.

MacLeod, C. M. (1991). Fifty years of the Stroop effect: An integrative review and reinterpretation of effects. *Psychological Bulletin, 114,* 376–390.

MacLeod, C. M., Dodd, M. D., Sheard, E. D., Wilson, D. E., & Bibi, U. (2003). In opposition to inhibition. In B. H. Ross (Ed.), *The psychology of learning and motivation* (pp. 163–214). San Diego: Academic Press.

MacLeod, D., & Prior, M. (1996). Attention deficits in adolescents with ADHD and other clinical groups. *Child Neuropsychology, 2,* 1–10.

Magnus, P., Gjessing, H. K., Skrondal, A., & Skjaerven, R. (2001). Paternal contribution to birth weight. *Journal of Epidemiology and Community Health, 55,* 873–877.

Magnússon, P., Smári, J., Grétarsdottir, H., & Prándardóttir, H. (1999). Attention-deficit/hyperactivity symptoms in Icelandic schoolchildren: Assessment with the Attention Deficit/Hyperactivity Rating Scale–IV. *Scandinavian Journal of Psychology, 40,* 301–306.

Maher, B. S., Marazita, M. L., Ferrell, R. E., & Vanyukov, M. M. (2002). Dopamine system genes and attention deficit hyperactivity disorder: A meta-analysis. *Psychiatric Genetics, 12,* 207–215.

Manassis, K., Tannock, R., & Barbosa, J. (2000). Dichotic listening and response inhibition in children with comorbid anxiety disorders and ADHD. *Journal of the American Academy of Child and Adolescent Psychiatry, 39,* 1152–1159.

Mannuzza, S., & Klein, R. G. (2000). Long-term prognosis in attention-deficit/hyperactivity disorder. *Child and Adolescent Psychiatric Clinics of North America, 9,* 711–726.

Manor, I., Eisenberg, J., Tyano, S., Sever, Y., Cohen, H., Ebstein, R. P., et al. (2001). Family-based association study of the serotonin transporter promoter region polymorphism (5-HTTLPR) in attention-deficit hyperactivity disorder. *American Journal of Medical Genetics, 105,* 91–95.

March, J. S., Parker, J. D., Sullivan, K., Stallings, P., & Conners, C. K. (1997). The Multidimensional Anxiety Scale for Children (MASC): Factor structure, reliability, and validity. *Journal of the American Academy of Child and Adolescent Psychiatry, 36,* 554–565.

Marcotte, A. C., Thacher, P. V., Butters, M., Bortz, J., Acebo, C., & Carskadon, M. A. (1998). Parental report of sleep problems in children with attentional and learning disorders. *Journal of Developmental and Behavioral Pediatrics, 19,* 178–186.

Marshall, P. (1989). Attention deficit disorder and allergy: A neurochemical model of the relation between illnesses. *Psychological Bulletin, 106,* 434–446.

Martel, M., & Nigg, J. T. (in press). Relations of ADHD to temperamental resiliency, emotionality, and control. *Journal of Child Psychology and Psychiatry*

Martinez-Frias, M. L., Bermejo, E., Rodriguez-Pinilla, E., & Frias, J. L. (2004). Risk for congenital anomalies associated with different sporadic and daily doses of alcohol consumption during pregnancy: A case–control study. *Birth Defects Research: Part A. Clinical and Molecular Teratology, 70,* 194–200.

Martinussen, R., Hayden, J., Hogg-Johnson, S., & Tannock, R. (2005). A meta-analysis of working memory impairments in children with attention-deficit/hyperactivity disorder. *Journal of the American Academy of Child and Adolescent Psychiatry, 44,* 377–384.

Mason, C. A., Scott, K. G., Chapman, D. A., & Tu, S. (2000). A review of some individual- and community-level effect size indices for the study of risk factors for child and adolescent development. *Educational and Psychological Measurement, 60,* 385–410.

Matthews, H. B., & Dedrick, R. L. (1984). Pharmacokinetics of PCBs. *Annual Review of Pharmacology and Toxicology, 24,* 85–103.

Matthys, W., van Goozen, S. H. M., de Vries, H., Cohen-Kettenis, P. T., & van Engeland, H. (1998). The dominance of behavioral activation over behavioral inhibition in conduct disordered boys with or without attention deficit hyperactivity disorder. *Journal of Child Psychology and Psychiatry, 39,* 643–651.

Mayr, U. (2002). Inhibition of action rules. *Psychonomic Bulletin and Review, 9,* 93–99.

McBurnett, K. (1992). Psychobiological approaches to personality and their applications to child psychopathology. In B. B. Lahey & A. E. Kazdin (Eds.), *Advances in clinical child psychology* (Vol. 14, pp. 107–164). New York: Plenum Press.

McBurnett, K., Pfiffner, L. J., & Frick, P. J. (2001). Symptom properties as a function of ADHD type: An argument for the continued study of sluggish cognitive tempo. *Journal of Abnormal Child Psychology, 29,* 207–213.

McCormick, D. A., & Bal, T. (1997). Sleep and arousal: Thalamocortical mechanisms. *Annual Review of Neuroscience, 20,* 185–215.

McCracken, J. T. (1991). A two-part model of stimulant action on attention-deficit hyperactivity disorder in children. *Journal of Neuropsychiatry and Clinical Neurosciences, 3,* 201–209.

McGee, R., Stanton, W. R., & Sears, M. R. (1993). Allergic disorders and attention deficit disorders in children. *Journal of Abnormal Child Psychology, 21,* 79–88.

McGuffin, P., Owen, M. J., O'Donovan, M. C., Thapar, A., & Gottesman, I. I. (1994). *Seminars in psychiatric genetics.* London: Gaskell.

McInness, A., Humphries, T., Hogg-Johnson, S., & Tannock, R. (2003). Listening comprehension and working memory are impaired in attention-deficit hyperactivity disorder irrespective of language impairments. *Journal of Abnormal Child Psychology, 31,* 427–444.

McIntyre, C., Blackwell, S., & Denton, C. (1978). Effect of noise distractibility on the spans of apprehension of hyperactive boys. *Journal of Abnormal Psychology, 6,* 483–492.

McKinney, J. D., & Waller, C. L. (1994). Polychlorinated biphenyls as hormonally active structural analogues. *Environmental Health Perspectives, 102*(3), 290–297.

McLeer, S. V., Callaghan, M., Henry, D., & Wallen, J. (1994). Psychiatric disorders in sexually abused children. *Journal of the American Academy of Child and Adolescent Psychiatry, 33,* 313–319.

Meaney, F. J., Miller, L. A., & FASSNET Team. (2003). A comparison of fetal alcohol syndrome surveillance network and birth defects surveillance methodology in determining prevalence rates of fetal alcohol syndrome. *Birth Defects Research: Part A. Clinical and Molecular Teratology, 67, 819–821.*

Medina, A. E., Krahe, T. E., & Ramoa, A. S. (2005). Early alcohol exposure induces persistent alteration of cortical columnar organization and reduced orientation selectivity in the visual cortex. *Journal of Neurophysiology, 93,* 1317–1325.

Meehl, P. E. (1972). Specific genetic etiology, psychodynamics, and therapeutic nihilism. *International Journal of Mental Health, 1,* 10–27.

Meehl, P. E. (1995). Bootstraps taxometrics: Solving the classification problem in psychopathology. *American Psychologist, 50,* 266–275.

Melvin, C. L., & Gaffney, C. A. (2004). Treating nicotine use and dependence of pregnant and parenting smokers: An update. *Nicotine and Tobacco Research, 6*(Suppl. 2), S107–S124.

Menzies, R. (1997). A sociological perspective on impulsivity: Some cautionary comments on the genesis of a clinical construct. In C. D. Webster & M. A.

Jackson (Eds.), *Impulsivity: Theory, assessment, and treatment* (pp. 42–62). New York: Guilford Press.

Meyer, A. (1998). Attention deficit/hyperactivity disorder among North Sotho speaking primary school children in South Africa: Prevalence and sex ratios. *Journal of Psychology in Africa, 8,* 186–195.

Meyer, P. A., Pivetz, T., Dignam, T. A., Homa, D. M., Schoonover, J., Brody, D., et al. (2003). Surveillance for elevated blood lead levels among children— United States, 1997–2001. *Morbidity and Mortality Weekly Report Surveillance Summary, 52*(10), 1–21.

Mezzacappa, E., Kindlon, D., Saul, J. P., & Earls, F. (1998). Executive and motivational control of performance task behavior, and autonomic heart-rate regulation in children: Physiologic validation of two-factor solution inhibitory control. *Journal of Child Psychology and Psychiatry, 39,* 525–531.

Mick, E., Biederman, J., Faraone, S. V., Sayer, J., & Kleinman, S. (2002a). Case–control study of attention-deficit hyperactivity disorder and maternal smoking, alcohol use, and drug use during pregnancy. *Journal of the American Academy of Child and Adolescent Psychiatry, 41,* 378–385.

Mick, E., Biederman, J., Prince, J., Fischer, M., & Faraone, S. V. (2002b). Impact of low birthweight on attention-deficit hyperactivity disorder. *Journal of Developmental and Behavioral Pediatrics, 23,* 16–22.

Middleton, F. A., & Strick, P. L. (2001). Cerebellar projections to the prefrontal cortex of the primate. *Journal of Neuroscience, 2,* 700–712.

Middleton, F. A., & Strick, P. L. (2002). Basal-ganglia 'projections' to the prefrontal cortex of the primate. *Cerebral Cortex, 9,* 926–935.

Milberger, S., Biederman, J., Faraone, S. V., Chen, L., & Jones, J. (1996). Is maternal smoking during pregnancy a risk factor for attention deficit hyperactivity disorder in children? *American Journal of Psychiatry, 153,* 1138–1142.

Milberger, S., Biederman, J., Faraone, S. V., Chen, L., & Jones, J. (1997a). ADHD is associated with early initiation of cigarette smoking in children and adolescents. *Journal of the American Academy of Child and Adolescent Psychiatry, 36,* 37–44.

Milberger, S., Biederman, J., Faraone, S. V., Guite, J., & Tsuang, M. T. (1997b). Pregnancy, delivery and infancy complications and attention deficit hyperactivity disorder: Issues of gene–environment interaction. *Biological Psychiatry, 41,* 65–75.

Milberger, S., Biederman, J., Faraone, S. V., & Jones, J. (1998). Further evidence of an association between maternal smoking during pregnancy and attention deficit hyperactivity disorder: Findings from a high-risk sample of siblings. *Journal of Clinical Child Psychology, 27,* 352–358.

Milich, R., Balentine, A., & Lynam, D. (2001). ADHD combined type and ADHD predominantly inattentive type are distinct and unrelated disorders. *Clinical Psychology: Science and Practice, 8,* 463–488.

Milich, R., Hartung, C. M., Martin, C. A., & Haigler, E. D. (1994). Behavioral disinhibition and underlying processes in adolescents with disruptive behavior disorders. In D. K. Routh (Ed.), *Disruptive behavior disorders in childhood* (pp. 109–138). New York: Plenum Press.

Milich, R., Wolraich, M., & Lindgren, S. (1986). Suger and hyperactivity: A critical review of empirical findings. *Clinical Psychology Review, 6*, 493–513.

Miller, D. C., Kavcic, V., & Leslie, J. E. (1996). ERP changes induced by methylphenidate in boys with attention deficit hyperactivity disorder. *Journal of Attention Disorders, 1*, 95–113.

Miller, G. A. (1996). How we think about cognition, emotion, and biology in psychopathology. *Psychophysiology, 33*, 615–628.

Miller, M. B., Chapman, J. P., Chapman, L. J., & Collins, J. (1995). Task difficulty and cognitive deficits in schizophrenia. *Journal of Abnormal Psychology, 104*, 251–258.

Minder, B., Das-Smaal, E. A., Brand, E. F., & Orlebeke, J. F. (1994). Exposure to lead and specific attentional problems in schoolchildren. *Journal of Learning Disabilities, 27*, 393–399.

Mirsky, A. F., Anthony, B. J., Duncan, C. C., Ahearn, M. B., & Kellham, S. G. (1991). Analysis of the elements of attention: A neuropsychological approach. *Neuropsychology Review, 2*, 109–145.

Mirsky, A. F., & Duncan, C. C. (2001). A nosology of disorders of attention. *Annals of the New York Academy of Sciences, 931*, 17–32.

Miyake, A., Friedman, N. P., Emerson, M. J., Witzki, A. H., & Howerter, A. (2000). The unity and diversity of executive functions and their contributions to complex "frontal lobe" tasks: A latent variable analysis. *Cognitive Psychology, 41*, 49–100.

Moffitt, A. Caspi, M. Rutter, M., & Silva, P. (2001). *Sex differences in antisocial behaviour.* Cambridge, UK: Cambridge University Press.

Moffitt, T. E. (1990). Juvenile delinquency and attention deficit disorder: Boys' developmental trajectories from age 3 to age 15. *Child Development, 61*, 893–910.

Moffitt, T. E. (1993). Adolescence-limited and life-course-persistent antisocial behavior: A developmental taxonomy. *Psychological Review, 100*, 674–701.

Moffitt, T. E. (2005). The new look of behavioral genetics in developmental psychopathology: Gene–environment interplay in antisocial behaviors. *Psychological Bulletin, 131*, 533–554.

Moffitt, T. E., Caspi, A., & Rutter, M. (2005). Strategy for investigating interactions between measured genes and measured environments. *Archives of General Psychiatry, 62*, 473–481.

Molina, B. S., Smith, B. H., & Pelham, W. E. (2001). Factor structure and criterion validity of secondary school teacher ratings of ADHD and ODD. *Journal of Abnormal Child Psychology, 29*, 71–82.

Monastra, V. J., Lubar, J. F., Linden, M., VanDeusen, P., Green, G., Wing, W., et al. (1999). Assessing attention deficit hyperactivity disorder via quantitative electroencephalography: An initial validation study. *Neuropsychology, 13*, 424–433.

Monsell, S. (2003). Task switching. *Trends in Cognitive Sciences, 7*, 134–140.

Monsell, S., & Driver, J. (1998). Banishing the control homunculus. In S. Monsell & J. Driver (Eds.), *Attention and performance: Vol. 18. Control of cognitive processes* (pp. 4–32). Cambridge, MA: MIT Press.

Mostofsky, S. H., Abrams, M. T., Shafer, J. G. B., Goldberg, M. C., Courtney, S.

M., Calhoun, V. D., et al. (2003a). fMRI evidence that the neural basis of response inhibition is task-dependent. *Cognitive Brain Research, 17,* 419–430.

Mostofsky, S. H., Newschaffer, C. J., & Denckla, M. B. (2003b). Overflow movements predict impaired response inhibition in children with ADHD. *Perceptual and Motor Skills, 97,* 1315–1331.

Munoz, D. P., Hampton, K. A., Moore, K. D., & Goldring, J. E. (1999). Control of purposive saccadic eye movements and visual fixation in children with attention-deficit hyperactivity disorder. In W. Becker, H. Deubel, & T. Mergner (Eds.), *Current oculomotor research: Psychological and physiological aspects.* New York: Plenum Press.

Myers, G. J., & Davidson, P. W. (2000). Does methylmercury have a role in causing developmental disabilities in children? *Environmental health perspectives, 108*(Suppl. 3), 413–420.

Nachtman, J. P., Tubben, R. E., & Commissaris, R. L. (1986). Behavioral effects of chronic manganese administration in rats: Locomotor activity studies. *Neurobehavioral Toxicology and Teratology, 8*(6), 711–715.

Nanson, J. L., & Hiscock, M. (1990). Attention deficits in children exposed to alcohol prenatally. *Alcoholism: Clinical and Experimental Research, 14,* 656–661.

National Academy of Sciences. (2000). *Toxicological effects of methylmercury.* Washington, DC: National Academy Press.

National Advisory Committee on Hyperkinesis and Food Additives. (1980). *Report.* New York: Nutritional Foundation.

National Institutes of Health. (1982). NIH Consensus Development Conference: Defined diets and childhood hyperactivity. *Clinical Pediatrics, 21,* 627–630.

Neale, M. C., & Stevenson, J. (1989). Rater bias in the EASI temperament scales: A twin study. *Journal of Personality and Social Psychology, 56,* 446–455.

Needleman, H. L. (1990). The future challenge of lead toxicity. *Environmental Health Perspectives, 89,* 85–89.

Needleman, H. L. (2004). Lead poisoning. *Annual Review of Medicine, 55,* 209–222.

Needleman, H. L., & Landrigan, P. J. (2004). What level of lead in blood is toxic for a child? *American Journal of Public Health, 94,* 8.

Needleman, H. L., McFarland, C., Ness, R. B., Fienberg, S. E., & Tobin, M. J. (2002). Bone lead levels in adjudicated delinquents: A case–control study. *Neurotoxicology and Teratology, 24,* 711–717.

Needleman, H. L., Riess, J. A., Tobin, M. J., Biesecker, G. E., & Greenhouse, J. B. (1996). Bone lead levels and delinquent behavior. *Journal of the American Medical Association, 275*(5), 363–369.

Nesaretman, K., Corcoran, D., Dils, R. R., & Darbre, P. (1996). 3,4,3′,4′-Tetrachlorobiphenyl acts as an extrogen *in vitro* and *in vivo. Molecular Endocrinology, 10,* 923–936.

Nestler, E. J. (2004). Molecular mechanisms of drug addiction. *Neuropharmacology, 47*(Suppl. 1), 24–32.

Neuman, R. J., Sitdhiraksa, N., Reich, W., Ji, T. H., Joyner, C. A., Sun, L. W., et al. (2005). Estimation of prevalence of DSM-IV and latent class-defined ADHD subtypes in a population-based sample of child and adolescent twins. *Twin Research and Human Genetics, 8*, 392–401.

Neuman, R. J., Todd, R. D., Heath, A. C., Reich, W., Hudziak, J. J., Bucholz, K. K., et al. (1999). Evaluation of ADHD typology in three contrasting samples: A latent class approach. *Journal of the American Academy of Child and Adolescent Psychiatry, 38*, 25–33.

Neuringer, M., Reisbeck, S., & Janowsky, J. (1994). The role of Ω-3 fatty acids in visual and cognitive development: Current evidence and methods of assessment. *Journal of Pediatrics, 125*, S39–S47.

Newman, J. P., & Wallace, J. F. (1993). Diverse pathways to deficient self-regulation: Implications for disinhibitory psychopathology in children. *Clinical Psychology Review, 13*, 690–720.

Nichols, S. L., & Waschbusch, D. A. (2004). A review of the validity of laboratory cognitive tasks used to assess symptoms of ADHD. *Child Psychiatry and Human Development, 34*, 297–315.

Nigg, J. T. (1999). The ADHD response inhibition deficit as measured by the stop task: Replication with DSMIV combined type, extension, and qualification. *Journal of Abnormal Child Psychology, 27*, 391400.

Nigg, J. T. (2000). On inhibition/disinhibition in developmental psychopathology: Views from cognitive and personality psychology and a working inhibition taxonomy. *Psychological Bulletin, 126*, 200–246.

Nigg, J. T. (2001). Is ADHD an inhibitory disorder? *Psychological Bulletin, 127*, 571–598.

Nigg, J. T. (2003a). ADHD: Guides for the perplexed reflect the state of the field. Book commentary. *Journal of Clinical Child and Adolescent Psychology, 32*, 302–308.

Nigg, J. T. (2003b). Response inhibition and disruptive behaviors: Toward a multi-process conception of etiological heterogeneity for ADHD combined type and conduct disorder early onset type. *Annals of the New York Academy of Sciences, 1008*, 170–182.

Nigg, J. T. (2005). Neuropsychologic theory and findings in ADHD: The state of the field and salient challenges for the coming decade. *Biological Psychiatry, 57*(11), 1424–1435.

Nigg, J. T. (2006). A third pathway to ADHD via family distress. Unpublished data, Michigan State University, Department of Psychology.

Nigg, J. T. (in press). Temperament and developmental psychopathology. *Journal of Child Psychology and Psychiatry*.

Nigg, J. T., & Casey, B. J. (2005). An integrative theory of attention-deficit/ hyperactivity disorder based on the cognitive and affective neurosciences. *Development and Psychopathology, 17*, 785–806.

Nigg, J. T., Blaskey, L. B., Huang-Pollock, C., & John, O. P. (2002a). ADHD and personality traits: Is ADHD an extreme personality trait? *The ADHD Report, 10* (1), 6–11.

Nigg, J. T., Blaskey, L., Huang-Pollock, C., & Rappley, M. D. (2002b). Neuropsychological executive functions and ADHD DSM-IV subtypes. *Journal of the American Academy of Child and Adolescent Psychiatry, 41*, 59–66.

Nigg, J. T., Blaskey, L., Stawicki, J., & Sachek, J. (2004a). Evaluating the endophenotype model of ADHD neuropsychological deficit: Results for parents and siblings of children with DSM-IV ADHD combined and inattentive subtypes. *Journal of Abnormal Psychology, 113,* 614–625.

Nigg, J. T., Butler, K. M., Huang-Pollock, C. L., & Henderson, J. M. (2002c). Inhibitory processes in adults with persistent childhood onset ADHD. *Journal of Consulting and Clinical Psychology, 70,* 153–157.

Nigg, J. T., Carte, E., Hinshaw, S. P., & Treuting, J. (1998). Neuropsychological correlates of antisocial behavior and comorbid disruptive behavior disorders in children with ADHD. *Journal of Abnormal Psychology, 107,* 468480.

Nigg, J. T., & Goldsmith, H. H. (1998). Recent developments in behavioral genetics and developmental psychopathology. *Human Biology, 70,* 387–412.

Nigg, J. T., Goldsmith, H. H., & Sachek, J. (2004b). Temperament and attention-deficit/hyperactivity disorder: The development of a multiple pathway model. *Journal of Clinical Child and Adolescent Psychology, 33,* 42–53

Nigg, J. T., & Hinshaw, S. P. (1998). Parent personality traits and psychopathology associated with antisocial behaviors in childhood attention-deficit hyperactivity disorder. *Journal of Child Psychology and Psychiatry, 39,* 145–159.

Nigg, J. T., Hinshaw, S. P., & Halperin, J. (1996). Continuous performance test in boys with attention deficit hyperactivity disorder: Methylphenidate dose response and relations with observed behaviors. *Journal of Clinical Child Psychology, 25,* 330–340.

Nigg, J. T., Hinshaw, S. P., & Huang-Pollack, C. (2006). Disorders of attention and impulse regulation. In D. Cicchetti & D. Cohen (Eds.), *Developmental psychopathology* (2nd ed.). New York: Wiley.

Nigg, J. T., & Huang-Pollock, C. L. (2003). An early onset model of the role of executive functions and intelligence in conduct disorder/delinquency. In B. B. Lahey, T. Moffitt, & A. Caspi (Eds.), *Causes of conduct disorder and serious juvenile delinquency* (pp. 227–253). New York: Guilford Press.

Nigg, J. T., John, O. J., Blaskey, L., Huang-Pollock, C., Willcutt, E., Hinshaw, S. H., et al. (2002d). Big Five dimensions and ADHD symptoms: Links between personality traits and clinical symptoms. *Journal of Personality and Social Psychology, 83,* 451–469.

Nigg, J. T., Silk, K., Stavro, G., & Miller, T. (2005c). An inhibition perspective on borderline personality disorder. *Development and Psychopathology, 17,* 1129–1150.

Nigg, J. T., Stavro, G., Ettenhofer, M., Hambrick, D., Miller, T., & Henderson, J. M. (2005a). Executive functions and ADHD in adults: Evidence for selective effects on ADHD symptom domains. *Journal of Abnormal Psychology,* in press.

Nigg, J. T., Swanson, J., & Hinshaw, S. P. (1997). Covert visual attention in boys with attention deficit hyperactivity disorder: Lateral effects, methylphenidate response, and results for parents. *Neuropsychologia, 35,* 165–176.

Nigg, J. T., Willcutt, E., Doyle, A. E., & Sonuga-Barke, J. S. (2005b). Causal heterogeneity in attention deficit hyperactivity disorder: Do we need neuropsychologically impaired subtypes? *Biological Psychiatry, 57*(11), 1224–1230.

Nolan, E. E., Gadow, K. D., & Sprafkin, J. (2001). Teacher reports of DSM-IV ADHD, ODD and CD symptoms in schoolchildren. *Journal of the American Academy of Child and Adolescent Psychiatry, 40,* 241–249.

Norman, D. A., & Shallice, T. (1986). Attention to action: Willed and automatic control of behavior. In R. J. Davidson, G. E. Schwartz, & D. Shapiro (Eds.), *Consciousness and self-regulation* (pp. 1–18). New York: Plenum Press.

O'Brian, B. S., Frick, P. J., & Lyman, R. D. (1994). Reward dominance among children with disruptive behavior disorders. *Journal of Psychopathology and Behavioral Assessment, 16,* 131–145.

O'Brien, L. M., & Gozal D. (2004). Sleep in children with attention deficit/hyperactivity disorder. *Minerva Pediatrica, 56*(6), 585–601.

O'Brien, L. M., Holbrook, C. R., Mervis, C. B., Klaus, C. J., Bruner, J. L., Raffield, T. J., et al. (2003). Sleep and neurobehavioral characteristics of 5- to 7-year-old children with parentally reported symptoms of attention-deficit/hyperactivity disorder. *Pediatrics, 111,* 554–563.

O'Callaghan, M. J., & Harvey, J. M. (1997). Biological predictors and comorbidity of attention deficit and hyperactivity disorder in extremely low birth weight infants at school. *Journal of Pediatric and Child Health, 33,* 491–496.

O'Connor, T. G., Heron, J., Golding, J., Beveridge, M., & Glover, V. (2002). Maternal antenatal anxiety and children's behavioral/emotional problems at 4 years: Report from the Avon Longitudinal Study of Parents and Children. *British Journal of Psychiatry, 180, 502–508.*

O'Connor, T. G., & Rutter, M. (2000). Attachment disorder behavior following early severe deprivation: Extension and longitudinal follow-up. English and Romanian Adoptees Study Team. *Journal of the American Academy of Child and Adolescent Psychiatry, 39,* 703–712.

O'Connor, T. G., Rutter, M., Beckett, C., Keaveney, L., Kreppner, J. M. . & English and Romanian Adoptees Study Team. (2000). The effects of global severe privation on cognitive competence: Extension and longitudinal follow-up. *Child Development, 71,* 376–390.

Ogdie, M. N., Bakker, S. C., Fisher, S. E., Francks, C., Yang, M. H., Cantor, R. M., et al. (2006). Pooled genome-wide linkage data on 424 ADHD ASPs suggests genetic heterogeneity and a common risk locus at 5p13. *Molecular Psychiatry, 11,* 5–8.

Ogdie, M. N., Fisher, S. E., Yang, M., Ishii, J., Francks, C., Loo, S. K., et al. (2004). Attention deficit hyperactivity disorder: Fine mapping supports linkage to 5p13, 6q12, 16p13, and 17p11. *American Journal of Human Genetics, 75,* 661–668.

Ogdie, M. N., Macphie, I. L., Minassian, S. L., Yang, M., Fisher, S. E., Francks, C., et al. (2003). A genomewide scan for attention-deficit/hyperactivity disorder in an extended sample: Suggestive linkage on 17p11. *American Journal of Human Genetics, 72,* 1268–1279.

Øie, M., Rund, B., & Sundet, K. (1998). Covert visual attention in patients with early-onset schizophrenia. *Schizophrenia Research, 34,* 195–205.

Okagaki, L., & French, P. A. (1996). Effects of video game playing on measures of spatial performance: Gender effects in late adolescence. *Applied Developmental Psychology, 15,* 33–58.

O'Keefe, M. J., O'Callaghan, M., Williams, G. M., Najman, J. M., & Bor, W. (2003). Learning, cognitive, and attentional problems in adolescents born small for gestational age. *Pediatrics, 112*, 301–307.

O'Leary, C. M. (2004). Fetal alcohol syndrome: Diagnosis, epidemiology, and developmental outcomes. *Journal of Pedatrics and Child Health, 40*, 2–7.

O'Leary, S. G., Slep, A. M., & Reid, M. J. (1999). A longitudinal study of mothers' overreactive discipline and toddlers' externalizing behavior. *Journal of Abnormal Child Psychology, 27*, 331–341.

Olson, H. C., Feldman, J. J., Streissguth, A. P., Sampson, P. D., & Bookstein, P. L. (1998). Neuropsychological deficits in adolescents with fetal alcohol syndrome: Clinical findings. *Alcoholism: Clinical and Experimental Research, 22*, 1998–2012.

O'Malley, K. D., & Nanson, J. (2002). Clinical implications of a link between fetal alcohol spectrum disorder and attention-deficit hyperactivity disorder. *Canadian Journal of Psychiatry, 47*, 349–354.

Oosterlaan, J., Logan, G. D., & Sergeant, J. A. (1998). Response inhibition in AD/HD, CD, comorbid AD/HD + CD, anxious, and control children: A meta-analysis of studies with the stop task. *Journal of Child Psychology and Psychiatry, 39*, 411–425.

Oosterlaan, J., & Sergeant, J. A. (1998a). Response inhibition and response re-engagement in attention-deficit/hyperactivity disorder, disruptive, anxious and normal children. *Behavioural Brain Research, 94*, 33–43.

Oosterlaan, J., & Sergeant, J. A. (1998b). Effects of reward and response cost on response inhibition in AD/HD, disruptive, anxious, and normal children. *Journal of Abnormal Child Psychology, 26*, 161–174.

Osius, N., Karmaus, W., Kruse, H., & Witten, J. (1999). Exposure to polychlorinated biphenyls and levels of thyroid hormones in children. *Environmental Health Perspectives, 107*, 843–849.

Parasuraman, R., Warm, J. S., & See, J. E. (1998). Brain systems of vigilance. In R. Parasuraman (Ed.), *The attentive brain* (pp. 221–256). Cambridge, MA: MIT Press.

Park, L., Nigg, J. T., Waldman, I., Nummy, K. A., Huang-Pollock, C., Rappley, M., et al. (2005). Association and linkage of ?-2A adrenergic receptor gene polymorphisms with childhood ADHD. *Molecular Psychiatry, 10*, 572–580.

Pashler, H. (1998). Task switching and multi-task performance. In S. Monsell & J. Driver (Eds.), *Attention and performance: Vol. 18. Control of cognitive processes* (pp. 277–307). Cambridge, MA: MIT Press.

Passarotti, A., Banich, M. T., Sood, R. K., & Wang, J. M. (2002). A generalized role of interhemispheric interaction under attentionally demanding conditions: Evidence from the auditory and tactile modality. *Neuropsychologia, 40*, 1082–1096.

Pastandin, S., Lantin, C. I., Mulder, P. G. H., Boersma, E. R., Sauer, P. J. J., & Weisglas-Kuperus, N. (1999). Effects of environmental exposure to polychlorinated biphenyls and dioxins on cognitive abilities in Dutch children at 42 months of age. *Journal of Pediatrics, 134*, 33–41.

Patterson, C. M., & Newman, J. P. (1993). Reflectivity and learning from aversive events: Toward a psychological mechanism for the syndromes of disin-hibition. *Psychological Review, 100,* 716–736.

Patterson, G. R. (1986). Performance models for antisocial boys. *American Psychologist, 41,* 432–44.

Patterson, G. R., DeGarmo, D. S., & Knutson, N. (2000). Hyperactive and anti-social behavior: Comorbid or two points in the same process? *Development and Psychopathology, 12,* 91–106.

Patterson, G. R., Forgatch, M. S., Yoerger, K. L., & Stoolmiller, M. (1998). Variables that initiate and maintain an early-onset trajectory for juvenile offending. *Development and Psychopathology, 10,* 531–547.

Patterson, G. R., & Reid, J. B. (1973). Intervention for families of aggressive boys: A replication study. *Behaviour Research and Therapy, 11,* 383–394.

Pelham, W. E., Fabiano, G. A., & Massetti, G. M. (2005). Evidence-based assessment of attention deficit hyperactivity disorder in children and adolescents. *Journal of Clinical Child and Adolescent Psychology, 34,* 449–476.

Pelham, W. E., Jr. (2001). Are ADHD/I and ADHD/C the same or different? Does it matter? *Clinical Psychology: Science and Practice, 8,* 502–506.

Pelham, W. E., Jr., Wheeler, T., & Chronis, A. (1998). Empirically supported psychosocial treatments for attention deficit hyperactivity disorder. *Journal of Clinical Child Psychology, 27,* 190–205.

Pennington, B. F. (1991). *Diagnosing learning disorders: A neuropsychological framework.* New York: Guilford Press.

Pennington, B. F. (1997). Dimensions of executive functions in normal and abnormal development. In N. A. Krasnegor, G. R. Lyon, & P. S. Goldman-Rakic (Eds.), *Development of the prefrontal cortex: Evolution, neurobiology, and behavior* (pp. 265–281). Baltimore: Brookes.

Pennington, B. F. (2002). *The development of psychopathology.* New York: Guilford Press.

Pennington, B. F., Groisser, D., & Welsh, M. C. (1993). Contrasting cognitive deficits in attention-deficit hyperactivity disorder versus reading disability. *Developmental Psychology, 29,* 511–523.

Pennington, B. F., & Ozonoff, S. (1996). Executive functions and developmental psychopathology. *Journal of Child Psychology and Psychiatry, 37,* 51–87.

Perchet, C., Revol, O., Fourneret, P., Mauguiere, F., & Garcia-Larrea, L. (2001). Attention shifts and anticipatory mechanics in hyperactive children: An ERP study using the Posner paradigm. *Biological Psychiatry, 50,* 44–57.

Pereira, H. S., Eliasson, A. C., & Forssberg, H. (2000). Determintal neural control of precision grip lifts in children with ADHD. *Developmental Medicine and Child Neurology, 42,* 545–553.

Pereira, H. S., Landgren, M., Gilberg, C., & Forssberg, H. (2001). Parametric control of fingertip forces during precision grip lifts in children with DCD (developmental coordination disorder) and DAMP (deficits in attention motor control and perception). *Neuropsychologia, 39,* 478–488.

Picchietti, D. L., England, S. J. , Walters, A. S., Willis, K., & Verrico, T. (1998). Periodic limb movement disorder and restless legs syndrome in children with attention-deficit hyperactivity disorder. *Journal of Child Neurology, 13*(12), 588–594.

Pickering, A. D., & Gray, J. A. (1999). The neuroscience of personality. In L. A. Pervin & O. P. John (Eds.), *Handbook of personality: Theory and research* (2nd ed., pp. 277–299). New York: Guilford Press.

Piek, J. P., Dyke, M. J., Nieman, A., Anderson, M., Hay, D. A., Smith, L. M., et al. (2004). The relationship between motor coordination, executive functioning, and attention in school-aged children. *Archives of Clinical Neuropsychology, 19*, 1063–1076.

Piek, J. P., Pitcher, T. M., & Hay, D. A. (1999). Motor coordination and kinaesthesia in boys with attention deficit-hyperactivity disorder. *Developmental Medicine and Child Neurology, 37*, 976–984.

Pihl, R. O., & Parkes, M. (1977). Hair element content in learning disabled children. *Science, 198*, 204–206.

Pillow, D. R., Pelham, W. E., Jr., Hoza, B., Molina, B. S., & Stultz, C. H. (1998). Confirmatory factor analyses examining attention deficit hyperactivity disorder symptoms and other childhood disruptive behaviors. *Journal of Abnormal Child Psychology, 2*, 293–309.

Pineda, D. A., Ardila, A., & Rosselli, M. (1999). Neuropsychological and behavioral assessment of ADHD in seven- to twelve-year-old children: A discriminant analysis. *Journal of Learning Disabilities, 32*, 159–173.

Pineda, D. A., Ardila, A., Rosselli, M., Cadavid, C., Mancheno, S., & Mejia, S. (1993). Executive dysfunctions in children with attention deficit hyperactivity disorder. *International Journal of Neuroscience, 96*, 177–196.

Pineda, D. A., Lopera, F., Palacio, J. D., Ramirez, D., & Henao, G. C. (2003). Prevalence estimations of attention-deficit/hyperactivity disorder: Differential diagnosis and comorbidities in a Colombian sample. *International Journal of Neuroscience, 113*, 49–71.

Pinto-Martin, J., Whitaker, A., Feldman, J., Cnaan, A., Zhao, H., Bosen-Bloch, J., et al. (2004). Special education services and school performance in a regional cohort of low-birthweight infants at age nine. *Pediatric and Perinatal Epidemiology, 18*, 120–129.

Pitcher, T. M., Piek, J. P., & Hay, D. A. (2003). Fine and gross motor ability in males with ADHD. *Developmental Medicine and Child Neurology, 45*, 525–535.

Pliszka, S. R. (2005). Recent developments in neuroimaging of ADHD. *The ADHD Report, 13*(2), 1–5.

Pliszka, S. R., Borcherding, S. H., Spratley, K., Leon, S., & Irick, S. (1997). Measuring inhibitory control in children. *Journal of Developmental Pediatrics, 18*, 254–259.

Pliszka, S. R., Carlson, C. L., & Swanson, J. M. (1999). *ADHD with comorbid disorders*. New York: Guilford Press.

Pliszka, S. R., Hatch, J. P., Borcherding, S. H., & Rogeness, G. A. (1993). Classical conditioning in children with attention deficit hyperactivity disorder (ADHD) and anxiety disorders: A test of Quay's model. *Journal of Abnormal Child Psychology, 21*, 411–423.

Pliszka, S. R., Liotti, M., & Woldorff, M. G. (2000). Inhibitory control in children with attention-deficit/hyperactivity disorder: Event related potentials identify the processing component and timing of an impaired right-frontal response-inhibition mechanism. *Biological Psychiatry, 48*, 238–246.

Podolski, C. L., & Nigg, J. T. (2001). Parent stress and coping in relation to child ADHD severity and associated child disruptive behavior problems. *Journal of Clinical Child Psychology, 30,* 501–511.

Pollack, C. P., & Bright, D. (2003). Caffeine consumption and weekly sleep patterns in U.S. seventh-, eighth-, and ninth-graders. *Pediatrics, 111,* 42–46.

Pollak, S. D., Cicchetti, D., Klorman, R., & Brumaghim, J. T. (1997). Cognitive brain event-related potentials and emotion processing in maltreated children. *Child Development, 68,* 773–787.

Pomerleau, C. S., Downey, K. K., Snedecor, S. M., Mehringer, A. M., Marks, J. L., & Pomerleau, O. F. (2003). Smoking patterns and abstinence effects in smokers with no ADHD, childhood ADHD, and adult ADHD symptomatology. *Addiction and Behavior, 28,* 1149–1157.

Posner, M. I., & DiGirolamo, G. J. (1998). Executive attention: Conflict, target detection, and cognitive control. In R. Parasuraman (Ed.), *The attentive brain* (pp. 401–423). Cambridge, MA: MIT Press.

Posner, M. I., & Petersen, S. (1990). The attention system of the human brain. *Annual Review of Neuroscience, 13,* 25–42.

Posner, M. I., & Raichle, M. (1994). *Images of mind.* New York: Scientific American Library.

Posner, M. I., & Rothbart, M. K. (2000). Developing mechanisms of self-regulation. *Development and Psychopathology, 12,* 427–441.

Posner, M. I., Walker, J., Friederich, F., & Rafal, R. (1987). How do the parietal lobes direct covert attention? *Neuropsychologia, 25,* 135–145.

Potgeiter, S., Vervisch, J., & Lagae, L. (2003). Event related potentials during attention tasks in VLBW children with and without attention deficit disorder. *Clinical Neurophysiology, 114,* 1841–1849.

Potter, A. S., & Newhouse, P. A. (2004). Effects of acute nicotine administration on behavioral inhibition in adolescents with attention-deficit/hyperactivity disorder. *Psychopharmacology, 176,* 182–194.

Prendergast, M., Taylor, E., Rapoport, J. L., Bartko, J., Donnelly, M., Zametkin, A., et al. (1988). The diagnosis of childhood hyperactivity: A U. S.–U. K. cross-national study of DSM-III and ICD-9. *Journal of Child Psychology and Psychiatry, 29,* 289–300.

Pribram, K. H., & McGuinness, D. (1975). Arousal, activation, and effort in the control of attention. *Psychological Review, 82,* 116–149.

Purcell, S. (2002). Variance components models for gene–environment interaction in twin analysis. *Twin Research, 5,* 554–471.

Purvis, K., & Tannock, R. (2000). Response inhibition in ADHD and reading disorder. *Journal of the American Academy of Child and Adolescent Psychiatry, 39,* 485–494.

Putnam, S. P., Ellis, L. K., & Rothbart, M. K. (2001). The structure of temperament from infancy through adolescence. In A. Eliasz & A. Anglietner (Eds.), *Advances in research on temperament* (pp. 164–182). Lengerich, Germany: Pabst Science.

Quay, H. C. (1988). Attention-deficit disorder and the behavioral inhibition system: The relevance of the neuropsychological theory of Jeffrey A. Gray. In L. M. Bloomingdale & J. Sergeant (Eds.), *Attention-deficit disorder: Criteria, cognition, intervention* (pp. 117–126). New York: Pergamon Press.

Quay, H. C. (1997). Inhibition and attention deficit hyperactivity disorder. *Journal of Abnormal Child Psychology, 25,* 7–13.

Rafal, R., & Posner, M. I. (1987). Deficits in human visual spatial attention following thalamic lesions. *Proceedings of the National Academy of Sciences USA, 84,* 7349–7353.

Raine, A. (1996). Autonomic nervous system factors underlying disinhibited, antisocial, and violent behavior. *Annals of the New York Academy of Sciences, 794,* 46–59.

Raine, A. (2002). Biosocial studies of antisocial and violent behavior in children and adults: A review. *Journal of Abnormal Child Psychology, 30,* 311–326.

Rappley, M. D., Gardiner, J. C., Jetton, J. R., & Houang, R. T. (1995). The use of methylphenidate in Michigan. *Archives of Pediatrics and Adolescent Medicine, 149,* 675–679.

Rasmussen, E. R., Neuman, R. J., Heath, A. C., Levy, F., Hay, D. A., & Todd, R. D. (2004). Familial clustering of latent class and DSM-IV defined attention-deficit/hyperactivity disorder (ADHD) subtypes. *Journal of Child Psychology Psychiatry, 45,* 589–598.

Relman, A. S. (1980). The new medical–industrial complex. *New England Journal of Medicine, 303,* 963–970.

Rice, D. C. (1997a). Effect of postnatal exposure to a PCB mixture in monkeys on multiple fixed interval-fixed ratio performance. *Neurotoxicology and Teratology, 19,* 429–434.

Rice, D. C. (1997b). Neurotoxicity produced by developmental exposure to PCBs. *Mental Retardation and Developmental Disabilities Research Reviews, 3,* 223–229.

Rice, D. C. (1998). Effects of postnatal exposure of monkeys to a PCB mixture on spatial discrimination reversal and DRL performance. *Neurotoxicology and Teratology, 20,* 391–400.

Rice, D. C. (1999). Behavioral impairment produced by low-level postnatal PCB exposure in monkeys. *Environmental Research, 80*(2, Pt. 2), S113–S121.

Rice, D. C. (2000). Parallels between attention deficit hyperactivity disorder and behavioral deficits produced by neurotoxic exposure in monkeys. *Environmental Health Perspectives, 108*(Suppl. 3), 405–408.

Rice, D. C., & Haward, S. (1997). Effects of postnatal exposure to a PCB mixture in monkeys on nonspatial discrimination reversal and delayed alternation performance. *Neurotoxicology, 18,* 479–494.

Richardson, A. J., & Puri, B. K. (2000). The potential role of fatty acids in attention-deficit/hyperactivity disorder. *Prostoglandins, Leukotrienes and Essential Fatty Acids, 63,* 79–87.

Richardson, A. J., & Puri, B. K. (2002). A randomized double-blind, placebo-controlled study of the effects of supplementation with highly unsaturated fatty acids on ADHD-related symptoms in children with specific learning disabilities. *Progress in Neuro-Psychopharmacology and Biological Psychiatry, 26,* 233–239.

Richters, J. E., & Hinshaw, S. P. (1999). The abduction of disorder in psychiatry. *Journal of Abnormal Psychology, 108,* 438–445.

Rietveld, M. J., Hudziak, J. J., Bartels, M., van Beijsterveldt, C. E., & Boomsma, D. I. (2003). Heritability of attention problems in children: I. Cross-sectional results from a study of twins, age 3–12 years. *American Journal of Medical Genetics, 117B*(1), 102–113.

Rietveld, M. J., Hudziak, J. J., Bartels, M., van Beijsterveldt, C. E., & Boomsma, D. I. (2004). Heritability of attention problems in children: Longitudinal results from a study of twins, age 3 to 12. *Journal of Child Psychology and Psychiatry, 45*, 577–588.

Riggins-Caspers, K. M., Cadoret, R. J., Knutson, J. F., & Langbehn, D. (2003). Biology–environment interaction and evocative biology–environment correlation: Contributions of harsh discipline and parental psychopathology to problem adolescent behaviors. *Behavior Genetics, 33*, 205–220.

Rinne, T., Westenberg, H., den Boer, J. A., & van den Brink, W. (2000). Serotonergic blunting to meta-chlorphenylpiperazine (m-CPP) highly correlates with sustained child abuse in impulsive and autoaggressive female borderline patients. *Biological Psychiatry, 47*, 548–556.

Risch, N., & Botstein, D. (1996). A manic–depressive history. *Nature Genetics, 12*, 351–353.

Robins, T. R., & Rogers, R. D. (1998). Functioning of frontostriatal anatomical "loops" in mechanisms of cognitive control. In S. Monsell & J. Driver (Eds.), *Attention and performance: Vol. 18. Control of cognitive processes* (pp. 475–510). Cambridge, MA: MIT Press.

Robison, L. M., Sclar, D. A., Skaer, T. L., & Galin, R. S. (1999). National trends in the prevalence of attention-deficit/hyperactivity disorder and the prescribing of methylphenidate among school age children: 1990–1995. *Clinical Pediatrics, 38*, 209–217.

Rodriguez-Fornells, A., Lorenzo-Seva, U., & Andres-Pueyo, A. (2002). Are high-impulsive and high risk-taking people more motor disinhibited in the presence of incentive? *Personality and Individual Differences, 32*, 661–683.

Rogan, W. J., Gladen, B. C., McKinney, J. D., Carreras, N., Hardy, P., Thullen, J., et al. (1986). Neonatal effects of transplacental exposure to PCBs and DDE. *Journal of Pediatrics, 109*, 335–341.

Rohde, L. A., Biederman, J., Busnello, E. A., Zimmermann, H., Schmitz, M., Martins, S., et al. (1999). ADHD in a school sample of Brazilian adolescents: A study of prevalence, comorbid conditions, and impairments. *Journal of the American Academy of Child and Adolescent Psychiatry, 38*, 716–722.

Rojas, N. L., & Chan, E. (2005). Old and new controversies in the alternative treatment of attention-deficit hyperactivity disorder. *Mental Retardation and Developmental Disabilities Research Reviews, 11*(2), 116–130.

Ross, R. G., Harris, J. G., Olincy, A., & Radant, A. (2000). Eye movement task measures inhibition and spatial working memory in adults with schizophrenia, ADHD, and a normal comparison group. *Psychiatry Research, 95*, 35–42.

Rothbart, M. K., & Ahadi, S. A. (1994). Temperament and the development of personality. *Journal of Abnormal Psychology, 103*, 55–66.

Rothbart, M. K., Ahadi, S. A., Hershey, K. L., & Fisher, P. (2001). Investigations of temperament at three to seven years: the Children's Behavior Questionnaire. *Child Development, 72*, 1394–1408.

Rothbart, M. K., & Bates, J. E. (1998). Temperament. In W. Damon (Series Ed.) & N. Eisenberg (Vol. Ed.), *Handbook of child psychology: Vol. 3. Social, emotional, and personality development* (5th ed., pp. 105–176). New York: Wiley.

Rothbart, M. K., Posner, M. I., & Rosicky, J. (1994). Orienting in normal and pathological development. *Development and Psychopathology, 6,* 635–652.

Rothlind, J. C., Posner, M. I., & Schaughency, E. A. (1991). Lateralized control of eye movements in attention deficit hyperactivity disorder. *Journal of Cognitive Neuroscience, 3,* 374–393.

Rourke, B. P., Ahmad, S. A., Collins, D. W., Hayman-Abello, B. A., Hayman-Abello, S. A., & Warriner, E. M. (2002). Child clinical/pediatric neuropsychology: Some recent advances. *Annual Review of Psychology, 53,* 309–339.

Rowland, A. S., Umbach, D. M., Stallone, L., Naftel, A. J., Bohlig, E. M., & Sandler, D. P. (2002). Prevalence of medication treatment for attention deficit-hyperactivity disorder among elementary school children in Johnstone County, North Carolina. *American Journal of Public Health, 92,* 232–234.

Rubia, K., Oosterlaan, J., Sergeant, J. A., Brandeis, D., & Leeuwen, T. V. (1998). Inhibitory dysfunction in hyperactive boys. *Behavioural Brain Research, 94,* 25–32.

Rubia, K., Overmeyer, S., Taylor, E., Brammer, M., Williams, S. C. R., Simmons, A., et al. (1999). Hypofrontality in attention deficit hyperactivity disorder during higher order motor control: A study with functional MRI. *American Journal of Psychiatry, 156,* 891–896.

Rubia, K., Smith, A. B., Brammer, M. J., & Taylor, E. (2003). Right inferior prefrontal cortex mediates response inhibition while mesial frontal cortex is responsible for error detection. *NeuroImage, 20,* 351–358.

Rucklidge, J. J., & Tannock, R. (2002). Neuropsychological profiles of adolescents with ADHD: effects of reading difficulties and gender. *Journal of Child Psychology and Psychiatry, 43,* 988–1003.

Russell, T. V., Crawford, M. A., & Woodby, L. L. (2004). Measurements for active cigarette smoke exposure in prevalence and cessation studies: Why simply asking pregnant women isn't enough. *Nicotine and Tobacco Research,* 6(Suppl. 2), S141–S151.

Rutter, M. (2001). Child psychiatry in the era following sequencing the genome. In F. Levy & D.A. Hay (Eds.), *Attention, genes, and attention deficit hyperactivity disorder* (pp. 225–248). Philadelphia: Taylor & Francis.

Rutter, M. (2005). Environmentally mediated risks for psychopathology: Research strategies and findings. *Journal of the American Academy of Child and Adolescent Psychiatry, 44,* 3–18.

Rutter, M., Kreppner, J. M., O'Connor, T. G., & English and Romanian Adoptees (ERA) Study Team. (2001). Specificity and heterogeneity in children's responses to profound institutional privation. *British Journal of Psychiatry, 179,* 97–103.

Rutter, M., & Silberg, J. (2002). Gene–environment interplay in relation to emotional and behavioral disturbance. *Annual Review of Psychology, 53,* 463–490.

Safer, D. J., & Krager, J. M. (1992). Effect of a media blitz and a threatened lawsuit on stimulant treatment. *Journal of the American Medical Association,* *268,* 1004–1007.

Safer, D. J., & Zito, J. M. (1999). Psychotropic medication for ADHD. *Mental Retardation and Developmental Disabilities Research Reviews, 5,* 237–242.

Sagvolden, T. (2001). The spontaneously hypertensive rat as a model of ADHD. In M. V. Solanto, A. F. T. Arnsten, & F. X. Castellanos (Eds.), *Stimulant drugs and ADHD: Basic and clinical neuroscience* (pp. 221–237). New York: Oxford University Press.

Sagvolden, T., Aase, H., Zeiner, P., & Berger, D. F. (1998). Altered reinforcement mechanisms in attention deficit/hyperactivity disorder. *Behavioural Brain Research, 94,* 61–71.

Sagvolden, T., Johansen, E. B., Aase, H., & Russell, V. A. (2005). A dynamic developmental theory of attention-deficit/hyperactivity disorder (ADHD) predominantly hyperactive/impulsive and combined subtypes. *Behavioral and Brain Sciences, 28,* 397–419.

Sampson, P. D., Streissguth, A. P., Bookstein, F. L., Little, R. E., Clarren, S. K., Dehaene, P., et al. (1997). Incidence of fetal alcohol syndrome and prevalence of alcohol-related neurodevelopmental disorder. *Teratology, 56*(5), 317–326.

Satterfield, J. H., Cantwell, D. P., & Satterfield, B. T. (1974). Pathophysiology of the hyperactive child syndrome. *Archives of General Psychiatry, 31,* 839–844.

Satterfield, J. H., & Dawson, M. E. (1971). Electrodermal correlates of hyperactivity in children. *Psychophysiology, 8,* 191–197.

Satterfield, J. H., & Schell, A. M. (1984). Childhood brain function differences in delinquent and non-delinquent hyperactive boys. *Electroencephalography and Clinical Neurophysiology, 57,* 199–207.

Satterfield, J. H., Schell, A. M., Backs, R. W., & Hidaka, K. C. (1984). A cross-sectional and longitudinal study of age effects of electrophysiological measures in hyperactive and normal children. *Biological Psychiatry, 19,* 973–990.

Satterfield, J. H., Schell, A. M., & Nicholas, T. (1994). Preferential neural processing of attended stimuli in attention-deficit hyperactivity disorder and normal boys. *Psychophysiology, 31,* 1–10.

Saudino, K. J. (2003a). Parent ratings of infant temperament: Lessons from twin studies. *Infant Behavior and Development, 26,* 100–107.

Saudino, K. J. (2003b). The need to consider contrast effects in parent-rated temperament. *Infant Behavior and Development, 26,* 118–120.

Saudino, K. J., Cherny, S. S., & Plomin, R. (2000). Parent ratings of temperament in twins: Explaining the "too low" DZ correlations. *Twin Research, 3,* 224–233.

Scadding, J. G. (1967). Diagnosis: The clinician and the computer. *Lancet, ii,* 877–882.

Scarr, S., & McCartney, K. (1983). How people make their own environments: A theory of genotype greater than environment effects. *Child Development, 54,* 424–435.

Schab, D. W., & Trinh, N. T. (2004). Do artificial food colors promote hyperactivity in children with hyperactive syndromes?: A meta-analysis of double-blind placebo-controlled trials. *Journal of Developmental and Behavioral Pediatrics, 25,* 423–434.

Schachar, R., Mota, V. L., Logan, G. D., Tannock, R., & Klim, P. (2000). Confirmation of an inhibitory control deficit in attention-deficit/hyperactivity disorder. *Journal of Abnormal Child Psychology, 28,* 227–235.

Schachar, R., Tannock, R., & Logan, G. (1993). Inhibitory control, impulsiveness, and attention deficit hyperactivity disorder. *Clinical Psychology Review, 13,* 721–739.

Schachar, R., Tannock, R., Marriott, M., & Logan, G. (1995). Deficient inhibitory control in attention deficit hyperactivity disorder. *Journal of Abnormal Child Psychology, 23,* 411–437.

Schachar, R. J., Crosbie, J., Barr, C. L., Ornstein, T. J., Kennedy, J., Malone, M., et al. (2005). Inhibition of motor responses in siblings concordant and discordant for attention deficit hyperactivity disorder. *American Journal of Psychiatry, 162,* 1076–1082.

Schantz, S. L., Widholm, J. J., & Rice, D. C. (2003). Effects of PCB exposure on neuropsychological function in children. *Environmental Health Perspectives, 111,* 357–376.

Schecter, A. J., & Piskac, A. L. (2001). PCBs, dioxins, and dibenzofurans: Measured levels and toxic equivalents in blood, milk, and food from various countries. In L. W. Robertson & L. G. Hansen (Eds.), *PCBs: Recent advances in environmental toxicology and health effects* (pp. 161–168). Lexington: University Press of Kentucky.

Scheres, A., Oosterlaan, J., & Sergeant, J. A. (2001). Response inhibition with DSM-IV subtypes of AD/HD and related disruptive disorders: The role of reward. *Child Neuropsychology, 7,* 172–189.

Schettler, T. (2001). Toxic threats to neurological development of children. *Environmental Health Perspectives, 109*(Suppl. 6), 813–816.

Schmidt, M. H., Mocks, P., Lay, B., Hisert, H. G., Fojkar, R., Fritz-Sigmund, D., et al. (1997). Does oligoantigenic diet influence hyperactive/conduct-disordered children?: A controlled trial. *European Journal of Child and Adolescent Psychiatry, 6,* 88–95.

Schmitz, M., Cadore, L., Paczko, M., Kipper, L., Chaves, M., Rohde, L. A., et al. (2002). Neuropsychological performance in DSM-IV ADHD subtypes: An exploratory study with untreated adolescents. *Canadian Journal of Psychiatry, 47,* 863–869.

Schmitz, S., Saudino, K. J., Plomin, R., Fulker, D. W., & DeFries, J. C. (1996). Genetic and environmental influences on temperament in middle childhood: Analyses of teacher and tester ratings. *Child Development, 67,* 409422.

Schneider, W., & Shiffrin, R. M. (1977). Controlled and automatic human information processing: I. Detection, search, and attention. *Psychological Review, 84,* 1–66.

Schultz, W., Tremblay, L., & Hollerman, J. B. (2000). Reward processing in primate orbitofrontal cortex and basal ganglia. *Cerebral Cortex, 10,* 272–283.

Schwartz, P. M., Jacobson, S. W., Fein, G., Jacobson, J. L., & Price, H. A. (1983).

Lake Michigan fish consumption as a source of polychlorinated biphenyls in human cord serum, maternal serum, and milk. *American Journal of Public Health, 73*, 293–296.

Searight, H. R., & McLaren, A. L. (1998). Attentiondeficit hyperactivity disorder: The medicalization of misbehavior. *Journal of Clinical Psychology in Medical Settings, 5*, 467495.

Sedgwick, P. (1982). *Psycho politics*. New York: Harper & Row.

Seegal, R. F., Brosch, K. O., & Okoniewski, R. J. (1997). Effects of *in utero* and lactational exposure of the laboratory rat to 2,4,2',4'- and 3,4,3',4'-tetrachlorobiphenyl on dopamine function. *Toxicology and Applied Pharmacology, 146*, 95–103.

Seeger, G., Schloss, P., & Schmidt, M. H. (2001). Functional polymorphisms within the promoter of the serotonin transporter gene is associated with severe hyperkinetic disorders. *Molecular Psychiatry, 6*, 235–238.

Seguin, J. R., Boulerice, B., Harden, P. W., Tremblay, R. E., & Pihl, R. O. (1999). Executive functions and physical aggression after controlling for attention deficit hyperactivity disorder, general memory, and IQ. *Journal of Child Psychology and Psychiatry, 40*, 1197–1208.

Seguin, J. R., Nagin, D., Assaad, J. M., & Tremblay, R. E. (2004). Cognitive-neuropsychological function in chronic physical aggression and hyperactivity. *Journal of Abnormal Psychology, 113*, 603–613.

Seidman, L. J., Biederman, J., Faraone, S. V., Milberger, S., Norman, D., Seiverd, K., et al. (1995). Effects of family history and comorbidity on the neuropsychological performance of children with ADHD: Preliminary findings. *Journal of the American Academy of Child and Adolescent Psychiatry, 34*, 1015–1024.

Seidman, L. J., Valera, E. M., Makris, N. (2005). Structural brain imaging of attention-deficit/hyperactivity disorder. *Biological Psychiatry, 57*, 1263–1272.

Seligman, L. D., Ollendick, T. H., Langley, A. K., & Baldacci, H. B. (2004). The utility of measures of child and adolescent anxiety: A meta-analytic review of the Revised Children's Manifest Anxiety Scale, the State–Trait Anxiety Inventory for Children, and the Child Behavior Checklist. *Journal of Clinical Child and Adolescent Psychology, 33*, 557–565.

Serences, J., Shomstein, S., Leber, A., Egeth, H., & Yantis, S. (2005). Coordination of voluntary and stimulus-driven attentional control in human cortex. *Psychological Science, 16*, 114–122.

Sergeant, J. A. (2005). Modeling attention-deficit/hyperactivity disorder: A critical appraisal of the cognitive-energetic model. *Biological Psychiatry, 57*, 1248–1255.

Sergeant, J. A., Geurts, H., & Oosterlaan, J. (2002). How specific is a deficit of executive functioning for attention-deficit/hyperactivity disorder? *Behavioural Brain Research, 130*, 3–28.

Sergeant, J. A., Oosterlaan, J., & van der Meere, J. (1999). Information processing and energetic factors in attention-deficit/hyperactivity disorder. In H. C. Quay & A. E. Hogan (Eds.), *Handbook of disruptive behavior disorders* (pp. 75–104). New York: Kluwer Academic/Plenum.

Sergeant, J. A., & Scholten, C. A. (1985). On data limitations in hyperactivity. *Journal of Child Psychology and Psychiatry, 26*, 111–124.

Sergeant, J. A., & van der Meere, J. J. (1988). What happens after a hyperactive child commits an error? *Psychological Research, 24*, 157–164.

Sergeant, J. A., & van der Meere, J. J. (1990). Additive factor methodology applied to psychopathology with special reference to hyperactivity. *Acta Psychologica, 74*, 277–295.

Shapiro, K. L., & Raymond, J. E. (1994). Temporal allocation of visual attention: Inhibition or interference? In D. Dagenbach & T. H. Carr (Eds.), *Inhibitory processes in attention, memory, and language* (pp. 151–188). San Diego, CA: Academic Press.

Shapiro, S. K., & Herod, L. A. (1994). Combining visual and auditory tasks in the assessment of attention-deficit hyperactivity disorder. In D. K. Routh (Ed.), *Disruptive behavior disorders of childhood* (pp. 87–107). New York: Plenum Press.

Shapiro, S. K., Quay, H. C., Hogan, A. E., & Schwartz, K. P. (1988). Response perseveration and delayed responding in undersocialized aggressive conduct disorder. *Journal of Abnormal Psychology, 97*, 371373.

Sharma, V., Halperin, J., Newcorn, J., & Wolf, L. (1991). The dimension of focussed attention: Relationship to behavior and cognitive functioning in children. *Perceptual and Motor Skills, 72*, 787–793.

Sherman, D. K., Iacono, W. G., & McGue, M. K. (1997a). Attention-deficit hyperactivity disorder dimensions: A twin study of inattention and impulsivity–hyperactivity. *Journal of the American Academy of Child and Adolescent Psychiatry, 36*, 745–753.

Sherman, D. K., McGue, M., & Iacono, W. (1997b). Twin concordance for attention deficit hyperactivity disorder: Comparison of teachers' and mothers' reports. *American Journal of Psychiatry, 154*, 532535.

Shiner, R., & Caspi, A. (2003). Personality differences in childhood and adolescence: Measurement, development, and consequences. *Journal of Child Psychology and Psychiatry, 44*, 2–32.

Shomstein, S., & Yantis, S. (2006). Parietal cortex mediates voluntary control of spatial and nonspatial auditory attention. *Journal of Neuroscience, 26*, 435–439.

Silberg, J. L., Parr, T., Neale, M. C., Rutter, M., Angold, A., & Eaves, L. J. (2003). Maternal smoking during pregnancy and risk to boys' conduct disturbance: An examination of the causal hypothesis. *Biological Psychiatry, 53*, 130–135.

Silberg, J. L., Rutter, M., Meyer, J., Maes, H. H., Hewitt, J. K., Simonoff, E., et al. (1996). Genetic and environmental influences on the covariation between hyperactivity and conduct disturbance in juvenile twins. *Journal of Child Psychology and Psychiatry, 37*, 803–816.

Silberstein, R. B., Farrow, M., Levy, F., Pipingas, A., Hay, D. A., & Jarman, F. C. (1998). Functional brain electrical activity mapping in boys with attention-deficit/hyperactivity disorder. *Archives of General Psychiatry, 55*, 1105–1112.

Simmons, S. L., Cummings, J. A., Clemens, L. G., & Nunez, A. A. (2005). Exposure to PCB 77 affects maternal behavior of rats. *Physiology and Behavior, 84,* 81–86.

Simonoff, E., Pickles, A., Hervas, A., Silberg, J. L., Rutter, M., & Eaves, L. (1998). Genetic influences on childhood hyperactivity: Contrast effects imply parental rating bias, not sibling interaction. *Psychological Medicine, 28,* 825837.

Smith, E. E., & Jonides, J. (1999). Storage and executive processes in the frontal lobes. *Science, 283,* 1657–1661.

Smith, T. A., & Kronick, R. F. (1979). The policy culture of drugs: Ritalin, methadone, and the control of deviant behavior. *International Journal of the Addictions, 14,* 933–946.

Snyder, J., Reid, J., & Patterson, G. R. (2003). A social learning model of child and adolescent antisocial behavior. In B. B. Lahey, T. E. Moffitt, & A. Caspi (Eds.), *Causes of conduct disorder and juvenile delinquency* (pp. 27–48). New York: Guilford Press.

Sohlberg, M. M., & Mateer, C. A. (2001). Improving attention and managing attentional problems: Adapting rehabilitation techniques to adults with ADD. *Annals of the New York Academy of Sciences, 931,* 359–375.

Sokol, R. J., Delaney-Black, V., & Nordstrom, B. (2003). Fetal alcohol spectrum disorder. *Journal of the American Medical Association, 290,* 2996–2999.

Solanto, M. V., Abikoff, H., Sonuga-Barke, E., Schachar, R., Logan, G. D., Wigal, T., (2001a). The ecological validity of delay aversion and response inhibition as measures of impulsivity in AD/HD: A supplement to the NIMH Multimodal Treatment Study of AD/HD. *Journal of Abnormal Child Psychology, 29,* 215–228.

Solanto, M. V., Arnsten, A. F. T., & Castellanos, F. X. (Eds.). (2001b). *Stimulant drugs and ADHD: Basic and clinical neuroscience.* Oxford: Oxford University Press.

Sonuga-Barke, E. J. S. (2002). Psychological heterogeneity in AD/HD: A dual pathways model of motivation and cognition. *Behavioural Brain Research, 130,* 29–36.

Sonuga-Barke, E. J. S. (2003). The dual-pathway model of ADHD: An elaboration of neuro-developmental characteristics. *Neuroscience and Behavior Review, 27,* 593–604.

Sonuga-Barke, E. J. S. (2005). Causal models of attention-deficit/hyperactivity disorder: From common simple deficits to multiple developmental pathways. *Biological Psychiatry, 57,* 1231–1238.

Sonuga-Barke, E. J. S., Dalen, L., Daley, D., & Remington, B. (2002). Are planning, working memory, and inhibition associated with individual differences in preschool ADHD symptoms? *Developmental Neuropsychology, 21,* 255–272.

Sonuga-Barke, E. J. S., Dalen, L., & Remington, R. E. (2003). Do delay aversion and inhibitory deficits make distinct contributions to pre-school AD/HD? *Journal of the American Academy of Child and Adolescent Psychiatry, 42,* 1335–1342.

Sonuga-Barke, E. J. S., Daley, D., Thompson, M., Laver-Bradbury, C., & Weeks, A. (2001). Parent-based therapies for preschool attention-deficit/hyperactivity disorder: a randomized, controlled trial with a community sample. *Journal of the American Academy of Child and Adolescent Psychiatry, 40,* 402–408.

Spencer, P. S., & Schaumburg, H. H. (2000). *Experimental and clinical neurotoxicology* (2nd Ed.). New York: Oxford University Press.

Spitzer, R. L. (1999). Harmful dysfunction and the DSM definition of mental disorder. *Journal of Abnormal Psychology, 108,* 430–432.

Spitzer, R. L., & Endicott, J. (1978). Medical and mental disorder: Proposed definition and criteria. R. Spitzer & D. F. Klein (Eds.), *Critical issues in psychiatric diagnosis* (pp. 15–39). New York: Raven Press.

Stawicki, J. A., Nigg, J. T., & von Eye, A. (in press). Family psychiatric history evidence on the nosological relations of DSM-IV ADHD Combined and Inattentive subtypes: New data and meta-analysis. *Journal of Child Psychology and Psychiatry.*

Steger, J., Imhof, K., Coutts, E., Gudelfinger, R., Steinhausen, H., & Brandeis, D. (2001). Attentional and neuromotor deficits in ADHD. *Developmental Medicine and Child Neurology, 43,* 172–179.

Stein, J., Schettler, T., Wallinga, D., & Valenti, M. (2002). In harm's way: Toxic threats to child development. *Journal of Developmental and Behavioral Pediatrics, 23*(1, Suppl.), S13–S22.

Stevens, L. J., Zentall, S. S., Abate, M. L., Kuczeck, T., & Burgess, J. R. (1996). Omega-3 fatty acids in boys with behavior, learning, and health problems. *Physiology and Behavior, 59,* 915–920.

Stevenson, J. (1992). Evidence for genetic aetiology in hyperactivity in children. *Behavior Genetics, 22,* 337–344.

Stewart, P., Fitzgerald, S., Reihman, J., Gump, B., Lonky, E., Darvill, T., et al. (2003). Prenatal PCB exposure, the corpus callosum, and response inhibition. *Environmental Health Perspectives, 111,* 1670–1677.

Stoll, A. L. (2001). *The omega-3 connection.* New York: Simon & Schuster.

Stone, B. M., & Reynolds, C. R. (2003). Can the National Health and Nutrition Examination Survey III (NHANES III) data help resolve the controversy over low blood lead levels and neuropsychological development in children? *Archives of Clinical Neuropsychology, 18,* 219–244.

Stratton, K., Howe, C., & Battaglia, F. C. (1996). *Fetal alcohol syndrome: Diagnosis, epidemiology, prevention, and treatment.* Washington, DC: Institute of Medicine and National Academy Press.

Streissguth, A. P., Barr, H. M., Sampson, P. D., & Bookstein, F. L. (1994a). Prenatal alcohol and offspring development: The first fourteen years. *Drug and Alcohol Dependence, 36,* 89–99.

Streissguth, A. P., Sampson, P. D., Barr, H. M., Bookstein, F. L., & Carmichael-Olson, H. (1994b). The effects of prenatal exposure to alcohol and tobacco: Contributions from the Seattle Longitudinal Prospective Study and Implications for Public Policy. In H. L. Needleman & D. Bellinger (Eds.), *Prenatal exposure to toxicants: Developmental consequences* (pp. 148–183). Baltimore: Johns Hopkins University Press.

Swanson, J. M., Casey, B. J., Nigg, J. T., Castellanos, F. X., Volkow, N. D., & Taylor, E. (2004). Clinical and cognitive definitions of attention deficits in children with attention-deficit/hyperactivity disorder. In M. I. Posner (Ed.), *Cognitive neuroscience of attention* (pp. 430–446). New York: Guilford Press.

Swanson, J. M., & Castellanos, F. X. (2002). Biological bases of ADHD: Neuroanatomy, genetics, and pathophysiology. In P. S. Jensen & J R. Cooper (Eds.), *Attention-deficit hyperactivity disorder: State of the science, best practices* (pp. 7-1–7-20). Kingston, NJ: Civic Research Institute.

Swanson, J. M., Castellanos, F. X., Frith, U., Pennington, B. F., Steinfer, D., Spitzer, M., et al. (2001a). Psychopathology. *Developmental Science, 4*, 345–357.

Swanson, J. M., Flodman, P., Kennedy, J., Spence, M. A., Moyzis, R., Schuck, S., et al. (2000a). Dopamine genes and ADHD. *Neuroscience and Biobehavioral Reviews, 24*, 21–25.

Swanson, J. M., Kraemer, H. C., Hinshaw, S. P., Arnold, L. E., Conners, C. K., Abikoff, H. B., et al. (2001b). Clinical relevance of the primary findings of the MTA: Success rates based on severity of ADHD and ODD symptoms at the end of treatment. *Journal of the American Academy of Child and Adolescent Psychiatry, 40*, 168–179.

Swanson, J. M., Oosterlaan, J., Murias, M., Shuck, S., Flodman, P., Spence, A., et al. (2000b). Attention deficit/hyperactivity disorder in children with a 7–repeat allele of the dopamine receptor D4 gene have extreme behavior but normal performance on critical neuropsychological tests of attention. *Proceedings of the National Academy of Sciences USA, 97*, 4754–4759.

Swanson, J. M., Posner, M., Potkin, S., Bonforte, S., Youpa, D., & Fiore, C. (1991). Activating tasks for the study of visual–spatial attention in ADHD children: A cognitive anatomic approach. *Journal of Child Neurology, 6*, S119–S127.

Swanson, J. M., Sergeant, J. A., Taylor, E., Sonuga-Barke, E. J. S., Jensen, P. S., & Cantwell, D. P. (1998). Attention-deficit hyperactivity disorder and hyperkinetic disorder. *Lancet, 351*, 429–433.

Szasz, T. S. (1974). *The myth of mental illness: Foundations of a theory of personal conduct* (rev. ed.). New York: Harper & Row.

Szatmari, P., Offord, D. R., & Boyle, M. H. (1989). Correlates, associated impairments, and patterns of service utilization of children with attention deficit disorder: Findings from the Ontario Child Health Study. *Journal of Child Psychology and Psychiatry, 39*, 65–99.

Szatmari, P., Saigal, S., Rosebaum, P., & Cambell, D. (1993). Psychopathology and adaptive functioning among extremely low birthweight children at eight years of age. *Development and Psychopathology, 5*, 345–357.

Szatmari, P., Saigal, S., Rosebaum, P., Cambell, D., & King, S. (1990). Psychiatric disorders at five years among children with birthweight less than 1000 g: A regional perspective. *Developmental Medicine and Child Neurology, 32*, 954–962.

Tannock, R. (1998). Attention deficit hyperactivity disorder: Advances in cognitive, neurobiological, and genetic research. *Journal of Child Psychology and Psychiatry, 39*, 65–99.

Tannock, R., Ickowicz, A., & Schachar, R. (1995). Differential effects of methylphenidate on working memory in ADHD children with and without comorbid anxiety. *Journal of the American Academy of Child and Adolescent Psychiatry, 34,* 886–896.

Tannock, R., & Schachar, R. (1996). Executive dysfunction as an underlying mechanism of behavior and language problems in attention deficit hyperactivity disorder. In J. H. Beitchman, N. J. Cohen, M. M. Konstantareas, & R. Tannock (Eds.), *Language, learning, and behavior disorders* (pp. 128–155). Cambridge, UK: Cambridge University Press.

Tarnowski, K., Prinz, R., & Nay, S. (1986). Comparative analysis of attentional deficits in hyperactive and learning-disabled children. *Journal of Abnormal Psychology, 95,* 341–345.

Taylor, E., Sandberg, S., Thorley, G., & Giles, S. (1991). *The epidemiology of childhood hyperactivity.* London: Oxford University Press.

Taylor, F. K. (1971). A logical analysis of the medico-psychological concept of disease. *Psychological Medicine, 1,* 356–364.

Taylor, M., Sunohara, G., Khan, S., & Malone, M. (1997). Parallel and serial attentional processes in ADHD: ERP evidence. *Developmental Neuropsychology, 13,* 531–540.

Teicher, M. H., Andersen, S. L., Polcari, A., Anderson, C. M., & Navalta, C. P. (2002). Developmental neurobiology of childhood stress and trauma. *Psychiatric Clinics of North America, 25*(2), 397–426.

Teicher, M. H., Andersen, S. L., Polcari, A., Anderson, C. M.. Navalta, C. P., & Kim, D. M. (2003). The neurobiological consequences of early stress and childhood maltreatment. *Neuroscience & Biobehavioral Reviews, 27,* 33–44.

Tellegen, A. (1985). Structures of mood and personality and their relevance to assessing anxiety, with an emphasis on self-report. In A. H. Tuma & J. Maser (Eds.), *Anxiety and the anxiety disorders* (pp. 681–706). Hillsdale, NJ: Erlbaum.

Tercyak, K. P., Lerman, C., & Audrain, J. (2002). Association of attention-deficit/hyperactivity disorder symptoms with levels of cigarette smoking in a community sample of adolescents. *Journal of the American Academy of Child and Adolescent Psychiatry, 41,* 799–805.

Thapar, A., Fowler, T., Rice, F., Scourfield, J., van den Bree, M., Thomas, H., et al. (2003). Maternal smoking during pregnancy and attention deficit hyperactivity disorder symptoms in offspring. *American Journal of Psychiatry, 160,* 1985–1989.

Thapar, A., Harrington, R., Ross, K., & McGuffin, P. (2000). Does the definition of ADHD affect heritability? *Journal of the American Academy of Child and Adolescent Psychiatry, 39*(12), 1528–1536.

Theuwes, J., Atchley, P., & Kramer, A. F. (1998). On the time course of top-down and bottom-up control of visual attention. In S. Monsell & J. Driver (Eds.), *Attention and performance: Vol. 18. Control of cognitive processes* (pp. 105–124). Cambridge, MA: MIT Press.

Thomas, A., & Chess, S. (1977). *Temperament and development.* New York: Brunner/Mazel.

Thomson, G. O., Raab, G. M., Hepburn, W. S., Hunter, R., Fulton, M., & Laxen, D. P. (1989). Blood-lead levels and children's behavior: Results from the Edinburgh Lead Study. *Journal of Child Psychology and Psychiatry, 30,* 515–528.

Toplak, M. E., Dockstader, C., & Tannock, R. (in press). Temporal information processing in ADHD: Findings to date and new methods. *Journal of Neuroscience Methods.*

Toplak, M. E., Rucklidge, J. J., Hetherington, R., John, S. C. F, & Tannock, R. (2003). Time perception deficits in attention-deficit/hyperactivity disorder and comorbid reading difficulties in child and adolescent samples. *Journal of Child Psychology and Psychiatry, 44,* 1–16.

Tran, T. T., Chowanadisai, W., Crinella, F. M., Chicz-DeMet, A., & Lonnerdal, B. (2002a). Effect of high dietary manganese intake of neonatal rats on tissue mineral accumulation, striatal dopamine levels, and neurodevelopmental status. *Neurotoxicology, 23,* 635–643.

Tran, T. T., Chowanadisai, W., Lonnerdal, B., Le, L., Parker, M., Chicz-Demet, A., et al. (2002b). Effects of neonatal dietary manganese exposure on brain dopamine levels and neurocognitive functions. *Neurotoxicology, 23,* 645–651.

Triesman, A., & Gelade, G. (1980). A feature integration theory of attention. *Cognitive Psychology, 12,* 97–136.

Tripp, G., & Alsop, B. (1999). Sensitivity to reward frequency in boys with attention deficit hyperactivity disorder. *Journal of Clinical Child Psychology, 28,* 366–375.

Trommer, B. L., Hoeppner, J. B., & Zecker, S. G. (1991). The go–no go test in attention deficit disorder is sensitive to methylphenidate. *Journal of Child Neurology, 6,* S128–S131.

Tu, S. (2003). Developmental epidemiology: A review of three key measures of effect. *Journal of Clinical Child and Adolescent Psychology, 32,* 187–192.

Tucker, D. M., & Williamson, P. A. (1984). Asymmetric neural control systems in human self-regulation. *Psychological Review, 91,* 185–215.

Tully, L. A., Arseneault, L., Caspi, A., Moffitt, T. E., & Morgan, J. (2004). Does maternal warmth moderate the effects of birth weight on twins' attention-deficit/hyperactivity disorder (ADHD) symptoms and low IQ? *Journal of Consulting and Clinical Psychology, 72,* 218–226.

Turkheimer, E. (1998). Heritability and biological explanation. *Psychological Review, 105,* 782–791.

Turkheimer, E., D'Onofrio, M. M., Maes, H., & Eaves, L. J. (2005). Analysis and interpretation of twin studies including measures of shared environment. *Child Development, 76,* 1217–1233.

Turkheimer, E., Haley, A., Waldron, M., D'Onofrio, B., & Gottesman, I. I. (2003). Socioeconomic status modifies heritability of IQ in young children. *Psychological Science, 14,* 623–628.

Tuthill, R. W. (1996). Hair lead levels related to children's classroom attention-deficit behavior. *Archives of Environmental Health, 51,* 214–220.

Uhlig, T., Merkenschlager, A., Brandmaier, R., & Egger, J. (1997). Topgraphic mapping of brain electrical activity in children with food-induced attention deficit hyperkinetic disorder. *Neuropediatrics, 156,* 557–561.

U.S. Department of Health and Human Services. (2001). *Youth violence: A report of the Surgeon General.* Rockville, MD: Author.

Vaidya, C. J., Austin, G., Kirkorian, G., Ridlehuber, H. W., Desmond, J. E., Glover, G. H., et al. (1998). Selective effects of methyplhenidate in attention deficit hyperactivity disorder: A functional magnetic resonance study. *Proceedings of the National Academy of Sciences USA, 95,* 14494–14499.

van den Bergh, B. R., & Marcoen, A. (2004). High antenatal maternal anxiety is related to ADHD symptoms, externalizing problems, and anxiety in 8- and 9-year-olds. *Child Development, 75,* 1085–1097.

van der Meere, J. J. (2002). The role of attention. In S. Sandberg (Ed.), *Hyperactivity and attention disorders of childhood* (2nd ed., pp. 162–213). Cambridge, UK: Cambridge University Press.

van der Meere, J. J., Shalev, R. S., Borger, N., & Gross-Tsur, V. (1995). Sustained attention, activation, and MPH in ADHD. *Journal of Child Psychology and Psychiatry, 36,* 697–703.

van der Meere, J. J., & Stermerdink, N. (1999). The development of state regulation in normal children: An indirect comparison with children with ADHD. *Developmental Neuropsychology, 16,* 213–225.

van Mourik, R., Oosterlaan, J., & Sergeant, J. A. (2005). The Stroop revisited: A meta–analysis of interference control in AD/HD. *Journal of Child Psychology and Psychiatry, 46,* 150–165.

Vermiglio, F., Lo Presti, V. P., Moleti, M., Sidoti, M., Tortorella, G., Scaffidi, G., et al. (2004). Attention deficit and hyperactivity disorders in the offspring of mothers exposed to mild–moderate iodine deficiency: A possible novel iodine deficiency disorder in developed countries. *Journal of Clinical Endocrinology and Metabolism, 89,* 6054–6060.

Vitale, J. E., Newman, J. P., Bates, J. E., Goodnight, J., Dodge, K. A., & Pettit, G. S. (2005). Deficient behavioral inhibition and anomalous selective attention in a community sample of adolescents with psychopathic traits and low anxiety traits. *Journal of Abnormal Child Psychology, 33,* 461–470.

Voigt, R. G., Llorente, A. M., Jensen, C. L., Fraley, J. K., Berretta, M. C., & Heird, W. C. (2001). A randomized, double-blind, placebo-controlled trial of docosahexaenoic acid supplementation in children with attention-deficit/hyperactivity disorder. *Journal of Pediatrics, 139,* 189–196.

Vreugdenhil, H. J. K., Mulder, P. G. H., Emmen, H. H., & Weisglas-Kuperus, N. (2004). Effects of perinatal exposure to PCBs on neuropsychological functions in the Rotterdam cohort at 9 years of age. *Neuropsychology, 18,* 185–193.

Wakefield, J. C. (1992). The concept of mental disorder: On the boundary between biological facts and social values. *American Psychologist, 47,* 373–388.

Wakefield, J. C. (1999). Evolutionary versus prototype analyses of the concept of disorder. *Journal of Abnormal Psychology, 108,* 374–399.

Waldman, I. D., Rowe, D. C., Abramowitz, A., Kozel, S. T., Mohr, J. H., Sherman, S. L., et al. (1998). Association and linkage of the dopamine transporter gene and attention-deficit hyperactivity disorder in children: Heterogeneity owing to diagnostic subtype and severity. *American Journal of Human Genetics, 63,* 1767–1776.

Walkawiak, J., Wiener, J. A., Fastabend, A., Heinzow, B., Kramer, U., Schmidt, E., et al. (2001). Environmental exposure to polychlorinated biphenyls and quality of the home environment: Effects on psychodevelopment in early childhood. *Lancet, 358,* 1602–1607.

Waller, N. G., & Meehl, P. E. (1998). *Advanced quantitative techniques in the social sciences: Vol. 9. Multivariate taxometric procedures: Distinguishing types from continua.* Thousand Oaks, CA: Sage.

Wasserstein, J., & Lynn, A. (2001). Metacognitive remediation in adult ADHD: Treating executive function deficits via executive functions. *Annals of the New York Academy of Sciences, 931,* (pp. 376–384).

Wasserstein, J., Wolf, L. E., & Lefever, F. F. (Eds.). (2001). Adult attention deficit disorder: Brain mechanisms and life outcomes. *Annals of the New York Academy of Sciences, 931.*

Watson, D., Kotov, R., & Gamez, W. (2006). Basic dimensions of temperament in relation to personality and psychopathology. In R. F. Krueger & J. Tackett (Eds.), *Personality and psychopathology* (pp. 7–38). New York: Guilford Press.

Weinberg, W. A., & Harper, C. R. (1993). Vigilance and its disorders. *Neurologic Clinics, 11,* 59–78.

Weinstein, D., Staffelbach, D., & Biaggio, M. (2000). Attention-deficit hyperactivity disorder and posttraumatic stress disorder: Differential diagnosis in childhood sexual abuse. *Clinical Psychology Review, 20,* 359–378.

Weiss, B. (1994). The developmental neurotoxicity of mercury. In H. L. Needleman & D. Bellinger (Eds.), *Prenatal exposure to toxicants* (pp. 112–129). Baltimore: Johns Hopkins University Press.

Weiss, B. (2000). Vulnerability of children and the developing brain to neurotoxic hazards. *Environmental Health Perspectives, 108*(Suppl. 3), 375–381.

Weiss, G., & Hechtman, L. T. (1993). *Hyperactive children grown up* (2nd ed). New York: Guilford Press.

Weissman, M. M., Warner, V., Wickramaratne, P. J., & Kandel, D. B. (1999). Maternal smoking during pregnancy and psychopathology in offspring followed to adulthood. *Journal of the American Academy of Child and Adolescent Psychiatry, 38,* 892–899.

Wells, K. C., & Egan, J. (1988). Social learning and systems family therapy for childhood oppositional disorder: Comparative treatment outcome. *Comprehensive Psychiatry, 29,* 138–146.

Wender, P. H. (1995). *Attention-deficit hyperactivity disorder in adults.* New York: Oxford University Press.

Wender, P. H. (2000). *ADHD: Attention deficit hyperactivity disorder in children and adults.* New York: Oxford University Press.

Wessels, D., Barr, D. B., & Mendola, P. (2003). Use of biomarkers to indicate exposure of children to organophosphate pesticides: Implications for a longitudinal study of children's environmental health. *Environmental Health Perspectives, 111,* 1939–1946.

Whalen, C. K., Jamner, L. D., Henker, B., Delfino, R. J., & Lozano, J. M. (2002). The ADHD spectrum and everyday life: Experience sampling of adolescent moods, activities, smoking, and drinking. *Child Development, 73,* 209–227.

Whalen, C. K., Jamner, L. D., Henker, B., Gehricke, J. G., & King, P. S. (2003). Is there a link between adolescent cigarette smoking and pharmacotherapy for ADHD? *Psychology of Addictive Behaviors, 17,* 332–335.

Whitaker, A. H., Van Rossem, R., Feldman, J. F., Schonfeld, I. S., Pinto-Martin, J. A., & Paneth, N. (1997). Psychiatric outcomes in low birthweight children at age 6 years: Relation to neonatal cranial ultrasound abnormalities. *Archives of General Psychiatry, 54,* 847–855.

Wigal, S. B., Nemet, D., Swanson, J. M., Regino, R., Trampush, J., Ziegler, M. G., Cooper, D. M. (2003). Catecholamine response to exercise in children with attention deficit hyperactivity disorder. *Pediatric Research, 53,* 756–761.

Wilens, T. E., Faraone, S. V., & Biederman, J. (2005). Attention deficit/hyperactivity disorder in adults. *Journal of the American Medical Association, 292,* 619–623.

Willcutt, E. G., Brodsky, K., Chhabildas, N., Shanahan, M., Yerys, B., Scott, A., et al. (2005a). The neuropsychology of ADHD: Validity of the executive function hypothesis. In D. Gozal & D. Molfese (Eds.), *Attention deficit hyperactivity disorder: from genes to practice* (pp. 185–213). Totowa, NJ: Humana Press.

Willcutt, E. G., Doyle, A. E., Nigg, J. T., Faraone, S. V., & Pennington, B. F. (2005b). Validity of the executive function theory of attention deficit hyperactivity disorder: A meta-analytic review. *Biological Psychiatry, 57*(11), 1336–1346.

Willcutt, E. G., Pennington, B. F., Boada, R., Ogline, J. S., Tunick, R. A., Chhabildas, N. A., et al. (2001). A comparison of the cognitive deficits in reading disability and attention-deficit/hyperactivity disorder. *Journal of Abnormal Psychology, 110,* 157–172.

Willcutt, E. G., Pennington, B. F., & DeFries, J. C. (2000). Etiology of inattention and hyperactivity/impulsivity in a community sample of twins with learning difficulties. *Journal of Abnormal Child Psychology, 28,* 149–159.

Williams, B. R., Ponesse, J. S., Schachar, R. J., Logan, G. D., & Tannock, R. (1999). Development of inhibitory control across the life-span. *Developmental Psychology, 35,* 205–213.

Williams, G. M., O'Callaghan, M., Najman, J. M., Bor, W., Anderson, M. J., Richards, D., et al. (1998). Maternal cigarette smoking and child psychiatric morbidity: A longitudinal study. *Pediatrics, 102,* e11.

Winrow, C. J., Hemming, M. L., Allen, D. M., Quistad, G. B., Casida, J. E., & Barlow, C. (2003). Loss of neuropathy target esterase in mice links organophosphate exposure to hyperactivity. *Nature Genetics, 33,* 477–485.

Wolf, J. M. (1998). Visual search. In H. Pashler (Ed.), *Attention* (pp. 13–73). London: Psychology Press.

Wolfe, S. M. (2003). Profitably inventing new diseases. *Public Citizen Health Research Group Health Letter, 19*(8), 1–3.

Wolraich, M. L., Hannah, J. N., Baumgaertel, A., & Feurer, I. D. (1998). Examination of DSM-IV criteria for attention deficit/hyperactivity disorder in a county-wide sample. *Journal of Developmental and Behavioral Pediatrics, 19,* 162–168.

Wolraich, M. L., Hannah, J. N., Pinnock, T. Y., Baumgaertel, A., & Brown, J. (1996). Comparison of diagnostic criteria for attention-deficit/hyperactivity disorder in a county-wide sample. *Journal of the American Academy of Child and Adolescent Psychiatry, 35,* 319–324.

Wolraich, M. L., Wilson, D. B., & White, J. W. (1985). The effect of sugar on behavior or cognition in children: A meta-analysis. *Journal of the American Medical Association, 274,* 1617–1621.

World Health Organization (WHO). (1993). *The ICD-10 classification of mental and behavioral disorders: Clinical descriptions and diagnostic guidelines (1992) and diagnostic criteria for research.* Geneva: World Health Organization.

Worman, H. J., & Courvalin, J. C. (2004). How do mutations in lamins A and C cause disease? *Journal of Clinical Investigation, 113,* 349–351.

Wright, J. C., Huston, A. C., Vandewater, E. A., Bickham, D. S., Scantlin, R. M., Kotler, J. A., et al. (2001). American children's use of electronic media in 1997: A national survey. *Applied Developmental Psychology, 22,* 31–47.

Yanez, L., Ortiz, D., Calderon, J., Batres, L., Carrizales, L., Mejia, J., et al. (2002). Overview of human health and chemical mixtures: Problems facing developing countries. *Environmental Health Perspectives, 110*(Suppl. 6), 901–909.

Yan, J. H., & Thomas, J. R. (2002). Arm movement control: Differences between children with and without attention deficit hyperactivity disorder. *Research Quarterly for Exercise and Sport, 73,* 10–18.

Yantis, S. (1998). Goal-directed and stimulus-driven determinants of attentional control. In S. Monsell & J. Driver (Eds.), *Attention and performance: Vol. 18. Control of cognitive processes* (pp. 73–103). Cambridge, MA: MIT Press.

Yong, L. G., Robaey, P., Karayanidis, F., Bourassa, M., Pelletier, G., & Geoffroy, G. (2000). ERPs and behavioral inhibition in a go/no-go task in children with attentiondeficit hyperactivity disorder. *Brain and Cognition, 43,* 215220.

Yu, M. L., Hsu, C. C., Gladen, B. C., & Rogan, W. J. (1991). *In utero* PCB/PCDF exposure: Relation of developmental delay to dysmorphology and dose. *Neurotoxicology and Teratology, 13,* 195–202.

Zacks, R. T., & Hasher, L. (1994). Directed ignoring: Inhibitory regulation of working memory. In D. Dagenbach & T. H. Carr (Eds.), *Inhibitory processes in attention, memory, and language* (pp. 241–264). San Diego, CA: Academic Press.

Zametkin, A. J., & Rapoport, J. L. (1987). Neurobiology of attention deficit disorder with hyperactivity: Where have we come in 50 years? *Journal of the American Academy of Child and Adolescent Psychiatry, 26,* 676–686.

Zelazo, P. D., Muller, U., Frye, D., & Marcovitch, S. (2003). The development of executive function: Cognitive complexity and control—revised. *Monographs of the Society for Research in Child Development, 68*(3), 93–119.

Zentall, S., & Zentall, T. (1983). Optimal stimulation: A model of disordered activity and performance in normal and deviant children. *Psychological Bulletin, 94,* 446–471.

Zito, J. M., Safer, D. J., DosReis, S., Gardner, J. F., Magder, L., Soeken, K., et al.

(2003). Psychotropic practice patterns for youth: A 10-year perspective. *Archives of Pediatrics and Adolescent Medicine, 157,* 17–25.

Zoeller, R. T. (2001). Polychlorinated biphenyls as disruptors of thyroid hormone action. In L. W. Robertson & L. G. Hansen (Eds.), *PCBs: Recent advances in environmental toxicology and health effects* (pp. 265–271). Lexington: University Press of Kentucky.

Zuckerman, M. (1991). *Psychobiology of personality.* New York: Cambridge University Press.

Zuckerman, M. (2001). Adult temperament and its biological basis. In A. Eliasz & A. Anglietner (Eds.), *Advances in research on temperament* (pp. 42–57). Lengerich, Germany: Pabst Science.

Zuckerman, M., Kuhlman, D. M., Joireman, J., Teta, P., & Kraft, M. (1993). A comparison of three structural models for personality: The Big Three, the Big Five, and the Alternative Five. *Journal of Personality and Social Psychology, 65,* 757–768.

Index